WORLD HEALTH ORGANIZATION

The
WORLD
HEALTH
REPORT
2000

Health Systems:

Improving Performance

WHO Library Cataloguing in Publication Data

The World health report 2000 : health systems : improving performance.
1. World health 2. Health systems plans 3. Delivery of health care
4. Health services administration 5. Financing, Health 6. Health services
accessibility 7. Social justice 8. Health care evaluation mechanisms
I. Title: Health systems : improving performance

ISBN 92 4 156198 X   (NLM Classification: WA 540.1)
ISSN 1020-3311

The World Health Organization welcomes requests for permission to reproduce or translate its publications, in part or in full. Applications and enquiries should be addressed to the Office of Publications, World Health Organization, 1211 Geneva 27, Switzerland, which will be glad to provide the latest information on any changes made to the text, plans for new editions, and reprints and translations already available.

The designations employed and the presentation of the material in this publication, including tables and maps, do not imply the expression of any opinion whatsoever on the part of the Secretariat of the World Health Organization concerning the legal status of any country, territory, city or area or of its authorities, or concerning the delimitation of its frontiers or boundaries. Dotted lines on maps represent approximate border lines for which there may not yet be full agreement.

The mention of specific companies or of certain manufacturers' products does not imply that they are endorsed or recommended by the World Health Organization in preference to others of a similar nature that are not mentioned. Errors and omissions excepted, the names of proprietary products are distinguished by initial capital letters.

Information concerning this publication can be obtained from:
World Health Report
World Health Organization
1211 Geneva 27, Switzerland
Fax: (41-22) 791 4870
Email: whr@who.int

Copies of this publication can be ordered from: bookorders@who.int

The principal writers of this report were Philip Musgrove, Andrew Creese, Alex Preker, Christian Baeza, Anders Anell and Thomson Prentice, with contributions from Andrew Cassels, Debra Lipson, Dyna Arhin Tenkorang and Mark Wheeler. The report was directed by a steering committee formed by Julio Frenk (chair), Susan Holck, Christopher Murray, Orvill Adams, Andrew Creese, Dean Jamison, Kei Kawabata, Philip Musgrove and Thomson Prentice. Valuable input was received from an internal advisory group and a regional reference group, the members of which are listed in the Acknowledgements. Additional help and advice were gratefully received from regional directors, executive directors at WHO headquarters and senior policy advisers to the Director-General.

The conceptual framework that underpins the report was formulated by Christopher Murray and Julio Frenk. The development of new analytical methods and summary indicators, new international data collection efforts and extensive empirical analysis that form the basis for the report was undertaken by over 50 individuals, most of them from the WHO Global Programme on Evidence for Health Policy, organized in eleven working groups. These groups covered basic demography, cause of death, burden of disease, disability-adjusted life expectancy, health inequalities, responsiveness, fairness of financial contribution, health system preferences, national health accounts and profiles, performance analysis and basic economic data. Members of each working group are listed in the Acknowledgements. Managerial and technical leadership for the working groups was provided by Julio Frenk, Christopher Murray, Kei Kawabata, Alan Lopez and David Evans. A series of technical reports from each of the working groups provides details on the methods, data and results, beyond the explanations included in the Statistical Annex.

The general approach to this report was discussed at an international consultative meeting on health systems, and the measurement of responsiveness was facilitated by a meeting of key informants. Both meetings were held in Geneva in December 1999 and the participants are listed in the Acknowledgements.

The report was edited by Angela Haden, assisted by Barbara Campanini. Administrative and technical support for the World Health Report team were provided by Shelagh Probst, Michel Beusenberg, Amel Chaouachi and Chrissie Chitsulo. The index was prepared by Liza Weinkove.

The cover shows a photograph of a sculpture entitled "Ascending Horizon" by Rafael Barrios, in Caracas, Venezuela. The photograph by Mireille Vautier is reproduced with the kind permission of ANA Agence photographique de presse, Paris, France.

Design by Marilyn Langfeld. Layout by WHO Graphics
Printed in France
2000/12934 – Sadag – 30 000

CONTENTS

LIST OF MEMBER STATES BY WHO REGION AND MORTALITY STRATUM

ACKNOWLEDGEMENTS

INDEX

TABLES

FIGURES

BOXES

MESSAGE FROM
THE DIRECTOR-GENERAL

*W*hat makes for a good health system? What makes a health system fair? And how do we know whether a health system is performing as well as it could? These questions are the subject of public debate in most countries around the world.

Naturally, answers will depend on the perspective of the respondent. A minister of health defending the budget in parliament; a minister of finance attempting to balance multiple claims on the public purse; a harassed hospital superintendent under pressure to find more beds; a health centre doctor or nurse who has just run out of antibiotics; a news editor looking for a story; a mother seeking treatment for her sick two-year old child; a pressure group lobbying for better services – all will have their views. We in the World Health Organization need to help all involved to reach a balanced judgement.

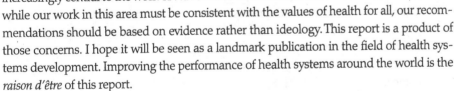

Whatever standard we apply, it is evident that health systems in some countries perform well, while others perform poorly. This is not due just to differences in income or expenditure: we know that performance can vary markedly, even in countries with very similar levels of health spending. The way health systems are designed, managed and financed affects people's lives and livelihoods. The difference between a well-performing health system and one that is failing can be measured in death, disability, impoverishment, humiliation and despair.

When I became Director-General in 1998, one of my prime concerns was that health systems development should become increasingly central to the work of WHO. I also took the view that

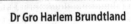

Dr Gro Harlem Brundtland

while our work in this area must be consistent with the values of health for all, our recommendations should be based on evidence rather than ideology. This report is a product of those concerns. I hope it will be seen as a landmark publication in the field of health systems development. Improving the performance of health systems around the world is the *raison d'être* of this report.

Our challenge is to gain a better understanding of the factors that make a difference. It has not been an easy task. We have debated how a health system should be defined in order to extend our field of concern beyond the provision of public and personal health services, and encompass other key areas of public policy that have an impact on people's health. This report suggests that the boundaries of health systems should encompass all actions whose primary intent is to improve health.

The report breaks new ground in the way that it helps us understand the goals of health systems. Clearly, their defining purpose is to improve and protect health – but they have other intrinsic goals. These are concerned with fairness in the way people pay for health care, and with how systems respond to people's expectations with regard to how they are treated. Where health and responsiveness are concerned, achieving a high average level is not good enough: the goals of a health system must also include reducing inequalities, in ways that improve the situation of the worst-off. In this report attainment in relation to these goals provides the basis for measuring the performance of health systems.

If policy-makers are to act on measures of performance, they need a clear understanding of the key functions that health systems have to undertake. The report defines four key functions: providing services; generating the human and physical resources that make service delivery possible; raising and pooling the resources used to pay for health care; and, most critically, the function of stewardship – setting and enforcing the rules of the game and providing strategic direction for all the different actors involved.

Undoubtedly, many of the concepts and measures used in the report require further refinement and development. To date, our knowledge about health systems has been hampered by the weakness of routine information systems and insufficient attention to research. This report has thus required a major effort to assemble data, collect new information, and carry out the required analysis and synthesis. It has also drawn on the views of a large number of respondents, within and outside WHO, concerning the interpretation of data and the relative importance of different goals.

The material in this report cannot provide definitive answers to every question about health systems performance. It does though bring together the best available evidence to date. It demonstrates that, despite the complexity of the topic and the limitations of the data, it is possible to get a reasonable approximation of the current situation, in a way that provides an exciting agenda for future work.

I hope that the report will contribute to work on how to assess and improve health systems. Performance assessment allows policy-makers, health providers and the population at large to see themselves in terms of the social arrangements they have constructed to improve health. It invites reflection on the forces that shape performance and the actions that can improve it.

For WHO, *The world health report 2000* is a milestone in a long-term process. The measurement of health systems performance will be a regular feature of all *World health reports* from now on – using improved and updated information and methods as they are developed.

Even though we are at an early stage in understanding a complex set of interactions, some important conclusions are clear.

- Ultimate responsibility for the performance of a country's health system lies with government. The careful and responsible management of the well-being of the population – stewardship – is the very essence of good government. The health of people is always a national priority: government responsibility for it is continuous and permanent.

- Dollar for dollar spent on health, many countries are falling short of their performance potential. The result is a large number of preventable deaths and lives stunted by disability. The impact of this failure is born disproportionately by the poor.

- Health systems are not just concerned with improving people's health but with protecting them against the financial costs of illness. The challenge facing governments in low income countries is to reduce the regressive burden of out-of-pocket payment for health by expanding prepayment schemes, which spread financial risk and reduce the spectre of catastrophic health care expenditures.
- Within governments, many health ministries focus on the public sector often disregarding the – frequently much larger – private finance and provision of care. A growing challenge is for governments to harness the energies of the private and voluntary sectors in achieving better levels of health systems performance, while offsetting the failures of private markets.
- Stewardship is ultimately concerned with *oversight* of the entire system, avoiding myopia, tunnel vision and the turning of a blind eye to a system's failings. This report is meant to make that task easier by bringing new evidence into sharp focus.

In conclusion, I hope this report will help policy-makers to make wise choices. If they do so, substantial gains will be possible for all countries, and the poor will be the principal beneficiaries.

Gro Harlem Brundtland
Geneva
June 2000

OVERVIEW

$\mathcal{T}$oday and every day, the lives of vast numbers of people lie in the hands of health systems. From the safe delivery of a healthy baby to the care with dignity of the frail elderly, health systems have a vital and continuing responsibility to people throughout the lifespan. They are crucial to the healthy development of individuals, families and societies everywhere.

In this report, health systems are defined as comprising all the organizations, institutions and resources that are devoted to producing health actions. A health action is defined as any effort, whether in personal health care, public health services or through intersectoral initiatives, whose primary purpose is to improve health.

But while improving health is clearly the main objective of a health system, it is not the only one. The objective of good health itself is really twofold: the best attainable average level – *goodness* – and the smallest feasible differences among individuals and groups – *fairness*. Goodness means a health system responding well to what people expect of it; fairness means it responds equally well to everyone, without discrimination. In *The world health report 2000*, devoted entirely to health systems, the World Health Organization expands its traditional concern for people's physical and mental well-being to emphasize these other elements of goodness and fairness.

To an unprecedented degree, it takes account of the roles people have as providers and consumers of health services, as financial contributors to health systems, as workers within them, and as citizens engaged in the responsible management, or stewardship, of them. And it looks at how well or how badly systems address inequalities, how they respond to people's expectations, and how much or how little they respect people's dignity, rights and freedoms.

The world health report 2000 also breaks new ground in presenting for the first time an index of national health systems' performance in trying to achieve three overall goals: *good health, responsiveness to the expectations of the population,* and *fairness of financial contribution*.

Progress towards them depends crucially on how well systems carry out four vital functions. These are: *service provision, resource generation, financing* and *stewardship*. The report devotes a chapter to each function, and reaches conclusions and makes policy recommendations on each. It places special emphasis on stewardship, which has a profound influence on the other three.

Many questions about health system performance have no clear or simple answers – because outcomes are hard to measure and it is hard to disentangle the health *system's* contribution from other factors. Building on valuable previous work, this report introduces WHO's framework for assessing health system performance. By clarifying and quantifying the goals of health systems and relating them to the essential functions, the framework is meant to help Member States measure their own performance, understand the factors that contribute to it, improve it, and respond better to the needs and expectations of the people they serve and represent. The analysis and synthesis of a wealth of information is summarized by a measure of overall achievement and by a performance index which should lead to much new research and policy development. The index will be a regular feature of forthcoming *World health reports* and will be improved and updated every year.

The framework was the basis for round table discussions entitled "*Addressing the major health system challenges*" among Ministers of Health at the 53rd World Health Assembly in Geneva in May 2000. The subject of these discussions is reflected throughout the report, and the outcome of the discussions will help orient future work on the framework.

Policy-makers need to know why health systems perform in certain ways and what they can do to improve the situation. All health systems carry out the functions of providing or delivering personal and non-personal health services; generating the necessary human and physical resources to make that possible; raising and pooling the revenues used to purchase services; and acting as the overall stewards of the resources, powers and expectations entrusted to them.

Comparing the way these functions are actually carried out provides a basis for understanding performance variations over time and among countries. Undoubtedly, many of the concepts and measures used in the report will require refinement. There is an important agenda of developing more and better data on goal attainment and on health system functions. Yet much can be learned from existing information. The report presents the best available evidence to date. In doing so, it seeks to push forward national and global development of the skills and information required to build a solid body of evidence on the level and determinants of performance, as a basis for improving how systems work.

"Improving performance" are therefore the key words and the *raison d'être* of this report. The overall mission of WHO is the attainment by all people of the highest possible level of health, with special emphasis on closing the gaps within and among countries. The Organization's ability to fulfil this mission depends greatly on the effectiveness of health systems in Member States – and strengthening those systems is one of WHO's four strategic directions. It connects very well with the other three: reducing the excess mortality of poor and marginalized populations; dealing effectively with the leading risk factors; and placing health at the centre of the broader development agenda.

Combating disease epidemics, striving to reduce infant mortality, and fighting for safer pregnancy are all WHO priorities. But the Organization will have very little impact in these and other battlegrounds unless it is equally concerned to strengthen the health systems through which the ammunition of life-saving and life-enhancing interventions are delivered to the front line.

This report asserts that the differing degrees of efficiency with which health systems organize and finance themselves, and react to the needs of their populations, explain much of the widening gap in death rates between the rich and poor, in countries and between countries, around the world. Even among countries with similar income levels, there are unacceptably large variations in health outcomes. The report finds that inequalities in life expectancy persist, and are strongly associated with socioeconomic class, even in countries that enjoy an average of quite good health. Furthermore the gap between rich and poor widens when life expectancy is divided into years in good health and years of disability. In effect, the poor not only have shorter lives than the non-poor, a bigger part of their lifetime is surrendered to disability.

In short, how health systems – and the estimated 35 million or more people they employ worldwide – perform makes a profound difference to the quality and value, as well as the length of the lives of the billions of people they serve.

HOW HEALTH SYSTEMS HAVE EVOLVED

This report's review of the evolution of modern health systems, and their various stages of reform, leaves little doubt that in general they have already contributed enormously to better health for most of the global population during the 20th century.

Today, health systems in all countries, rich and poor, play a bigger and more influential role in people's lives than ever before. Health systems of some sort have existed for as long as people have tried to protect their health and treat diseases. Traditional practices, often integrated with spiritual counselling and providing both preventive and curative care, have existed for thousands of years and often coexist today with modern medicine.

But 100 years ago, organized health systems in the modern sense barely existed. Few people alive then would ever visit a hospital. Most were born into large families and faced an infancy and childhood threatened by a host of potentially fatal diseases – measles, smallpox, malaria and poliomyelitis among them. Infant and child mortality rates were very high, as were maternal mortality rates. Life expectancy was short – even half a century ago it was a mere 48 years at birth. Birth itself invariably occurred at home, rarely with a physician present.

As a brief illustration of the contemporary role of health systems, one particular birth receives special attention in this report. Last year, United Nations experts calculated that the global population would reach six billion on 13 October 1999. On that day, in a maternity clinic in Sarajevo, a baby boy was designated as the sixth billionth person on the planet. He entered the world with a life expectancy of 73 years, the current Bosnian average.

He was born in a big city hospital, staffed by well-trained midwives, nurses, doctors and technicians. They were supported by high-technology equipment, drugs and medicines. The hospital is part of a sophisticated health service, connected in turn to a wide network of people and actions that in one way or another are concerned with measuring, maintaining and improving his health for the rest of his life – as for the rest of the population. Together, all these interested parties, whether they provide services, finance them or set policies to administer them, make up a health system.

Health systems have undergone overlapping generations of reforms in the past 100 years, including the founding of national health care systems and the extension of social insurance schemes. Later came the promotion of primary health care as a route to achieving affordable universal coverage – the goal of health for all. Despite its many virtues, a criticism of this route has been that it gave too little attention to people's *demand* for health care, and instead concentrated almost exclusively on their perceived *needs*. Systems have foundered when these two concepts did not match, because then the supply of services offered could not possibly align with both.

In the past decade or so there has been a gradual shift of vision towards what WHO calls the "new universalism". Rather than all possible care for everyone, or only the simplest and most basic care for the poor, this means delivery to all of high-quality essential care, defined mostly by criteria of effectiveness, cost and social acceptability. It implies explicit choice of priorities among interventions, respecting the ethical principle that it may be necessary and efficient to ration services, but that it is inadmissible to exclude whole groups of the population.

This shift has been partly due to the profound political and economic changes of the last 20 years or so. These include the transformation from centrally planned to market-oriented economies, reduced state intervention in national economies, fewer government controls, and more decentralization.

Ideologically, this has meant greater emphasis on individual choice and responsibility. Politically, it has meant limiting promises and expectations about what governments should do. But at the same time people's expectations of health systems are greater than ever before. Almost every day another new drug or treatment, or a further advance in medicine and health technology, is announced. This pace of progress is matched only by the rate at which the population seeks its share of the benefits.

The result is increasing demands and pressures on health systems, including both their public and private sectors, in all countries, rich or poor. Clearly, limits exist on what governments can finance and on what services they can deliver. This report means to stimulate public policies that acknowledge the constraints governments face. If services are to be provided for all, then not all services can be provided.

THE POTENTIAL TO IMPROVE

Within all systems there are many highly skilled, dedicated people working at all levels to improve the health of their communities. As the new century begins, health systems have the power and the potential to achieve further extraordinary improvements.

Unfortunately, health systems can also misuse their power and squander their potential. Poorly structured, badly led, inefficiently organized and inadequately funded health systems can do more harm than good.

This report finds that many countries are falling far short of their potential, and most are making inadequate efforts in terms of responsiveness and fairness of financial contribution. There are serious shortcomings in the performance of one or more functions in virtually all countries.

These failings result in very large numbers of preventable deaths and disabilities in each country; in unnecessary suffering; in injustice, inequality and denial of basic rights of individuals. The impact is most severe on the poor, who are driven deeper into poverty by lack of financial protection against ill-health. In trying to buy health from their own pockets, sometimes they only succeed in lining the pockets of others.

In this report, the poor also emerge as receiving the worst levels of responsiveness – they are treated with less respect for their dignity, given less choice of service providers and offered lower-quality amenities.

The ultimate responsibility for the overall performance of a country's health system lies with government, which in turn should involve all sectors of society in its stewardship. The careful and responsible management of the well-being of the population is the very essence of good government. For every country it means establishing the best and fairest health system possible with available resources. The health of the people is always a national priority: government responsibility for it is continuous and permanent. Ministries of health must therefore take on a large part of the stewardship of health systems.

Health policy and strategies need to cover the private provision of services and private financing, as well as state funding and activities. Only in this way can health systems as a whole be oriented towards achieving goals that are in the public interest. Stewardship encompasses the tasks of defining the vision and direction of health policy, exerting influence through regulation and advocacy, and collecting and using information. At the international level, stewardship means mobilizing the collective action of countries to generate global public goods such as research, while fostering a shared vision towards more equitable development across and within countries. It also means providing an evidence base to assist countries' efforts to improve the performance of their health systems.

But this report finds that some countries appear to have issued no national health policy statement in the past decade; in others, policy exists in the form of documents which gather dust and are never translated into action. Too often, health policy and strategic planning have envisaged unrealistic expansion of the publicly funded health care system, sometimes well in excess of national economic growth. Eventually, the policy and planning document is seen as infeasible and is ignored.

A policy framework should recognize all three health system goals and identify strategies to improve the attainment of each. But not all countries have explicit policies on the overall goodness and fairness of the health system. Public statements about the desired balance among health outcomes, system responsiveness and fairness in financial contribution are yet to be made in many countries. Policy should address the way in which the system's key functions are to be improved.

This report finds that, within governments, many health ministries are seriously shortsighted, focusing on the public sector and often disregarding the – frequently much larger – private provision of care. At worst, governments are capable of turning a blind eye to a "black market" in health, where widespread corruption, bribery, "moonlighting" and other illegal practices have flourished for years and are difficult to tackle successfully. Their vision does not extend far enough to help construct a healthier future.

Moreover, some health ministries are prone to losing sight completely of their most important target: the population at large. Patients and consumers may only come into view when rising public dissatisfaction forces them to the ministry's attention.

Many health ministries condone the evasion of regulations that they themselves have created or are supposed to implement in the public interest. Rules rarely enforced are invitations to abuse. A widespread example is the condoning of public employees charging illicit fees from patients and pocketing the proceeds, a practice known euphemistically as "informal charging". Such corruption deters poor people from using services they need, making health financing even more unfair, and it distorts overall health priorities.

PROVIDING BETTER SERVICES

Too many governments know far too little about what is happening in the provision of services to their people. In many countries, some if not most physicians work simultaneously for the government and in private practice. When public providers illegally use public facilities to provide special care to private patients, the public sector ends up subsidizing unofficial private practice. Health professionals are aware of practice-related laws but know that enforcement is weak or non-existent. Professional associations, nominally responsible for self-regulation, are too often ineffective.

Oversight and regulation of private sector providers and insurers must be placed high on national policy agendas. At the same time it is crucial to adopt incentives that are sensitive to performance. Good policy needs to differentiate between providers (public or private) who are contributing to health goals, and those who are doing damage, and encourage or sanction appropriately. Policies to change the balance between providers' autonomy and accountability need to be monitored closely in terms of their effect on health, responsiveness and the distribution of the financing burden.

Where particular practices and procedures are known to be harmful, the health ministry has a clear responsibility to combat them with public information and legal measures. Pharmaceutical sales by unregistered sellers, the dangers of excessive antibiotic prescription and of non-compliance with recommended dosages should all be objects of public stewardship, with active support from information campaigns targeted at patients, the providers in question and local health authorities.

Contrary to what might be expected, the share of private health financing tends to be larger in countries where income levels are lower. But poorer countries seldom have clear lines of policy towards the private sector. They thus have major steps to take in recognizing and communicating with the different groups of private providers, the better to influence and regulate them.

The private sector has the potential to play a positive role in improving the performance of the health system. But for this to happen, governments must fulfil the core public function of stewardship. Proper incentives and adequate information are two powerful tools to improve performance.

To move towards higher quality care, more and better information is commonly required on existing provision, on the interventions offered and on major constraints on service implementation. Local and national risk factors need to be understood. Information on numbers and types of providers is a basic – and often incompletely fulfilled – requirement. An understanding of provider market structure and utilization patterns is also needed, so that policy-makers know why this array of provision exists, as well as where it is growing.

An explicit, public process of priority setting should be undertaken to identify the contents of a benefit package which should be available to all, and which should reflect local disease priorities and cost effectiveness, among other criteria. Supporting mechanisms – clinical protocols, registration, training, licensing and accreditation processes – need to be brought up to date and used. There is a need for a regulatory strategy which distinguishes between the components of the private sector and includes the promotion of self-regulation.

Consumers need to be better informed about what is good and bad for their health, why not all of their expectations can be met, and that they have rights which all providers should respect. Aligning organizational structures and incentives with the overall objectives of policy is a task for stewardship, not just for service providers.

Monitoring is needed to assess behavioural change associated with decentralizing authority over resources and services, and the effects of different types of contractual relationships with public and private providers. Striking a balance between tight control and the independence needed to motivate providers is a delicate task, for which local solutions must be found. Experimentation and adaptation will be necessary in most settings. A supporting process for exchanging information will be necessary to create a 'virtual network' from a large set of semi-autonomous providers.

FINDING A BETTER BALANCE

The report says serious imbalances exist in many countries in terms of human and physical resources, technology and pharmaceuticals. Many countries have too few qualified health personnel, others have too many. Health system staff in many low-income nations are inadequately trained, poorly-paid and work in obsolete facilities with chronic shortages of equipment. One result is a "brain drain" of talented but demoralized professionals who either go abroad or move into private practice. Here again, the poor are most affected.

Overall, governments have too little information on financial flows and the generation of human and material resources. To rectify this, national health accounts (NHAs) should be much more widely calculated and used. They provide the essential information needed to monitor the ratio of capital to recurrent expenditure, or of any one input to the total, and to observe trends. NHAs capture foreign as well as domestic, public as well as private inputs and usefully assemble data on physical quantities – such as the numbers of nurses, medical equipment, district hospitals – as well as their costs.

NHAs in some form now exist for most countries, but they are still often rudimentary and are not yet widely used as tools of stewardship. NHA data allow the ministry of health to think critically about input purchases by all fundholders in the health system.

The concept of strategic purchasing, discussed in this report, does not only apply to the purchase of health care services: it applies equally to the purchase of health system inputs. Where inputs such as trained personnel, diagnostic equipment and vehicles are purchased directly with public funds, the ministry of health has a direct responsibility to ensure that value for money is obtained – not only in terms of good prices, but also in ensuring that effective use is made of the items purchased.

Where health system inputs are purchased by other agencies (such as private insurers, providers, households or other public agencies) the ministry's stewardship role consists of using its regulatory and persuasive influence to ensure that these purchases improve, rather than worsen, the efficiency of the input mix.

The central ministry may have to decide on major capital decisions, such as tertiary hospitals or medical schools. But regional and district health authorities should be entrusted with the larger number of lower-level purchasing decisions, using guidelines, criteria and procedures promoted by central government.

Ensuring a healthy balance between capital and recurrent spending in the health system requires analysis of trends in both public and private spending and a consideration of both domestic and foreign funds. A clear policy framework, incentives, regulation and public information need to be brought to bear on important capital decisions in the entire system to counter ad hoc decisions and political influence.

In terms of human resources, similar combinations of strategy have had some success in tackling the geographical imbalances common within countries. In general, the content of training needs to be reassessed in relation to workers' actual job content, and overall supply often needs to be adjusted to meet employment opportunities.

In some countries where the social return to medical training is negative, educational institutions are being considered for privatization or closure. Certainly, public subsidies for training institutions often need to be reconsidered in the light of strategic purchasing. Rebalancing the intake levels of different training facilities is often possible without closure, and might free resources which could be used to retrain in scarcer skills those health workers who are clearly surplus to requirements.

Major equipment purchases are an easy way for the health system to waste resources, when they are underused, yield little health gain, and use up staff time and recurrent budget. They are also difficult to control. All countries need access to information on technology assessment, though they do not necessarily need to produce this themselves. The stewardship role lies in ensuring that criteria for technology purchase in the public sector (which all countries need) are adhered to, and that the private sector does not receive incentives or public subsidy for its technology purchases unless these further the aim of national policy.

Providers frequently mobilize public support or subscriptions for technology purchase, and stewardship has to ensure that consumers understand why technology purchases have to be rationed like other services. Identifying the opportunity cost of additional technology in terms of other needed services may help to present the case to the public.

PROTECTING THE POOR

In the world's poorest countries, most people, particularly the poor, have to pay for health care from their own pockets at the very time they are sick and most in need of it. They are less likely to be members of job-based prepayment schemes, and have less access than better-off groups to subsidized services.

This report presents convincing evidence that prepayment is the best form of revenue collection, while out-of-pocket payment tends to be quite regressive and often impedes access to care. In poor countries, the poor often suffer twice – all of them have to pay an unfair share through taxes or insurance schemes, whether or not they use health services, and some of them have also to pay an even more unfair contribution from their pockets. Evidence from many health systems shows that prepayment through insurance schemes leads to greater financing fairness. The main challenge in revenue collection is to expand prepayment, in which public financing or mandatory insurance will play a central role. In the case of revenue pooling, creating as wide a pool as possible is critical to spreading financial risk for health care, and thus reducing individual risk and the spectre of impoverishment from health expenditures.

Insurance systems entail integration of resources from individual contributors or sources both to pool and to share risks across the population. Achieving greater fairness in financing is only achievable through risk pooling – that is, those who are healthy subsidize those who are sick, and those who are rich subsidize those who are poor. Strategies need to be designed for expansion of risk pooling so that progress can be made in such subsidies.

Raising the level of public finance for health is the most obvious route to increased prepayment. But the poorest countries raise less, in public revenue, as a percentage of national income than middle and upper income countries. Where there is no feasible organizational arrangement to boost prepayment levels, both donors and governments should explore ways of building enabling mechanisms for the development or consolidation of very large pools. Insurance schemes designed to expand membership among the poor would, moreover, be an attractive way to channel external assistance in health, alongside government revenue.

Many countries have employment-based schemes which increase benefits for their privileged membership – mainly employees in the formal sector of the economy – rather than widen them for a larger pool. Low income countries could encourage different forms of prepayment – job-based, community-based, or provider-based – as part of a preparatory process of consolidating small pools into larger ones. Governments need to promote community rating (i.e. each member of the community pays the same premium), a common benefit package and portability of benefits among insurance schemes, and public funds should pay for the inclusion of poor people in such schemes.

In middle income countries the policy route to fair prepaid systems is through strengthening the often substantial mandatory, income-based and risk-based insurance schemes, again ensuring increased public funding to include the poor. Although most industrialized countries already have very high levels of prepayment, some of these strategies are also relevant to them.

To ensure that prepaid finance obtains the best possible value for money, strategic purchasing needs to replace much of the traditional machinery linking budget holders to service providers. Budget holders will no longer be passive financial intermediaries. Strategic purchasing means ensuring a coherent set of incentives for providers, whether public or private, to encourage them to offer priority interventions efficiently. Selective contracting and the use of several payment mechanisms are needed to set incentives for better responsiveness and improved health outcomes.

In conclusion, this report sheds new light on what makes health systems behave in certain ways, and offers them better directions to follow in pursuit of their goals. WHO hopes it will help policy-makers weigh the many complex issues involved and make wise choices. If they do so, substantial gains will be possible for all countries; and the poor will be the principal beneficiaries.

CHAPTER ONE

Why do
Health Systems Matter?

Health systems consist of all the people and actions whose primary purpose is to improve health. They may be integrated and centrally directed, but often they are not. After centuries as small-scale, largely private or charitable, mostly ineffectual entities, they have grown explosively in this century as knowledge has been gained and applied. They have contributed enormously to better health, but their contribution could be greater still, especially for the poor. Failure to achieve that potential is due more to systemic failings than to technical limitations. It is therefore urgent to assess current performance and to judge how health systems can reach their potential.

1

Why do

Health Systems Matter?

The changing landscape

On 13 October 1999, in a maternity clinic in Sarajevo, Helac Fatima gave birth to a son. This was a special occasion, because United Nations demographers had calculated the global population would reach six billion on that day. The little Sarajevo boy was designated as the sixth billionth person on the planet.

Today there are four times as many people in the world as there were 100 years ago – there are now about 4000 babies born every minute of every day – and among the countless, bewildering changes that have occurred since then, some of the most profound have occurred in human health. For example, few if any of Helac Fatima's ancestors around 1899 were likely to have seen a hospital, far less been born in one.

The same was true for the great majority of the 1.5 billion people then alive. Throughout the world, childbirth invariably occurred at home, rarely with a physician present. Most people relied on traditional remedies and treatments, some of them thousands of years old. Most babies were born into large families and faced an infancy and childhood threatened by a host of potentially fatal diseases – measles, smallpox, malaria and poliomyelitis among them. Infant and child mortality rates were very high, as were maternal mortality rates. Life expectancy for adults was short – even half a century ago it was a mere 48 years at birth.

Last year the son of Helac Fatima entered the world with a life expectancy at birth of 73 years – the current Bosnian average. The global average is 66 years. He was born in a big city hospital staffed by well-trained midwives, nurses, doctors and technicians – who were supported by modern equipment, drugs and medicines. The hospital is part of a sophisticated health service. It is connected in turn to a wide network of people and actions that in one way or another are concerned with maintaining and improving his health for the rest of his life – as for the rest of the population. Together, all these interested parties, whether they provide services, finance them or set policies to administer them, make up a health system.

Health systems have played a part in the dramatic rise in life expectancy that occurred during the 20th century. They have contributed enormously to better health and influenced the lives and well-being of billions of men, women and children around the world. Their role has become increasingly important.

Enormous gaps remain, however, between the potential of health systems and their actual performance, and there is far too much variation in outcomes among countries which seem to have the same resources and possibilities. Why should this be so? Health systems would seem no different from other social systems in facing demands and incentives to perform as well as possible, and it might be expected that – with some degree of regulation by the state – their performance could be largely left to markets, just as with the provision of most other goods and services.

But health is fundamentally different from other things that people want, and the difference is rooted in biology. As eloquently expressed by Jonathan Miller, "Of all the objects in the world, the human body has a peculiar status: it is not only possessed by the person who has it, it also possesses and constitutes him. Our body is quite different from all the other things we claim as our own. We can lose money, books and even houses and still remain recognisably ourselves, but it is hard to give any intelligible sense to the idea of a disembodied person. Although we speak of our bodies as premises that we live in, it is a special form of tenancy: our body is where we can always be contacted" *(1)*. The person who seeks health care is of course a consumer – as with all other products and services – and may also be a co-producer of his or her health, in following good habits of diet, hygiene and exercise, and complying with medication or other recommendations of providers. But he or she is also the physical object to which all such care is directed.

Health, then, is a characteristic of an inalienable asset, and in this respect it somewhat resembles other forms of human capital, such as education, professional knowledge or athletic skills. But it still differs from them in crucial respects. It is subject to large and unpredictable risks, which are mostly independent of one another. And it cannot be accumulated as knowledge and skills can. These features are enough to make health radically unlike all other assets which people insure against loss or damage, and are the reason why health insurance is more complex than any other kind of insurance. If a car worth US$ 10 000 would cost $15 000 to repair after an accident, an insurer would only pay $10 000. The impossibility of replacing the body, and the consequent absence of a market value for it, precludes any such ceiling on health costs.

Since the poor are condemned to live in their bodies just as the rich are, they need protection against health risks fully as much. In contrast, where other assets such as housing are concerned, the need for such protection either does not arise, or arises only in proportion to income. This basic biological difference between health and other assets even exaggerates forms of market failure, such as moral hazard and imperfect and asymmetric information, that occur for other goods and services. Directly or indirectly, it explains much of the reason why markets work less well for health than for other things, why there is need for a more active and also more complicated role for the state, and in general why good performance cannot be taken for granted.

The physical integrity and dignity of the individual are recognized in international law, yet there have been shameful instances of the perversion of medical knowledge and skills, such as involuntary or uninformed participation in experiments, forced sterilization, or violent expropriation of organs. Health systems therefore have an additional responsibility to ensure that people are treated with respect, in accordance with human rights.

This report sets out to analyse the role of health systems and suggest how to make them more efficient and, most importantly, more accessible and responsive to the hundreds of millions of people presently excluded from benefiting fully from them. The denial of access to basic health care is fundamentally linked to poverty – the greatest blight on humanity's landscape. For all their achievements and good intentions, health systems have failed globally to narrow the health divide between rich and poor in the last 100 years. In fact, the gap is actually widening. Some such worsening often accompanies economic progress, as the already better-off are the first to benefit from it. But the means exist to accelerate the sharing by the poor in these benefits, and often at relatively low cost (see Box 1.1). Finding a successful new direction for health systems is therefore a powerful weapon in the fight against poverty to which WHO is dedicated. Not least for the children of the new century, countries need systems that protect all their citizens against both the health risks and the financial risks of illness.

WHAT IS A HEALTH SYSTEM?

In today's complex world, it can be difficult to say exactly what a health system is, what it consists of, and where it begins and ends. This report defines a health system to include *all the activities whose primary purpose is to promote, restore or maintain health.*

Formal health services, including the professional delivery of personal medical attention, are clearly within these boundaries. So are actions by traditional healers, and all use of medication, whether prescribed by a provider or not. So is home care of the sick, which is how somewhere between 70% and 90% of all sickness is managed *(2)*. Such traditional public health activities as health promotion and disease prevention, and other health-enhancing interventions like road and environmental safety improvement, are also part of the system. Beyond the boundaries of this definition are those activities whose primary purpose is something other than health – education, for example – even if these activities have a secondary, health-enhancing benefit. Hence, the general education system is outside the boundaries, but specifically health-related education is included. So are actions intended chiefly to improve health indirectly by influencing how non-health systems function – for example, actions to increase girls' school enrolment or change the curriculum to make students better future caregivers and consumers of health care.

Box 1.1 Poverty, ill-health and cost-effectiveness

The series of global estimates of the burden of disease do not distinguish between rich and poor, but an approximate breakdown can be derived by ranking countries by per capita income, aggregating from the lowest and highest incomes to form groups each constituting 20% of the world's population, and studying the distribution of deaths in each group, by age,[1] cause and sex.[2] These estimates show that in 1990, 70% of all deaths and fully 92% of deaths from communicable diseases in the poorest quintile were "excess" compared to the mortality that would have occurred at the death rates of the richest quintile. The figures for total losses of disability-adjusted life

years (DALYs) were similar, with a larger contribution from noncommunicable diseases. The large difference between the effects of communicable and noncommunicable diseases reflects the concentration of deaths and DALYs lost to communicable diseases among the global poor: about 60% of all ill-health for the poor versus 8–11 % among the richest quintile. This is strongly associated with differences in the age distribution of deaths: just over half of all deaths among the poor occur before 15 years of age, compared to only 4% among the rich. The difference between the poor and the rich is large even in a typical high-mortality African country, and much greater in a typical lower-mortality Latin American

country, where deaths at early ages have almost been eliminated among the wealthy.

There are relatively cost-effective interventions available against the diseases that account for most of these rich–poor differences, and particularly to combat deaths and health losses among young children.[3] Interventions costing an estimated $100 or less per DALY saved could deal with 8 or 9 of the 10 leading causes of ill-health under the age of 5 years, and 6 to 8 of the 10 main causes between the ages of 5 and 14 years. All of these are either communicable diseases or forms of malnutrition. Death and disability from these causes is projected to decline rapidly by 2020, roughly equalizing the health damage from

communicable and noncommunicable diseases among the poor. If the projected rate of decline of communicable disease damage could be doubled, the global rich would gain only 0.4 years of life expectancy, but the global poor would gain an additional 4.1 years, narrowing the difference between the two groups from 18.4 to 13.7 years. Doubling the pace of reduction of noncommunicable disease damage, in contrast, would preferentially benefit the well-off as well as costing considerably more. The association between poverty and cost-effectiveness is only partial, and probably transitory, but in today's epidemiological and economic conditions it is quite strong.

---

[1] Gwatkin DR. *The current state of knowledge about how well government health services reach the poor: implications for sector-wide approaches.* Washington, DC, The World Bank, 5 February 1998 (discussion draft).
[2] Gwatkin DR, Guillot M. *The burden of disease among the world's poor: current situation, future trends, and implications for policy.* Washington, DC, Human Development Network of The World Bank, 2000.
[3] *World development report 1993 – Investing in health.* New York, Oxford University Press for The World Bank, 1993: Tables B.6 and B.7.

This way of defining a system does not imply any particular degree of integration, nor that anyone is in overall charge of the activities that compose it. In this sense, every country has a health system, however fragmented it may be among different organizations or however unsystematically it may seem to operate. Integration and oversight do not determine the system, but they may greatly influence how well it performs.

Unfortunately, nearly all the information available about health systems refers only to the provision of, and investment in, health services: that is, the health *care* system, including preventive, curative and palliative interventions, whether directed to individuals or to populations. In most countries, these services account for the great bulk of employment, expenditure and activity that would be included in a broader notion of the health system, so it might seem that little is lost in concentrating on a narrower definition that fits the existing data. Those data have required great efforts to collect – and this report further offers several kinds of information and analysis, such as estimates of life expectancy adjusted for time lived with disability, assessments of how well health systems treat patients, national health accounts, and estimates of household contribution to financing.

Nonetheless, efforts are needed to quantify and assess those activities implied by the wider definition, so as to begin to gauge their relative cost and effectiveness in contributing to the goals of the system. To take one example, in the United States between 1966 and 1979 the introduction of a variety of safety features in automobile design (laminated windshields, collapsible steering columns, interior padding, lap and shoulder belts, side marker lights, head restraints, leak resistant fuel systems, stronger bumpers, increased side door strength and better brakes) helped reduce the vehicle accident fatality rate per mile travelled by 40%. Only three of these innovations added more than $10 to the price of a car, and in total they accounted for only 2% of the average price increase during 1975–1979 (3). From 1975 to 1998, seat belts saved an estimated 112 000 lives in the United States, and total traffic fatalities continued to fall. The potential health gains were even greater: in 1998 alone, 9000 people died because they did not use their belts (4).

The potential savings in other countries are very large. Road traffic accidents are increasing rapidly in poor countries and are projected to move from the ninth to third place in the worldwide ranking of burden of ill-health by the year 2020. Even in many middle income countries, the fatality rates per head or per vehicle mile are much higher than in the United States (5). Sub-Saharan Africa has the world's highest rate of fatalities per vehicle. The cost of improving vehicles may be high, relative to expenditure on health care, in low and middle income countries, so the effect of including such activities in the definition of the health system may be greater. Unsafe roads also contribute greatly to the vehicular toll in poorer countries, and the cost of improving roads could be much larger than the cost of making cars safer. But behavioural changes such as using seat belts once installed, and respecting speed limits, are nearly costless and could save many lives; they are very likely to be more cost-effective than treatment of crash victims.

Where information corresponding to a broader definition of health systems is not available, this report necessarily uses the available data that match the notion of the health care system. Even by this more limited definition, health systems today represent one of the largest sectors in the world economy. Global spending on health care was about $2985 billion (thousand million) in 1997, or almost 8% of world gross domestic product (GDP), and the International Labour Organisation estimates that there were about 35 million health workers worldwide a decade ago, while employment in health services now is likely to be substantially higher. These figures reflect how what was for thousands of years a basic, private relationship – in which one person with an illness was looked after by family members or religious caregivers, or sometimes paid a professional healer to treat him or her – has expanded over the past two centuries into the complex network of activities that now comprise a health system.

More than simple growth, the creation of modern health systems has involved increasing differentiation and specialization of skills and activities. It has also involved an immense shift in the economic burden of ill-health. Until recently, most of that burden took the form of lost productivity, as people died young or became and remained too sick to work at full strength. The cost of health care accounted for only a small part of the economic loss, because such care was relatively cheap and largely ineffective. Productivity losses are still substantial, especially in the poorest countries, but success in prolonging life and reducing disability has meant that more and more of the burden is borne by health systems. This includes the cost of drugs – for controlling diabetes, hypertension, and heart disease, for example – that allow people to stay active and productive. Part of the growth in resources used by health systems is a transfer from other ways of paying for the economic damage due to illness and early death.

The resources devoted to health systems are very unequally distributed, and not at all in proportion to the distribution of health problems. Low and middle income countries account for only 18% of world income and 11% of global health spending ($250 billion or 4% of GDP in those countries). Yet 84% of the world's population live in these countries, and they bear 93% of the world's disease burden. These countries face many difficult challenges in meeting the health needs of their populations, mobilizing sufficient financing in an equitable and affordable manner, and securing value for scarce resources.

Today in most developed countries – and many middle income countries – governments have become central to social policy and health care. Their involvement is justified on the grounds of both equity and efficiency. However, in low income countries – where total public revenues for all uses are scarce (often less than 20% of GDP) and institutional capacity in the public sector is weak – the financing and delivery of health services is largely in the hands of the private sector. In many of these countries, large segments of the poor still have no access to basic and effective care.

WHAT DO HEALTH SYSTEMS DO?

For rich and poor alike, health needs today are very different from those of 100 or even 50 years ago. There are growing expectations of access to health care in some form, and growing demands for measures to protect the sick, and their families, against the financial costs of ill-health. The circle in which health systems are required to function has been pushed yet wider by raised awareness of the impact on health of developments such as industrialization, road transport, environmental damage and the globalization of trade. People also now turn to health systems for help with a much wider variety of problems than before – not just for the relief of pain and treatment of physical limitations and emotional disorders but for advice on diet, child-rearing and sexual behaviour that they used to seek from other sources.

People typically come into direct contact with a health system as patients, attended by providers, only once or twice a year. More often their contact is as consumers of non-prescription medications and as recipients of health-related information and advice. They meet the system as contributors to paying for it, knowingly every time they buy care out of pocket or pay insurance premiums or social security contributions, and unknowingly whenever they pay taxes that are used in part to finance health. It matters very much how the system treats people's health needs and how it raises revenues from them, including how much protection it offers them from financial risk. But it also matters how it responds to their expectations. In particular, people have a right to expect that the health system will treat them with individual dignity. So far as possible, their needs should be promptly attended to, without long delays in waiting for diagnosis and treatment – not only for better health outcomes but also to respect the value of people's time and to reduce their anxiety. Patients also often expect confidentiality, and to be involved in choices about their own health, including where and from whom they receive care. They should not always be expected passively to receive services determined by the provider alone.

In summary, health systems have a responsibility not just to improve people's health but to protect them against the financial cost of illness – and to treat them with dignity. As is discussed in more detail in Chapter 2, health systems thus have three fundamental objectives. These are:

- improving the health of the population they serve;
- responding to people's expectations;
- providing financial protection against the costs of ill-health.

Because these objectives are not always met, public dissatisfaction with the way health services are run or financed is widespread, with accounts of errors, delays, rudeness, hostility and indifference on the part of health workers, and denial of care or exposure to calamitous financial risks by insurers and governments, on a grand scale.

Because better health is the most important objective of a health system, and because health status is worse in poor populations, one might assume that for a low income country, improving health is all that matters. Concern for the non-health outcomes of the system, for fairly sharing the burden of paying for health so that no one is exposed to great financial risk, and attending to people's wishes and expectations about how they are to be treated, would then be considered luxuries, gaining in importance only as income rises and health improves. But this view is mistaken, for several reasons. Poor people, as indicated earlier, need financial protection as much as or more than the well-off, since even small absolute risks may have catastrophic consequences for them. And the poor are just as entitled to respectful treatment as the rich, even if less can be done for them materially. Moreover, pursuing the objectives of responsiveness and financial protection does not necessarily take substantial resources away from activities to improve health. Much improvement in how a health system performs with respect to these responsibilities may often be had at little or no cost. So all three objectives matter in every country, independently of how rich or poor it is or how its health system is organized. Better ways of achieving these objectives, treated in later chapters, are similarly relevant for all countries and health systems, although the specific implications for policy will vary according to income level and the cultural and organizational features of the system.

WHY HEALTH SYSTEMS MATTER

The contribution that health systems make to improving health has been examined much more closely than how well they satisfy the other two objectives mentioned above, for which there is little comparable information and analysis. This report therefore develops measures corresponding to all three objectives, for assessing how systems perform. Even the contribution that health systems make to improved health is difficult to judge, because different kinds of evidence seem to give conflicting answers. At the level of interventions against particular diseases or conditions, there is now substantial and growing evidence that large improvements in health can be achieved at reasonable cost, for individuals and for large populations *(6)*. Such data are the basis for estimates that in poor countries, roughly one-third of the disease burden in 1990 might be averted at a total cost per person of only $12 *(7)*.

Even without progress in fundamental science, changes in the way currently available interventions are organized and delivered can reverse the spread of an epidemic and dramatically reduce the cost of saving a life. For example, in the Brazilian Amazon, greater emphasis on early malaria case detection and treatment, together with more focused efforts on mosquito control, turned around an epidemic and cut the cost of saving a life by case prevention from nearly $13 000 to only about $2000 *(8)*.

At the level of overall progress in health, as reported in *The world health report 1999*, the generation and utilization of knowledge – that is, scientific and technical progress – explained almost half of the reduction in mortality between 1960 and 1990 in a sample of 115 low and middle income countries, while income growth explained less than 20% and increases in the educational level of adult females less than 40%. Such estimates summarize progress in developing and applying interventions of many kinds against a large number of diseases. Prominent among these are antimalaria and immunization programmes, and the increasing use of antibiotics for the treatment of respiratory and other infectious diseases. Since it is the health system that develops and applies those interventions, two kinds of evidence, one detailed and the other aggregated, indicate clearly that health systems not only can but do make a large difference to health.

Taking a narrower focus on diseases for which there are effective treatments, numerous studies beginning in the 1970s *(9, 10)* have consistently found that preventable deaths, that is "deaths due to causes amenable to medical care" have fallen at a faster rate than other deaths. Similarly, a comparison of death rate differences between western Europe and formerly communist countries of eastern Europe attributed 24% of the difference in male life expectancy and 39% of that in female life expectancy to the availability of modern medical care. Such care is not guaranteed simply by the existence of medical facilities *(11)*.

At the same time, other evidence seems to show that health systems make little or no difference. This emerges from some other comparisons across countries rather than through time. Often these show that while per capita income is strongly related to some measure of health status – as are other factors such as female education, income inequality or cultural characteristics – there is little independent connection with inputs such as doctors or hospital beds *(12)*, with total health expenditure *(13)*, with expenditure only on conditions amenable to medical care *(14)*, or with public spending on health *(15)*. It is not surprising to find that these relations are weak in rich countries, since many causes of death and disability are already controlled and there are many different ways to spend health system resources, with quite varying effects on health status. But health system expenditure often seems to make little difference even in poor countries with high infant and child mortality, which it should be a priority to reduce.

Furthermore, health systems make costly, even fatal mistakes far too frequently. In the United States alone, medical errors in hospitals cause at least 44 000 needless deaths a year, with another 7000 occurring as a result of mistakes in prescribing or using medication, making these errors more deadly than such killers as motor vehicle accidents, breast cancer and AIDS *(16)*. The economic cost of these mistakes is at least $17 billion, of which health care costs are more than half. And even when no one makes errors, patients often acquire new infections in hospital, and the massive use of antibiotics promotes pathogen resistance to them, so that some part of ill-health is caused by the very efforts to treat it.

These conflicting kinds of evidence can be reconciled in two ways: first, by noting that while health systems account for much health progress through time, that progress is far from uniform among countries at any one time, even among countries with similar levels of income and health expenditure; and second, by recognizing that the errors of the system diminish but do not offset the good it accomplishes. Nonetheless, "there is an enormous gap between the apparent potential of public spending to improve health status and the actual performance" *(15)*, and the same is doubtless true of resource use in general. One measure of that gap is that many deaths of children under 5 years of age could be averted for $10 or less, as estimated from cost-effectiveness studies of particularly valuable interventions, but the average actual expenditure in poor countries per death prevented, as estimated from the overall relation between spending and mortality, is $50 000 or more. The overall relation between child mortality and income implies that in a poor country of two million population, total income would have to rise by roughly $1 million in order to avert a single death. This is several orders of magnitude higher than the average health expenditure needed to save a life. Per capita, these numbers imply health expenditure of only $0.025 versus an income increase of $0.50. Income differences may explain more of health variation among countries than do differences in health expenditure. But raising income is not on that account a cheaper or easier way to improve health.

Concerning the more distant past, historians debate whether declines in mortality rates in some European and Latin American countries in the 19th and 20th centuries owe more to such factors as an improving diet and other socioeconomic progress than to personal medical care. But health systems, defined broadly, include all of the non-personal, population-based or public health interventions such as the promotion of healthy lifestyles, insecticide spraying against vector-borne diseases, anti-tobacco campaigns and the protection of food and water. So even if personal services accounted for very little health gain until recently, the health system as defined in this report began to make a large difference more

---

Box 1.2 Health knowledge, not income, explains historical change in urban–rural health differences

In the first half of the 19th century, life expectancy was much shorter in London and Paris, respectively, than in the rural areas of England and Wales or of France; a similar difference prevailed between the urban and rural areas of Sweden in the first decades of the 20th century. Large cities were unhealthy because unclean personal habits did more to spread disease when people were crowded together and because garbage and even excrement were accumulated, drawing flies and rodents and contaminating the air and water.[1] Pollution was wors-

ened by burning soft coal and by discharges from factories.

Crowding and poverty produce many of the same problems in the large cities of poor countries today, which typically have more polluted air and water than urban areas in richer countries. Vehicular exhaust, unknown a century ago, is already a major health threat in such areas as Delhi and Mexico City. Rapid growth has made it hard to expand such services as piped water, sewerage facilities and garbage collection fast enough to keep pace. In slum areas, even if safe water is available, many households have no access to sani-

tary waste disposal, and much garbage is simply dumped or burned in the open. Nonetheless the health consequences are not so severe as in European cities 150 years ago. On one hand, increased knowledge of how diseases are caused and transmitted has led to valiant efforts to reduce contamination, control disease vectors and educate the population to take better care of their health. On the other hand, even very poor urban dwellers now have better access to effective personal health care than much of the rural population, adding to the inducements to migrate to the city. Slum

residents in Lima, for example, are as likely to immunize their children and to take them for medical care when sick as residents of better-off neighbourhoods, and much more likely to do so than people living in Peru's mountainous interior.[2] Both the public health and the personal care interventions have contributed to reversing the urban–rural differences in health status; better health among urban populations is due more to the application of improved knowledge than to higher incomes in cities.

[1] Easterlin RA. *How beneficient is the market? A look at the modern history of mortality.* Los Angeles, University of Southern California, 1998 (unpublished paper).
[2] Musgrove P. Measurement of equity in health. *World Health Statistics Quarterly*, 1986, 39(4).

than a century ago, chiefly through improvements in urban sanitation and personal hygiene. These changes – removing excrement and garbage, protecting water supplies, and washing one's hands – happened because of more understanding of how diseases are *spread*, even before there was any useful knowledge of how they are *caused*. Some improved individual hygienic practices are centuries old, while collective measures are generally more recent. Growth in income alone would not have improved health under the conditions of the time, and may even have worsened it because of urban filth and crowding; similar conditions often prevail in the cities of poor countries today, but the threat to health is better controlled (see Box 1.2).

So health systems *are* valuable and important, but they could accomplish much more with the available understanding of how to improve health. The failings which limit performance do not result primarily from lack of knowledge but from not fully applying what is already known: that is, from systemic rather than technical failures. This is true even of most medical errors, because "the problem is not bad people; the problem is that the system needs to be made safer" *(16)*. How to measure current performance and how to achieve the potential improvements in it are the subject of this report. Research to expand knowledge is crucial in the long run, as progress over the last two centuries shows; in the short run, much could be accomplished by wider and better application of existing knowledge. This can improve health more quickly than continued and more equally distributed socioeconomic progress, important as that is. The next sections discuss how modern health systems arose, and how they have been repeatedly subjected to reforms intended to make them work better in one way or another.

HOW MODERN HEALTH SYSTEMS EVOLVED

Health systems of some sort have existed for as long as people have tried deliberately to protect their health and treat diseases. Throughout the world, traditional practices based on herbal cures, often integrated with spiritual counselling, and providing both preventive and curative care, have existed for thousands of years, and often coexist today with modern medicine. Many of them are still the treatment of choice for some health conditions, or are resorted to because modern alternatives are not understood or trusted, or fail, or are too expensive. Traditional Chinese medicine can be traced back more than 3000 years, and still plays a huge role in the Chinese health system, as do its equally ancient equivalents in the Indian sub-continent and similar systems of belief and practice among indigenous African and American peoples. But until the modern growth of knowledge about disease, there were few cures for ailments and little effective prevention of disease.

With rare exceptions, even in industrialized countries, organized health systems in the modern sense, intended to benefit the population at large, barely existed a century ago. Although hospitals have a much longer history than complete systems in many countries, few people living 100 years ago would ever visit one – and that remains true for many millions of the poor today. Until well into the 19th century they were for the most part run by charitable organizations, and often were little more than refuges for the orphaned, the crippled, the destitute or the insane. And there was nothing like the modern practice of referrals from one level of the system to another, and little protection from financial risk apart from that offered by charity or by small-scale pooling of contributions among workers in the same occupation.

Towards the close of the 19th century, the industrial revolution was transforming the lives of people worldwide. At the same time societies began to recognize the huge toll of death, illness and disability occurring among workforces, whether from infectious diseases which killed many thousands during the construction of the Panama Canal or from industrial accidents and exposures. Once it was realized that mosquitoes transmitted malaria and yellow fever, control of the insects' breeding-sites became part of prevention efforts that also translated into benefits for surrounding communities. In addition to the human costs, the toll of illness and death meant great losses in productivity. In response, company owners began providing medical services to treat their workers. As the importance of clean water and sanitation became better understood, they also improved workers' basic living conditions. Wars were another influence – the American Civil War showed that soldiers on both sides were more likely to be killed by disease than by the enemy. The same message came home from the Crimean and Boer wars.

About the same time, workers' health was becoming a political issue in some European countries, but for quite different reasons. Bismarck, Chancellor of Germany, reasoned that government take-over of labour unions' sickness funds would remove a source of their support at a moment when socialist workers' movements were gaining strength, and also increase workers' economic security *(17)*. Thus, in 1883, Germany enacted a law requiring employer contributions to health coverage for low-wage workers in certain occupations, adding other classes of workers in subsequent years. This was the first example of a state-mandated social insurance model. The popularity of this law among workers led to the adoption of similar legislation in Belgium in 1894 and Norway in 1909. Until Britain followed suit in 1911, medical care for British wage-earners tended to be paid for by their subscriptions to trade unions or friendly societies, which in turn paid the providers. But only the worker, and not his family, had such coverage.

In the late 1800s, Russia had begun setting up a huge network of provincial medical stations and hospitals where treatment was free and supported by tax funds. After the Bolshevik revolution in 1917, it was decreed that free medical care should be provided for the entire population, and the resulting system was largely maintained for almost eight decades. This was the earliest example of a completely centralized and state-controlled model.

The influence of the German model began to spread outside Europe after the First World War. In 1922, Japan added health benefits to the other benefits for which workers were eligible, building on its tradition of managerial paternalism. In 1924, Chile brought all covered workers under the umbrella of a Ministry of Labour scheme. By 1935, a total of 90% of Denmark's population was covered by work-related health insurance. Social insurance was introduced in the Netherlands during the country's occupation in the Second World War.

Not least among its effects, the Second World War damaged or virtually destroyed health infrastructures in many countries and delayed their health system plans. Paradoxically, it also paved the way for the introduction of some others. Wartime Britain's national emergency service to deal with casualties was helpful in the construction of what became, in 1948, the National Health Service, perhaps the most widely influential model of a health system. The Beveridge Report of 1942 *(18)* had identified health care as one of the three basic prerequisites for a viable social security system. The government's White Paper of 1944 stated the policy that "Everybody, irrespective of means, age, sex or occupation shall have equal opportunity to benefit from the best and most up-to-date medical and allied services available", adding that those services should be comprehensive and free of charge and should promote good health, as well as treating sickness and disease. New Zealand had already become, in 1938, the first country to introduce a national health service. Almost simultaneously, Costa Rica laid the foundation for universal health insurance in 1941. In

Mexico, the Institute of Social Security and the Ministry of Health were both founded in 1943. A scheme for a national health service broadly similar to the British model was proposed in South Africa in 1944, comprising free health care and a network of community centres and general practitioners as part of a referral system, but was not implemented (19).

In the immediate post-war period, Japan and the Soviet Union also extended their limited national systems to cover most or all of the population, as did Norway and Sweden, Hungary and other communist states in Europe, and Chile. As former colonies gained independence, they also tried to adopt modern, comprehensive systems with heavy state participation. India developed ambitious five-year development plans for a health system, based on the Bhore Report of 1946 (20). The factors which made this period of system-building and expansion possible included realization of the power of the modern state, post-war movements towards reconciliation, stability and reconstruction, and collective solidarity stemming from the war effort. Newly acquired citizenship and the belief in a relatively effective and benevolent state which could promote development of all kinds led to a social and political environment in which "classical universalism", the concept of free access to all kinds of health care for all, could take root.

Today's health systems are modelled to varying degrees on one or more of a few basic designs that emerged and have been refined since the late 19th century. One of these aims to cover all or most citizens through mandated employer and employee payments to insurance or sickness funds, while providing care through both public and private providers. The earliest such social insurance systems usually evolved from small, initially voluntary, associations; later versions have sometimes been created *ex nihilo* by public action. Another, slightly more recent, model centralizes planning and financing, relying primarily on tax revenues and on public provision. Resources are traditionally distributed by budgets, sometimes on the basis of fixed ratios between populations and health workers or facilities. In a third model, state involvement is more limited but still substantial, sometimes providing coverage only for certain population groups and giving way for the rest of the populace to largely private finance, provision and ownership of facilities. Relatively pure examples, in which one or another model accounts for the bulk of resources or provision, are found mostly in rich countries; health systems in middle income countries, notably in Latin America, tend to be a mixture of two or even all three types (21). Much debate has centred on whether one way of organizing a health system is better than another, but what matters about a system's overall structure is how well it facilitates the performance of its key functions.

THREE GENERATIONS OF HEALTH SYSTEM REFORM

During the 20th century, there have been three overlapping generations of health system reforms. They have been prompted not only by perceived failures in health but also by a quest for greater efficiency, fairness and responsiveness to the expectations of the people that systems serve. The first generation saw the founding of national health care systems, and the extension to middle income nations of social insurance systems, mostly in the 1940s and 1950s in richer countries and somewhat later in poorer countries. By the late 1960s, many of the systems founded a decade or two earlier were under great stress. Costs were rising, especially as the volume and intensity of hospital-based care increased in developed and developing countries alike. Among systems that were nominally universal in coverage, health services still were used more heavily by the better-off, and efforts to reach the poor were often incomplete. Too many people continued to depend on their own resources to pay for health, and could often get only ineffective or poor quality care.

These problems were apparent, and increasingly acute, in poorer countries. Colonial powers in Africa and Asia, and governments in Latin America, had established health services that for the most part excluded indigenous populations. For example, where a European model of health care was implemented in the countries of Africa under British administration, it was primarily intended for colonial administrators and expatriates, with separate or second class provision made – if at all – for Africans. Charitable missions and public health programmes were relied on to provide some care for the majority, much as in parts of Europe. In these former colonies and low income countries, the health system had therefore never been able to deliver even the most basic services to people in rural areas. Health facilities and clinics had been built, but primarily in urban areas. In most developing countries, major urban hospitals received around two-thirds of all government health budgets, despite serving just 10% to 20% of the population. Studies of what hospitals actually did revealed that half or more of all inpatient spending went towards treating conditions that could often have been managed by ambulatory care, such as diarrhoea, malaria, tuberculosis and acute respiratory infections *(22)*.

There was, therefore, a need for radical change that would make systems more cost-efficient, equitable, and accessible. A second generation of reforms thus saw the promotion of primary health care as a route to achieving affordable universal coverage. This approach reflected experience with disease control projects in the 1940s in countries such as South Africa, the Islamic Republic of Iran, and former Yugoslavia. It also built on the successes and experiments of China, Cuba, Guatemala, Indonesia, Niger, the United Republic of Tanzania, and Maharashtra State in India *(23)*. Some of these countries, and others such as Costa Rica and Sri Lanka, achieved very good health outcomes at relatively little cost, adding 15 to 20 years to life expectancy at birth in a span of just two decades. In each case, there was a very strong commitment to assuring a minimum level for all of health services, food and education, along with an adequate supply of safe water and basic sanitation. These were the key elements, along with an emphasis on public health measures relative to clinical care, prevention relative to cure, essential drugs, and education of the public by community health workers. By adopting primary health care as the strategy for achieving the goal of "Health for All" at the Joint WHO/UNICEF International Conference on Primary Health Care held at Alma-Ata, USSR (now Almaty, Kazakhstan) in 1978, WHO reinvigorated efforts to bring basic health care to people everywhere.

The term "primary" quickly acquired a variety of connotations, some of them technical (referring to the first contact with the health system, or the first level of care, or simple treatments that could be delivered by relatively untrained providers, or interventions acting on primary causes of disease) and some political (depending on multisectoral action or community involvement). The multiplicity of meanings and their often contradictory implications for policy help explain why there is no one model of primary care, and why it has been difficult to follow the successful examples of the countries or states that provided the first evidence that a substantial improvement in health could be achieved at affordable cost. There was a substantial effort in many countries to train and use community health workers who could deliver basic, cost-effective services in simple rural facilities to populations that previously had little or no access to modern care. In India, for example, such workers were trained and placed in over 100 000 health posts, intended to serve nearly two-thirds of the population.

Despite these efforts, many such programmes were eventually considered at least partial failures. Funding was inadequate; the workers had little time to spend on prevention and community outreach; their training and equipment were insufficient for the problems they confronted; and quality of care was often so poor as to be characterized as "primitive" rather than "primary", particularly when primary care was limited to the poor and to only the simplest services. Referral systems, which are unique to health services and necessary to their proper performance, have proved particularly difficult to operate adequately *(24)*. Lower level services were often poorly utilized, and patients who could do so commonly bypassed the lower levels of the system to go directly to hospitals. Partly in consequence, countries continued to invest in tertiary, urban-based centres.

In developed countries, primary care has been better integrated into the whole system, perhaps because it has been more associated with general and family medical practice, and with lower-level providers such as nurse practitioners and physician assistants. Greater reliance on such practitioners forms the core of many developed countries' current reform agendas. Managed care, for example, revolves to a large extent around the strengthening of primary care and the avoidance of unnecessary treatment, especially hospitalization.

The approach emphasized in the primary health care movement can be criticized for giving too little attention to people's *demand* for health care, which is greatly influenced by perceived quality and responsiveness, and instead concentrating almost exclusively on their presumed *needs*. Systems fail when these two concepts do not match, because then the supply of services offered cannot possibly align with both. The inadequate attention to demand is reflected in the complete omission of private finance and provision of care from the Alma-Ata Declaration, except insofar as community participation is construed to include small-scale private financing.

Poverty is one reason why needs may not be expressed in demand, and that can be resolved by offering care at low enough cost, not only in money but also in time and non-medical expenses. But there are many other reasons for mismatches between what people need and what they want, and simply providing medical facilities and offering services may do nothing to resolve them. In general, both the first-generation and second-generation reforms have been quite supply-oriented. Concern with demand is more characteristic of changes in the third generation currently under way in many countries, which include such reforms as trying to make "money follow the patient" and shifting away from simply giving providers budgets, which in turn are often determined by supposed needs.

If the organizational basis and the quality of primary health care often failed to live up to their potential, much of the technical footing remains sound and has undergone continuous refinement. This development can be sketched as a gradual convergence towards what WHO calls the "new universalism"– high quality delivery of essential care, defined mostly by the criterion of cost-effectiveness, for everyone, rather than all possible care for the whole population or only the simplest and most basic care for the poor (see Figure 1.1).

Figure 1.1 Coverage of population and of interventions under different notions of primary health care

Interventions included	Population covered	
	Only the poor	Everyone
"Basic" or simple	"Primitive" health care	Original concept
"Essential" and cost-effective	"Selective" primary health care ⟶	New universalism
Everything medically useful	(Never seriously contemplated)	Classical universalism

Adapted from Frenk J. *Building on the legacy: primary health care and the new policy directions at WHO*. Address to the American Public Health Association, Chicago, IL, 8 November 1999.

The notions that health and nutrition interventions can make a substantial difference to the health of large populations *(25)* and of obtaining "good health at low cost" *(26)* by selectively concentrating efforts against diseases that account for large, avoidable burdens of ill-health, are the basis for packages of interventions, variously called "basic" or "essential" or "priority", that have been developed in several countries from epidemiological information and estimates of cost-effectiveness of interventions *(27, 28)*. And the common failures in diagnosis and treatment due to inadequate training and excessive separation among disease control efforts have led to the development of clusters of interventions and more thorough training to support their delivery, most notably in the integrated management of childhood illness *(29)*.

This evolution also implies an emphasis on public or publicly guaranteed and regulated finance, but not necessarily on public delivery of services. And it implies explicit choice of priorities among interventions, respecting the ethical principle that it may be necessary and efficient to ration services but that it is inadmissible to exclude whole groups of the population. However, it is easier to define a set of interventions that would preferentially benefit the poor if fully applied to the population, than it is to assure either that most of the poor actually do benefit, or that most of the beneficiaries are poor. Government health care services, although usually intended to reach the poor, often are used more by the rich. In 11 countries for which the distribution of benefits has been calculated from the distribution of public expenditure and utilization rates, the poorest quintile of the population never accounts for even its equal share (20%), and in seven of those countries the richest quintile takes 29% to 33% of the total benefit. This pro-rich bias is due largely to disproportionate use of hospital services by the well-off, who (with one exception) always account for at least 26% of the overall benefit. The distribution of primary care is almost always more beneficial to the poor than hospital care is, justifying the emphasis on the former as the way to reach the worst-off. Even so, the poor sometimes obtain less of the benefit of primary care than the rich *(30)*. The poor often obtain much of their personal ambulatory care – which accounts for the bulk of their use of the health system and their out-of-pocket expenditure, and offers the greatest opportunity for further health gains – from private providers *(31)*, and those services may be either more or less pro-poor than the care offered by the public sector.

The ideas of responding more to demand, trying harder to assure access for the poor, and emphasizing financing, including subsidies, rather than just provision within the public sector, are embodied in many of the current third-generation reforms. These efforts are more difficult to characterize than earlier reforms, because they arise for a greater variety of reasons and include more experimentation in approach. In part, they reflect the profound political and economic changes that have been taking place in the world. By the late 1980s, the transformation from communist to market-oriented economies was under way in China, central Europe, and the former Soviet Union. Heavy-handed state intervention in the economy was becoming discredited everywhere, leading to widespread divestiture of state enterprises, promotion of more competition both internally and externally, reduction in government regulation and control, and in general, much more reliance on market mechanisms. Ideologically, this meant greater emphasis on individual choice and responsibility. Politically, it meant limiting promises and expectations about what governments should do, particularly via general revenues, to conform better to their actual financial and organizational capacities.

Health systems have not been immune from these large-scale changes. One consequence has been a greatly increased interest in explicit insurance mechanisms, including privately financed insurance. Reforms including such changes have occurred in several Asian countries, universal health insurance being introduced to different degrees in the Republic of Korea, Malaysia, Singapore and China (Province of Taiwan). Reforms to consolidate, extend or merge insurance coverage for greater risk-sharing have also occurred in Argentina, Chile, Colombia and Mexico, and a mixture of insurance and out-of-pocket health care has replaced much of the public system throughout the former communist countries. In developed countries which already had essentially universal coverage, usually less drastic changes have taken place in how health care is financed. But there have been substantial changes in who determines how resources are used, and in the arrangements by which funds are pooled and paid to providers. General practitioners and primary care physicians, as 'gatekeepers' to the health system, have sometimes been made accountable "not only for their patients' health but also for the wider resource implications of any treatments prescribed. In some countries this role has been formalised through establishing 'budget holding' for general practitioners and primary care physicians, for example, through general practice 'fund holding' in the UK, Health Maintenance Organizations in the USA, and Independent Practice Associations in New Zealand" (*32*). And in the United States, there has been a great shift of power from providers to insurers, who now largely control the access of doctors and patients to one another.

FOCUSING ON PERFORMANCE

This report does not analyse the variety of current reform efforts and proposals in detail, nor offer a model of how to construct or reconstruct a health system. The world is currently experimenting with many variants, and there is no clearly best way to proceed. But there do seem to be some clear conclusions about the organizations, rules and incentives that best help a health system to use its resources to achieve its goals; these are the subject of Chapter 3. How much can be accomplished with currently available resources – people, buildings, equipment and knowledge – depends greatly on the past investment and training that created those resources. And mistakes in investment have long-lasting consequences. The questions of how best to create resources, and what mistakes to avoid, are the subject of Chapter 4. There are comparable conclusions about what is desirable in the financing of the system; these are treated in Chapter 5. Finally, the health system as a whole needs comprehensive oversight, to stay directed to its goals and to ensure that the tasks of financing, investing and delivering services are adequately carried out. Suggestions concerning this more general function are developed in Chapter 6. These subjects are emphasized partly because so much reform today aims to change such aspects, rather than simply expanding supply or determining which interventions to offer. And all changes, to be justified, need to improve the performance of the system.

How then can the potential of health systems be fulfilled? How can they perform better, so that besides protecting health, they respond to people's expectations, and protect them financially against the costs of ill-health? Chapter 2 sets out a framework for assessing health system performance and understanding the factors that contribute to it in the four key areas treated in subsequent chapters: providing services, developing the resources – human, material and conceptual – required for the system to work, mobilizing and channelling financing, and ensuring that the individuals and organizations that compose the system act as good stewards of the resources and trust given to their care.

REFERENCES

1. Miller J. *The body in question.* New York, Random House, 1978: 14.

2. Kleinman A. Concepts and a model for the comparison of medical systems as cultural systems. *Social Science and Medicine,* 1978, **12**: 85–93.

3. Claybrook J. Remarks at the Seventh Annual North Carolina Highway Safety Conference, 1980. On Bureau of Transportation Statistics, Transportation Research Board web site at http://www4.nas.edu/trb/crp.nsf/

4. US Department of Transportation. *Traffic safety facts 1998.* Washington, DC, National Highway Traffic Safety Administration, 1998.

5. OECD. *International road traffic and accident database.* Paris, Organisation for Economic Co-operation and Development, 1999.

6. Jamison DT et al. *Disease control priorities in developing countries.* New York, Oxford University Press for The World Bank, 1993.

7. *World development report 1993 – Investing in health.* New York, Oxford University Press for The World Bank, 1993: Table 5.3.

8. Akhavan D et al. Cost-effective malaria control in Brazil. Cost-effectiveness of a malaria control program in the Amazon Basin of Brazil, 1988–1996. *Social Science and Medicine,* 1999, **49**(10): 1385–99: Table 5.

9. Rutstein DD et al. Measuring the quality of medical care – a clinical method. *New England Journal of Medicine,* 1976, **294**(11): 582-588.

10. Charlton JR, Velez R. Some international comparisons of mortality amenable to medical intervention. *British Medical Journal,* 1986, **292**: 295–301.

11. Velkova A, Wolleswinkel-van den Bosch JH, Mackenbach JP. The East–West life expectancy gap: differences in mortality from conditions amenable to medical intervention. *International Journal of Epidemiology,* 1997, **26**(1): 75–84.

12. Cochrane AL, St Leger AS, Moore F. Health service 'input' and mortality 'output' in developed countries. *Journal of Epidemiology and Community Health,* 1978, **32**(3): 200–205.

13. Musgrove P. *Public and private roles in health: theory and financing patterns.* Washington, DC, The World Bank, 1996 (World Bank Discussion Paper No. 339).

14. Mackenbach JP. Health care expenditure and mortality from amenable conditions in the European Community. *Health Policy,* 1991, **19**: 245–255.

15. Filmer D, Pritchett L. The impact of public spending on health: does money matter? *Social Science and Medicine,* 1999, **49**(10): 1309–1323.

16. Kohn L, Corrigan J, Donaldson M, eds. *To err is human: building a safer health system.* Washington, DC, Institute of Medicine, National Academy of Sciences, 1999.

17. Taylor ASP. *Bismarck – the man and the statesman.* London, Penguin, 1995: 204.

18. *Social insurance and allied services. Report by Sir William Beveridge.* London, HMSO, 1942.

19. Savage M, Shisana O. Health service provision in a future South Africa. In: Spence J, ed. *Change in South Africa.* London, The Royal Institute of International Affairs, 1994.

20. Government of India. *Health Survey and Development Committee Report. Vol. 1–4.* New Delhi, Ministry of Health, 1946.

21. Londoño JL, Frenk J. Structured pluralism: towards an innovative model for health system reform in Latin America. *Health Policy,* 1997, **41**(1) :1–36.

22. Barnum H, Kutzin J. *Public hospitals in developing countries: resource use, cost, financing.* Baltimore, MD, The Johns Hopkins University Press, 1993.

23. Newell KN. *Health by the people.* Geneva, World Health Organization, 1975.

24. Sanders D et al. Zimbabwe's hospital referral system: does it work ? *Health Policy and Planning,* 1998, **13**: 359-370.

25. Gwatkin DR, Wilcox JR, Wray JD. The policy implications of field experiments in primary health nutrition care. *Social Science and Medicine,* 1980, **14**(2): 121–128.

26. Halstead SB, Walsh JA, Warren KS, eds. *Good health at low cost.* New York, Rockefeller Foundation, 1985.

27. **Bobadilla JL et al**. Design, content and financing of an essential national package of health services. *Bulletin of the World Health Organization*, 1994, **72**(4): 653–662.

28. **Bobadilla JL**. *Searching for essential health services in low- and middle-income countries*. Washington, DC, Inter-American Development Bank, 1998.

29. **Tullock J**. Integrated approach to child health in developing countries. *The Lancet*, 1999, **354**(Suppl. II): 16–20.

30. **Gwatkin DR**. *The current state of knowledge about how well government health services reach the poor: implications for sector-wide approaches*. Washington, DC, The World Bank, 5 February 1998 (discussion draft).

31. **Berman P.** The organization of ambulatory care provision: a critical determinant of health system performance in developing countries. *Bulletin of the World Health Organization*, 2000, **78**(6) (in press).

32. **Wilton P, Smith RD.** Primary care reform: a three country comparison of 'budget holding'. *Health Policy*, 1998, **44**(2): 149–166.

CHAPTER TWO

How Well do Health Systems Perform?

Better health is unquestionably the primary goal of a health system. But because health care can be catastrophically costly and the need for it unpredictable, mechanisms for sharing risk and providing financial protection are important. A second goal of health systems is therefore fairness in financial contribution. A third goal – responsiveness to people's expectations in regard to non-health matters – reflects the importance of respecting people's dignity, autonomy and the confidentiality of information. WHO has engaged in a major exercise to obtain and analyse data in order to assess how far health systems in WHO Member States are achieving these goals for which they should be accountable, and how efficiently they are using their resources in doing so. By focusing on a few universal functions that health systems undertake, this report provides an evidence base to assist policy-makers improve health system performance.

2

How Well do
Health Systems Perform?

Attainment and performance

*A*ssessing how well a health system does its job requires dealing with two large questions. The first is how to measure the outcomes of interest – that is, to determine what is achieved with respect to the three objectives of good health, responsiveness and fair financial contribution (*attainment*). The second is how to compare those attainments with what the system *should* be able to accomplish – that is, the best that could be achieved with the same resources (*performance*). Although progress is feasible against many of society's health problems, some of the causes lie completely outside even a broad notion of what health systems are. Health systems cannot be held responsible for influences such as the distribution of income and wealth, any more than for the impact of the climate. But avoidable deaths and illness from childbirth, measles, malaria or tobacco consumption can properly be laid at their door. A fair judgement of how much health damage it should be possible to avoid requires an estimate of the best that can be expected, and of the least that can be demanded, of a system. The same is true of progress towards the other two objectives, although much less is known about them *(1)*.

Goals and functions

Better health is of course the *raison d'être* of a health system, and unquestionably its primary or defining goal: if health systems did nothing to protect or improve health there would be no reason for them. Other systems in society may contribute greatly to the population's health, but not as their primary goal. For example, the education system makes a large difference to health, but its defining goal is to educate. Influence also flows the other way: better health makes children better able to learn, but that is not the defining purpose of the health system. In contrast, the goal of fair financing is common to all societal systems. This is obvious when the system is paid for socially, but it holds even when everything is financed purely by individual purchases. It is only the notion of fairness that may vary. "Getting what you pay for" is generally accepted as fair in market transactions, but seems much less fair where health services are concerned. Similarly, in any system, people have expectations which society regards as legitimate, as to how they should be treated, both physically and psychologically. Responsiveness is therefore always a social goal. Taking the education system as an example, fair financing means the right balance of contributions from households which do and those which do not have children in school, and enough subsidy that poor children are not denied schooling for financial reasons. Responsiveness includes respect for parents' wishes for their children, and avoiding abuse or humiliation of the students themselves.

The health system differs from other social systems such as education, and from the markets for most consumer goods and services, in two ways which make the goals of fair financing and responsiveness particularly significant. One is that health care can be catastrophically costly. Much of the need for care is unpredictable, so it is vital for people to be protected from having to choose between financial ruin and loss of health. Mechanisms for sharing risk and providing financial protection are more important even than in other cases where people buy insurance, as for physical assets like homes or vehicles, or against the financial risk to the family of a breadwinner dying young. The other peculiarity of health is that illness itself, and medical care as well, can threaten people's dignity and their ability to control what happens to them more than most other events to which they are exposed. Among other things, responsiveness means reducing the damage to one's dignity and autonomy, and the fear and shame that sickness often brings with it.

Systems are often charged to be affordable, equitable, accessible, sustainable, of good quality, and perhaps to have many other virtues as well. However, desiderata such as accessibility are really a means to an end; they are instrumental rather than final goals. The more accessible a system is, the more people should utilize it to improve their health. In contrast, the goals of health, fair financing, and responsiveness are each intrinsically valuable. Raising the achievement of any goal or combination of goals, without lowering the attainment of another, represents an improvement. So if the achievement of these goals can be measured, then instrumental goals such as accessibility become unnecessary as proxy measures of overall performance; they are relevant rather as explanations of good or bad outcomes.

It is certainly true that financing that is more fairly distributed may contribute to better health, by reducing the risk that people who need care do not get it because it would cost too much, or that paying for health care leaves them impoverished and exposed to more health problems. And a system that is more responsive to what people want and expect can also make for better health, because potential patients are more likely to utilize care if they anticipate being treated well. Both goals therefore are partly instrumental, in that they promote improvements in health status. But they would be valuable even if that did not happen. That is, paying equitably for the system is a good thing in itself. So is assuring that people are treated promptly, with respect for their dignity and their wishes, and that patients receive adequate physical and affective support while undergoing treatment. The three goals are separable, as is often shown by people's unhappiness with a system even when the health outcomes are satisfactory.

Comparing how health systems perform means looking at what they achieve and at what they *do* – how they carry out certain *functions* – in order to achieve anything (2). These functions could be classified and related to system objectives in many different ways. For example, the "Public health in the Americas" initiative led by the Pan American Health Organization describes 12 different "essential functions", and proposes between three and six sub-functions for each one (3). Many of these functions correspond to the task of stewardship which this report emphasizes, others to service provision and to resource generation. The four functions described in this chapter embrace these and other more specific activities. Figure 2.1 indicates how these functions – delivering personal and non-personal health services; raising, pooling and allocating the revenues to purchase those services; investing in people, buildings and equipment; and acting as the overall stewards of the resources, powers and expectations entrusted to them – are related to one another and to the objectives of the system. Stewardship occupies a special place because it involves oversight of all the other functions, and has direct or indirect effects on all the outcomes. Comparing the way these functions are actually carried out provides a basis for understanding performance variations over time and among countries. Some evidence about these functions, and how they influence the attainment of the fundamental objectives in different health systems, is examined in the next four chapters.

In the view of most people, the health system is simply those providers and organizations which deliver personal medical services. Defining the health system more broadly means that the people and organizations which deliver medical care are not the whole system; rather, they exercise one of the principal functions of the system. They also share, sometimes appropriately and sometimes less so, in the other functions of financing, investment and stewardship. The question of who should undertake which functions is one of the crucial issues treated in later chapters.

It is common to describe the struggle for good health in quasi-military terms, to talk of "fighting" malaria or AIDS, to refer to a "campaign" of immunization or the "conquest" of smallpox, to "free" a population or a geographical area of some disease, to worry about the "arms race" that constantly occurs between pathogens and the drugs to hold them in check, to hope for a "silver bullet" against cancer or diabetes. In those terms, the providers of direct health services – whether aimed at individuals, communities or the environment – can be considered the front-line troops defending society against illness. But just as with an army, the health system must be much more than the soldiers in the field if it is to win any battles. Behind them is an entire apparatus to ensure that the fighters are adequately trained, informed, financed, supplied, inspired and led. It is also crucial to treat decently the population they are supposed to protect, to teach the "civilians" in the struggle how to defend themselves and their families, and to share equitably the burden of financing the war.

Unless those functions are properly carried out, firepower will be much less effective than it might be, and casualties will be higher. The emphasis here on overall results and on the functions more distant from the front line does not mean any denigration of the importance of disease control. It means rather to step back and consider what it is that the system as a whole is trying to do, and how well it is succeeding. Success means, among other things, more effective control of diseases, through better performance.

Figure 2.1 Relations between functions and objectives of a health system

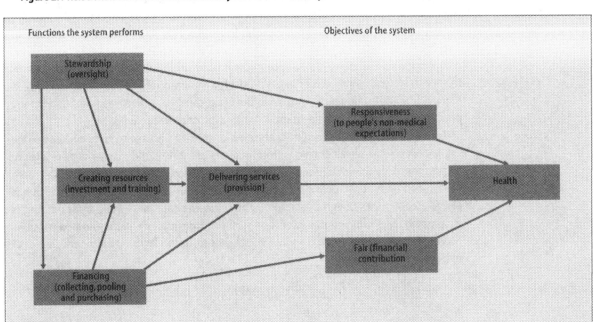

GOODNESS AND FAIRNESS:
BOTH LEVEL AND DISTRIBUTION MATTER

A good health system, above all, contributes to good health. But it is not always satisfactory to protect or improve the average health of the population, if at the same time inequality worsens or remains high because the gain accrues disproportionately to those already enjoying better health. The health system also has the responsibility to try to reduce inequalities by preferentially improving the health of the worse-off, wherever these inequalities are caused by conditions amenable to intervention. The objective of good health is really twofold: the best attainable average level – *goodness* – and the smallest feasible differences among individuals and groups – *fairness*. A gain in either one of these, with no change in the other, constitutes an improvement, but the two may be in conflict. The logic is somewhat parallel to that concerning the distribution of income in a population. It is desirable to raise the average level, to reduce inequality, or both, and sometimes to judge the relative values of one and the other goal (with the difference that there is no argument for taking health away from anyone – health, unlike income or nonhuman assets, cannot be directly redistributed).

The distinction between the overall level and how it is distributed in the population also applies to responsiveness. Goodness means the system responds well on average to what people expect of it, with respect to its non-health aspects. Fairness means that it responds equally well to everyone, without discrimination or differences in how people are treated. The distribution of responsiveness matters, just as the distribution of health does. Either one is valuable by itself.

In contrast to the objectives of good health and responsiveness, there is no overall notion of goodness related to financing. There are good and bad ways to raise the resources for a health system, of course, but they are more or less good primarily as they affect how fairly the financial burden is shared. Fair financing, as the name suggests, is concerned only with distribution. It is not related to the total resource bill, nor to how the funds are used. While it is unambiguously preferable to have better health or a higher level of responsiveness, it is not always better to spend more on health because at high levels of expenditure there may be little additional health gain from more resources. The objectives of the health system do not include any particular level of total spending, either absolutely or relative to income. This is because, at all levels of spending, the resources devoted to health have competing uses, and it is a social choice – with no correct answer – how much to allocate to the health system. Nonetheless there is probably a minimum level of expenditure required to provide a whole population with a handful of the most cost-effective services, and many poor countries are currently spending too little even to assure that *(4)*.

In countries where most health financing is private, and is largely out of pocket, no one makes this choice overall; it results from millions of individual decisions. As the level of prepayment rises, there are fewer and larger decisions, because spending is more and more determined by the policies and budgets of public entities and insurance funds. The public budget decision has the greatest effect in high income countries where most funding is government controlled or mandated, but in all countries it is one of the most basic public decisions. It is something that can be directly chosen, as the level of health outcome or of responsiveness cannot be.

MEASURING GOAL ACHIEVEMENT

To assess a health system, one must measure five things: the overall level of health; the distribution of health in the population; the overall level of responsiveness; the distribution of responsiveness; and the distribution of financial contribution. For each one, WHO has used existing sources or newly generated data to calculate measures of attainment for the countries where information could be obtained. These data were also used to estimate values when particular numbers were judged unreliable, and to estimate attainment and performance for all other Member States. Several of these measures are novel and are explained in detail in the Statistical Annex, where all the estimates are given, along with intervals expressing the uncertainty or degree of confidence in the point estimate. The correct value for any indicator is estimated to have an 80% probability of falling within the uncertainty interval, with chances of 10% each of falling below the low value or above the high one. This recognition of inexactness underscores the importance of getting more and better data on all the basic indicators of population health, responsiveness and fairness in financial contribution, a task which forms part of WHO's continuing programme of work.

The achievements with respect to each objective are used to rank countries, as are the overall measures of achievement and performance described below. Since a given country or health system may have very different ranks on different attainments, Annex Table 1 shows the complete ranking for all Member States on all the measures. In several subsequent tables, countries are ranked in order of achievement or performance, and the order varies from one table to another. Since the ranking is based on estimates which include uncertainty as to the exact values, the rank assigned also includes uncertainty: a health system is not always assigned a specific position relative to all others but is estimated to lie somewhere within a narrower or broader range, depending on the uncertainties in the calculation. The ranks of different health systems therefore sometimes overlap to a greater or lesser degree, and two or more countries may have the same rank.

Health is the defining objective for the health system. This means making the health status of the entire population as good as possible over people's whole life cycle, taking account of both premature mortality and disability. Annex Table 2 presents three conventional and partial measures of health status, by country, without ranking: these are the probability of dying before age five years or between ages 15 and 59 years, and life expectancy at birth. For the first time, these measures are presented with estimates of uncertainty, and these uncertainties carry over to subsequent calculations. On the basis of the mortality figures, five strata are identified, ranging from low child and adult mortality to high child mortality and very high adult death rates. Combining these strata with the six WHO Regions gives 14 subregions defined geographically and epidemiologically (see the list of Member States by WHO Region and mortality stratum). Annex Table 3 presents estimates of mortality by cause and sex in 1999 in each of these subregions (not by country), and Annex Table 4 combines these death rates with information about disability to create estimates of one measure of overall population health: the burden of disease, that is, the numbers of disability-adjusted life years (DALYs) lost.

To assess overall population health and thus to judge how well the objective of good health is being achieved, WHO has chosen to use disability-adjusted life expectancy (DALE), which has the advantage of being directly comparable to life expectancy estimated from mortality alone and is readily compared across populations. Annex Table 5 provides estimates for all countries of disability-adjusted life expectancy. DALE is estimated to equal or exceed 70 years in 24 countries, and 60 years in over half the Member States of WHO. At the other extreme are 32 countries where disability-adjusted life expectancy is estimated to be less than 40 years. Many of these are countries with major epidemics of HIV/AIDS, among other causes. Box 2.1 describes how these summary measures of population health are constructed and how they are related.

Figure 2.2 summarizes the relation between DALE and life expectancy without adjustment, for each of the 14 subregions, for both men and women. The adjustment is nearly uniform, at about seven years of healthy life equivalent lost to disability. Both absolutely and relatively this loss is slightly less for richer, low-mortality subregions, despite the fact that people live longer there and so have more opportunity to acquire non-fatal disabilities. Disability makes a substantial difference in poorer countries because some limitations – injury, blindness, paralysis and the debilitating effects of several tropical diseases such as malaria and schistosomiasis – strike children and young adults. Separating life expectancy into years in good health and years lived with disability therefore widens rather than narrows the difference in health status between richer and poorer populations. This is most evident in the share of life expectancy which is lost to disability: it ranges from less than 9% in the healthiest subregions to more than 14% in the least healthy. Annex Table 5 shows these shares for individual countries, where the range is even wider.

Annex Table 5 also provides estimates of health inequality. The distributional measure of health ranges from 1 for the case of perfect equality to zero for extreme inequality, which corresponds to a fraction of the population having an expectancy of 100 years and the rest

---

Box 2.1 Summary measures of population health

No measure is perfect for the purpose of summing up the health of a population; each way of estimating it violates one or another desirable criterion. The two principal approaches are the burden of disease, which measures losses of good health compared to a long life free of disability, and some measure of life expectancy, adjusted to take account of time lived with a disability. Both ways of summarizing health use the same information about mortality and disability, and both are related to a survivorship curve, such as the bold line between the areas labelled *Disability* and *Mortality* in the figure.

The area labelled *Mortality* represents losses due to death, compared to a high standard of life expectancy: the burden of disease corresponds to all of that area plus a fraction of the area corresponding to time lived with disability. The fraction depends on the disability weights assigned to various states between death and perfect health. Life expectancy without any adjustment corresponds to the areas labelled *Survival free of disability* and *Disability* together, the whole area under the survivorship curve. Disability-adjusted life expectancy (DALE) then corresponds to the area for sur-

vival plus part of that for disability.

DALE is estimated from three kinds of information: the fraction of the population surviving to each age, calculated from birth and death rates; the prevalence of each type of disability at each age; and the weight assigned to each type of disability, which may or may not vary with age. Survival at each age is adjusted downward by the sum of all the disability effects, each of which is the product of a weight and the complement of a prevalence (the share of the population not suffering that disability). These adjusted survival shares are then divided by the initial population, before any mortality occurred, to give the average number of equivalent healthy life years that a newborn member of the population could expect to live.

One important difference between the burden of disease estimation using disability-adjusted life years (DALYs) and that of DALE is that the former do, but the latter do not, distinguish the contribution of each disease to the overall result. DALE has the advantage that it does not require as many choices of parameters for the calculation, and it is directly comparable to the more familiar notion of life expectancy without adjustment.

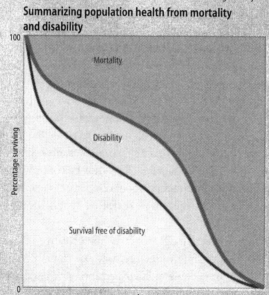

Summarizing population health from mortality and disability

Source: Murray CJL, Salomon JA, Mathers C. *A critical examination of summary measures of population health.* Geneva, World Health Organization, 1999 (GPE Discussion paper No. 12).

having no expectation of surviving infancy. *If everyone had the same life expectancy, adjusted for disability, the system would be perfectly fair with respect to health, even though people would actually die at different ages.* For a small number of countries it has been possible to estimate the distribution of life expectancy within the population using information on both child

Figure 2.2 Life expectancy and disability-adjusted life expectancy for males and females, by WHO Region and stratum defined by child mortality and adult mortality, 1999

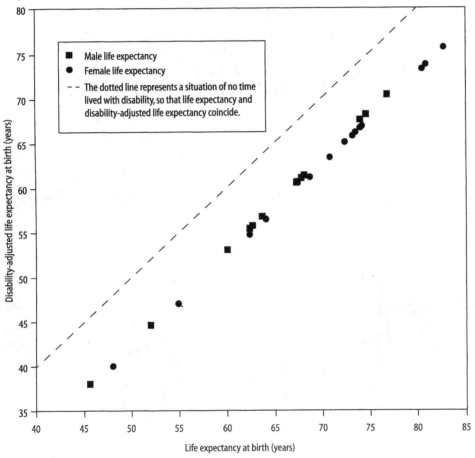

WHO Region	Mortality stratum		Males		Females	
	Child	Adult	Life expectancy	Disability adjusted	Life expectancy	Disability adjusted
AFR	High	High	52.0	44.6	54.9	47.0
	High	Very high	45.6	38.0	48.0	40.0
AMR	Very low	Very low	73.9	67.5	80.4	73.2
	Low	Low	67.3	60.6	74.1	66.8
	High	High	63.6	56.7	68.6	61.1
EMR	Low	Low	67.7	61.0	70.7	63.3
	High	High	60.0	53.0	62.3	54.7
EUR	Very low	Very low	74.5	68.1	80.8	73.7
	Low	Low	67.3	60.6	73.9	66.6
	Low	High	62.3	55.4	73.4	66.1
SEAR	Low	Low	67.2	60.5	73.1	65.7
	High	High	62.6	55.7	64.0	56.4
WPR	Very low	Very low	76.7	70.3	82.7	75.6
	Low	Low	68.0	61.3	72.3	65.0

and adult mortality; these results are presented below. For most countries, however, it has so far been possible to use only child mortality data. Because high-income countries have largely eliminated child mortality, the highest ranking countries in Annex Table 5 nearly all have relatively high incomes; most are European. A few Latin American countries which

Figure 2.3 Inequality in life expectancy at birth, by sex, in six countries

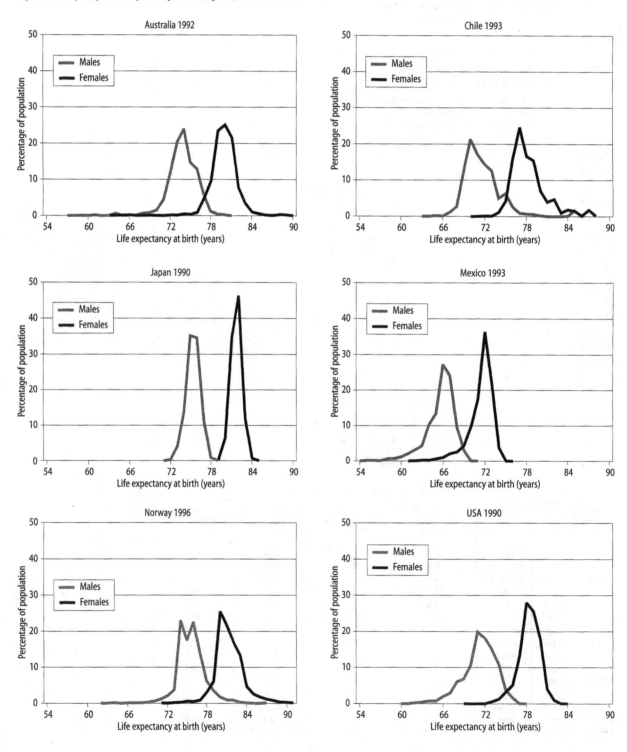

have made great progress in controlling child deaths also show considerable equality of health. Except for Afghanistan and Pakistan, all the countries ranked lowest on child health equality are in sub-Saharan Africa, where child mortality is still relatively high. When more complete data are available on inequalities in adult mortality they will be used in future WHO estimates, and these rankings will change, because high income countries differ more in adult than in child death rates.

Inequalities in life expectancy persist, and are strongly associated with socioeconomic class, even in countries with quite good health status on average (5). Figure 2.3 illustrates these inequalities for six countries, showing the distribution of life expectancy at birth for both men and women, using data on adult as well as child mortality, estimated from large numbers of small-area studies which cover the entire country. Among these six countries, health is most equally distributed in Japan. Both distributions of life expectancy are sharply peaked, concentrating the whole population of either men or women in a range of only about six years. There is far more inequality in Mexico and in the United States, and in both cases that arises because part of the population has a much lower expectation than the rest, after age five years. The inequality is particularly marked for men. An opposite pattern characterizes Chile, which shows very high equality in child health: the degree of adult inequality is about the same as for Mexico and the United States, but it arises because part of the population has an unusually high life expectancy. Australia and Norway both show more symmetric distributions. These results emphasize the value of judging health system achievement not only by averages or overall levels but by seeing whether everyone has about the same expectation of life.

Responsiveness is not a measure of how the system responds to health needs, which shows up in health outcomes, but of how the system performs relative to non-health aspects, meeting or not meeting a population's expectations of how it should be treated by providers of prevention, care or non-personal services. (The last category is least important, since individuals normally do not come into personal contact with such interventions. However, even public health measures such as vector control can be conducted with more or less respect for people and their wishes. Assessing the responsiveness of providers of non-personal services is a particular challenge.)

Some systems are highly unresponsive. The Soviet health system prior to 1990 had become highly impersonal and inhuman in the way it processed people. A common complaint in many countries about public sector health workers focuses on their rudeness and arrogance in relations with patients (6, 7). Waiting times for non-emergency surgery vary considerably among industrialized countries (8) and are the subject of much criticism of ministries of health (9). Recognizing responsiveness as an intrinsic goal of health systems establishes that these systems are there to serve people, and involves more than an assessment of people's satisfaction with the purely medical care they receive.

The general notion of responsiveness can be decomposed in many ways. One basic distinction is between elements related to respect for human beings as persons – which are largely subjective and judged primarily by the patient – and more objective elements related to how a system meets certain commonly expressed concerns of patients and their families as clients of health systems, some of which can be directly observed at health facilities. Subdividing these two categories leads to seven distinct elements or aspects of responsiveness.

Respect for persons includes:

- Respect for the dignity of the person. At the extreme, this means not sterilizing individuals with a genetic disorder or locking up people with communicable diseases, which would violate basic human rights. More generally, it means not humiliating or demeaning patients.
- Confidentiality, or the right to determine who has access to one's personal health information.
- Autonomy to participate in choices about one's own health. This includes helping choose what treatment to receive or not to receive.

Client orientation includes:

- Prompt attention: immediate attention in emergencies, and reasonable waiting times for non-emergencies.
- Amenities of adequate quality, such as cleanliness, space, and hospital food.
- Access to social support networks – family and friends – for people receiving care.
- Choice of provider, or freedom to select which individual or organization delivers one's care.

In general, responsiveness contributes to health by promoting utilization, but that is not always the case. Greater autonomy can mean that people do not take up an intervention because they perceive the individual benefit to be small or the risk to be substantial, and do not value the collective or population benefit. This is particularly likely for immunization, especially if there is fear of adverse reactions. Individual freedom to choose whether or not to be immunized is in conflict with the public health objective of high coverage to prevent epidemics. Such conflict has occurred, for example, in the United Kingdom for pertussis and in Greece for rubella vaccine *(10)*. The overall performance of a health system may therefore involve trade-offs among objectives.

Opinions on how well a health system performs on such subjective dimensions as responsiveness might be influenced by any of a number of features of the systems themselves, or of the respondents. Since poor people may expect less than rich people, and be more satisfied with unresponsive services, measures of responsiveness should correct for

---

Box 2.2 How important are the different elements of responsiveness ?

The key informant survey, consisting of 1791 interviews in 35 countries, yielded scores (from 0 to 10) on each element of responsiveness, as well as overall scores. A second, Internet-based survey of 1006 participants (half from within WHO) generated opinions about the relative importance of the elements, which were used to combine the element scores into an overall score instead of just taking the mean or using the key informants' overall responses.

Respondents were asked to rank the seven elements in order of importance, and the weights were derived from the frequencies with which an element was ranked first, second, and so on. Respect for persons and client orientation were rated as equally important overall, and the three elements of respect for persons were also regarded as all about equally important. The four elements of

Respect for persons	
Total	50%
Respect for dignity	16.7%
Confidentiality	16.7%
Autonomy	16.7%
Client orientation	
Total	50%
Prompt attention	20%
Quality of amenities	15%
Access to social support networks	10%
Choice of provider	5%

client orientation received different rankings and therefore unequal weights. The final weights are shown in the table.

Analysis of the element scores themselves, as estimated by the key informants, showed three consistent biases: for the same country, women respondents gave lower scores than men, and government officials gave higher scores than more independent informants; and all informants' scores tended to be higher for countries with less political freedom, as measured by a composite index. The data were adjusted to make the scores comparable across countries by removing the influence of these factors, so that all the scores are estimates of the ratings that would be given in a politically free country, by respondents who did not work for the government, half of whom were women.

these differences, as well as for cultural differences among countries *(11)*. Even without such adjustment, comparisons of how knowledgeable observers rate health system achievements can reveal on which aspects of responsiveness a system seems to satisfy its users best. Judgements about average level and inequality of the components of responsiveness were developed in each of 35 countries by a network of 50 or more key informants. A separate survey of over a thousand respondents was used to develop weights for combining these scores into an overall rating. Box 2.2 describes the results of this exercise. Estimates for other Member States were derived from the 35 observations, adjusted for differences among countries and informant groups. Surveys of population opinion and direct observation of health provision can both be used to complement these judgements.

Figure 2.4 illustrates in detail the scores of the seven individual elements, relative to the overall score, within each of 13 countries chosen to reflect all WHO Regions and typical of the entire set of countries studied. The health systems examined always appear to perform relatively well on the two dimensions of access to social support networks and confidentiality, sometimes very much better than on other aspects. The systematically high rating for social support may reflect a trade-off against the quality of amenities, because a health care facility that cannot, for lack of resources, offer good quality food or non-medical attention can compensate for that by allowing relatives and friends to attend to patients' needs. One reason why confidentiality seems not to be a problem in these countries may be that there is little private insurance and therefore little risk of coverage being denied because a provider reveals some information about a patient. There is somewhat less consistency at the other end of the scale, but autonomy is among the three lowest-rated elements of responsiveness 34 times out of 35 – and the lowest ranked element almost half the time – and performance is also often poor with respect to choice of provider and promptness of care.

As with health status, it is not only overall responsiveness that matters, if some people are treated with courtesy while others are humiliated or disdained. *A perfectly fair health system would make no such distinctions, and would receive the same rating of responsiveness on every element, for every group in the population.* In almost every country where key informants were surveyed, the poor were identified as the main disadvantaged group. In particular, they were considered to be treated with less respect for their dignity, to have less choice of providers and to be offered poorer quality amenities than the non-poor. In nearly as many cases, rural populations – among whom the poor are concentrated – were regarded as being treated worse than urban dwellers, suffering especially from less prompt attention, less choice of providers and lower quality of amenities. Some respondents in one or several countries also identified women, children or adolescents, indigenous or tribal groups or others as receiving worse treatment than the rest of the population.

The elements of client orientation, where the poor and the rural population are less well treated, all have economic implications: it generally costs more to assure quick attention and to offer high quality food, more space and well-kept facilities. It also makes cost control harder if people are allowed to choose their providers, and costs differ among them. The strongest associations occur for quality of basic amenities and promptness of attention. The former is closely related to income per head and to the share of private expenditure in total health spending; the latter is closely related to average years of schooling of the population, which is also associated with income. In contrast, the elements of respect for persons can be costless, apart perhaps from some training of providers and administrators. These elements – respect for dignity, autonomy, and confidentiality – show no relation to health system spending. There is scope for improving health system performance in these respects without taking any resources away from the primary objective of better health. This

Figure 2.4 Relative scores of health system responsiveness elements, in 13 countries, 1999

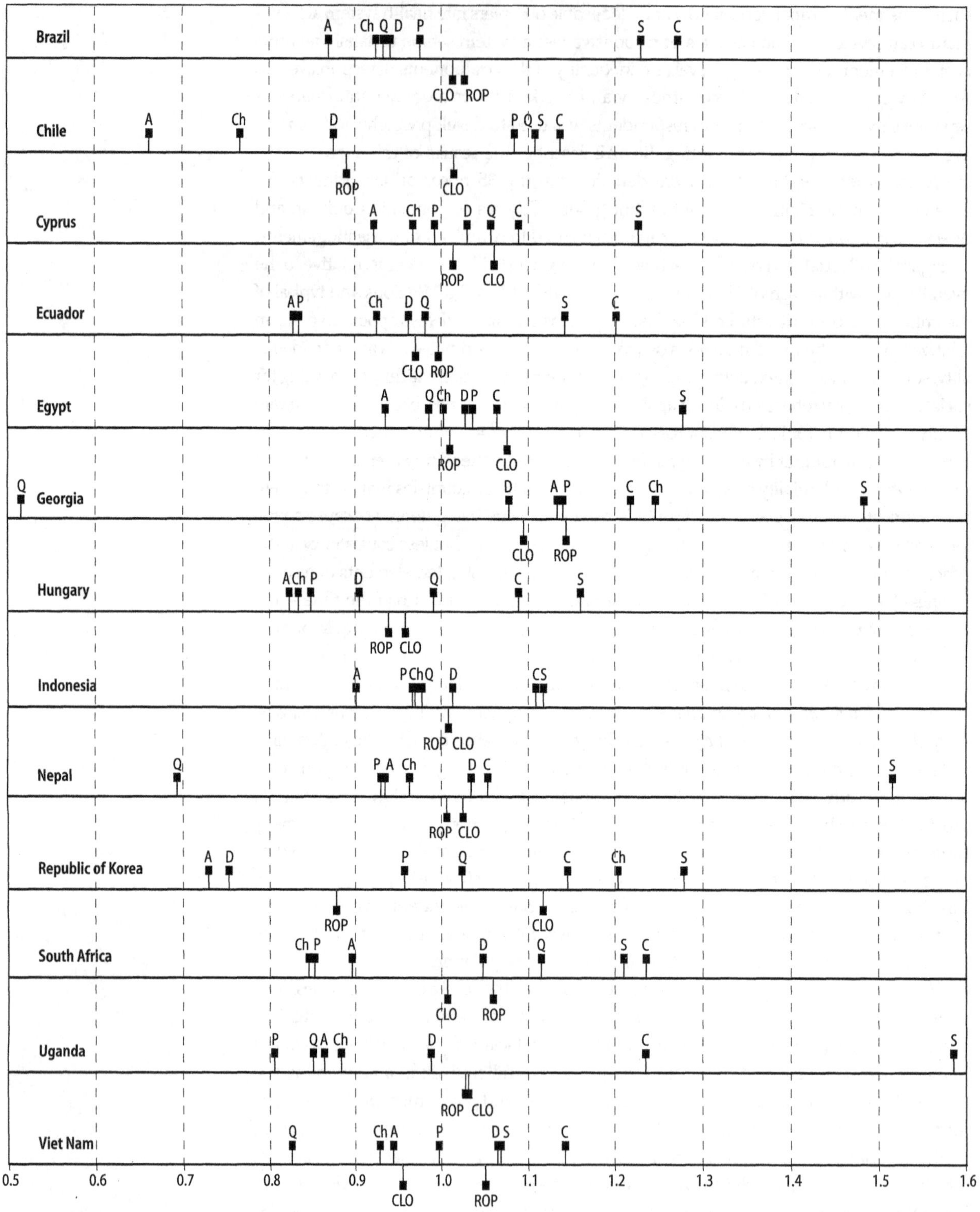

All scores are normalized relative to the average overall country responsiveness score = 1.
A = autonomy, C = confidentiality, Ch = choice of provider or facility, D = dignity, P= promptness, Q = quality of basic amenities, S = access to social support networks, ROP = respect of persons, CLO = client orientation.

is particularly the case for autonomy, where performance is often poorly rated.

Annex Table 6 reports adjusted scores for overall responsiveness, as well as a measure of fairness based on the informants' views as to which groups are most often discriminated against in a country's population and on how large those groups are. Either a larger group being affected, or more informants agreeing on that group's being treated worse than some others, implies more inequality of responsiveness and therefore less achievement of fairness. Since some elements of responsiveness are costly, it is not surprising that most of the highest ranked countries spend relatively large amounts on health. They are also often countries where a large share of provision is private, even if much of the financing for it is public or publicly mandated. However, the association with a country's income or health expenditure is less marked than it is for health status. Several poor African and Asian countries rank fairly high on the level of responsiveness. And countries that perform well on average for responding to people's expectations may nonetheless rank much lower on the distributional index.

Fair financing in health systems means that the risks each household faces due to the costs of the health system are distributed according to ability to pay rather than to the risk of illness: a fairly financed system ensures financial protection for everyone. A health system in which individuals or households are sometimes forced into poverty through their purchase of needed care, or forced to do without it because of the cost, is unfair. This situation characterizes most poorer countries and some middle and high income ones, in which at least part of the population is inadequately protected from financial risks *(12)*.

Paying for health care can be unfair in two different ways. It can expose families to large *unexpected* expenses, that is, costs that could not be foreseen and have to be paid out of pocket at the moment of utilization of services rather than being covered by some kind of prepayment. Or it can impose *regressive* payments, in which those least able to contribute pay proportionately more than the better-off. The first problem is solved by minimizing the share of out-of-pocket financing of the system, so as to rely as fully as possible on more predictable prepayment that is unrelated to illness or utilization. The second is solved by assuring that each form of prepayment – through taxes of all kinds, social insurance, or voluntary insurance – is progressive or at least neutral with respect to income, being related to capacity to pay rather than to health risk.

Out-of-pocket payments are generally regressive but they can, in principle, be neutral or progressive. When this happens, and out-of-pocket expenses are not too large, they need not impoverish anyone or deter the poor from obtaining care. However, of all the forms of financing they are the most difficult to make progressive. Arrangements that exempt the destitute from user fees at public facilities, or impose a sliding scale based on socioeconomic characteristics, are attempts to reduce the risk associated with out-of-pocket payments *(13, 14)*. Except when private practitioners know their clientele well enough to discriminate among them in fees – and the better-off accept that their charges will subsidize the worse-off – such arrangements are limited to public facilities, which often account for only a small share of utilization in poor countries. And even then, such schemes require relatively high administrative costs to distinguish among users, and typically affect only a small amount of total risk-related payments.

For this reason, financial fairness is best served by more, as well as by more progressive, prepayment in place of out-of-pocket expenditure. And the latter should be small not only in the aggregate, but relative to households' ability to pay. Prepayment that is closely related to *ex ante* risk, as judged from observable characteristics – risk-related insurance premiums, for example – is still preferable to out-of-pocket payment because it is more predictable, and may be justified to the extent that the risks are under a person's control. However, the ideal is largely to disconnect a household's financial contribution to the health system from its health risks, and separate it almost entirely from the use of needed services. The question of how far insurance prepayments may be related to risks, and how such premiums should be financed, including subsidies for those unable to pay, is treated in Chapter 5.

Ex post, the burden of health financing on a particular household is the share that its actual health expenses are of its capacity to pay. The numerator includes all costs attributable to the household, including those it is not even aware of paying, such as the share of sales or value-added taxes it pays on consumption, which governments then devote to health, and the contribution via insurance provided, and partly financed, by employers.

The denominator is a measure of the household's capacity to pay. In poor households, a large share goes for basic necessities, particularly food, whereas richer households have more margin for other spending, including spending on health care. Food spending is treated as an approximation to expenditure on basic needs. Total non-food spending is taken as an approximation of the household's discretionary and relatively permanent income, which is less volatile than recorded income (15) and a better measure of what a household can afford to spend on health and other non-food needs.

In sum, *the way health care is financed is perfectly fair if the ratio of total health contribution to total non-food spending is identical for all households, independently of their income, their health status or their use of the health system.* This indicator expresses the trenchant view of Aneurin Bevan, that "The essence of a satisfactory health service is that the rich and the poor are treated alike, that poverty is not a disability, and wealth is not advantaged." (16). Clearly the financing would be unfair if poor households spent a larger share than rich ones, either because they were less protected by prepayment systems and so had to pay relatively more out of pocket, or because the prepayment arrangements were regressive. But to identify fairness with equality means that the system is also regarded as unfair if *rich* households pay more, as a share of their capacity. Simply by paying the same fraction as poor households, they would be subsidizing those with lower capacity to pay. It is true that well-off households might choose to pay still more, particularly by buying more insurance, but that can be considered equitable only if the extra spending is prepaid and if the choice is entirely voluntary and not determined by the system of taxes or mandatory insurance contributions.

Families that spend 50% or more of their non-food expenditure on health are likely to be impoverished as a result. Detailed household surveys show that in Brazil, Bulgaria, Jamaica, Kyrgyzstan, Mexico, Nepal, Nicaragua, Paraguay, Peru, the Russian Federation, Viet Nam and Zambia more than 1% of all households had to spend on health half or more of their full monthly capacity to pay, which means that in large countries millions of families are at risk of impoverishment. Invariably the reason is high out-of-pocket spending. This high potential for financial catastrophe has much to do with how the health system is financed, and not only with the overall level of spending or the income of the country.

The fairness of the distribution of financial contribution is summarized in an index which is inversely related to the inequality in the distribution, and presented in Annex Table 7. The index runs from zero (extreme inequality) to 1 (perfect equality). For most countries, and particularly for most high income countries, the value is not far from 1, but great inequality characterizes a few countries in which nearly all health spending is out-of-pocket, notably China, Nepal and Viet Nam. However, in some countries where most spending is out-of-

Figure 2.5 Household contributions to financing health, as percentage of capacity to pay, in eight countries

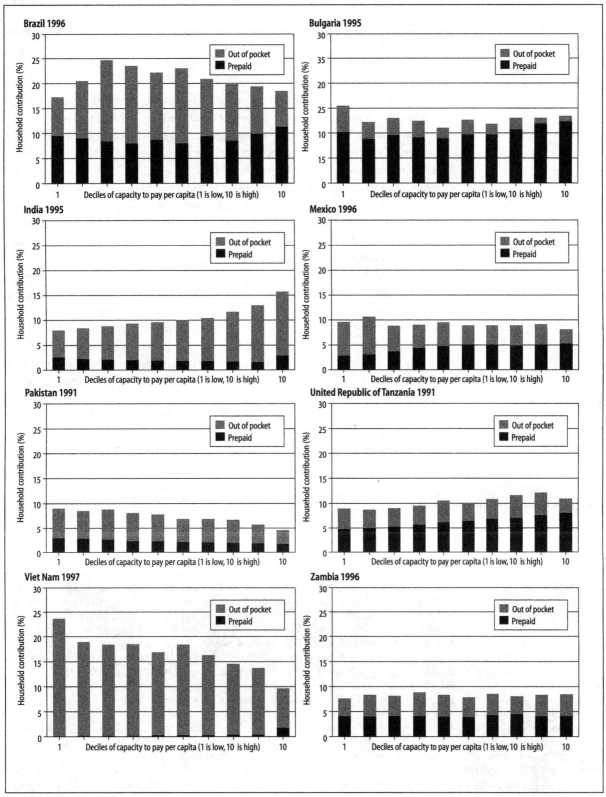

pocket, there is nonetheless little inequality because that spending is relatively progressive and few families spend as much as half their non-food expenditure on health. Bangladesh and India are examples. Generally, high values of equality are associated with predominantly prepaid financing, but Brazil shows extreme inequality despite a high share of prepayment, because of the great inequality in incomes and the large number of families at risk of impoverishment.

The summary measure of fairness does not distinguish poor from rich households. Figure 2.5 introduces this distinction, by showing how the burden is distributed across deciles of capacity to pay, and divided between prepayment and out-of-pocket spending, in eight low and middle income countries. Prepayment is clearly progressive – the rich contribute a larger share – in Mexico and the United Republic of Tanzania, and also in Bangladesh and Colombia (not shown). It is actually regressive in India and Pakistan, and also in Guyana, Kyrgyzstan, Nepal, Peru and the Russian Federation (not shown). In other countries – Brazil, Bulgaria, Jamaica, Nicaragua, Paraguay, Romania and Zambia – the prepaid contribution is distributed more or less neutrally or varies irregularly. Out-of-pocket spending shows more variation, as might be expected; for example, it is progressive in India and quite regressive in Pakistan and Viet Nam, where there is almost no prepaid financing at all.

Total non-food spending also includes whatever the household spends out of pocket on health care. That spending is largely unpredictable or transitory, so to include it may overstate the family's capacity to pay. If out-of-pocket expenditure is small, it makes no difference; but if it is large, it may have been financed by selling assets, going into debt, requiring more family members to work or for some to take on more hours or other employments, or even temporarily reducing consumption of necessities. If household capacity to pay is defined as non-food spending *less* out-of-pocket health spending, then families with large out-of-pocket expenditures are classified as poor, instead of being scattered throughout the population. The way the health system is financed then looks systematically less fair in most countries, and the culprit is always the large share of out-of-pocket spending. Pre-

Box 2.3 What does fair contribution measure and not measure ?

The way fair contribution to health care finance is measured is strictly *ex post*, referring to what households actually contribute rather than to their *ex ante* risks of needing health care. That means that there is no need to estimate the "coverage" of the population by different risk-sharing schemes. Coverage in financial rather than nominal terms – how much people are really protected, not simply whether they have insurance or participate in social security – is hard to estimate beforehand, and in any case such coverage is, like accessibility, an instrumental rather than a final goal. Nominal coverage does provide people with a sense of security which also

affects their spending and saving decisions, but that is not a goal in itself.

People who do not use care when they need it, because they cannot afford the out-of-pocket cost, appear to spend less than they really need to. Estimating what they *would* have spent if they could afford it would give a different distribution of contributions, and would almost surely show even more unfairness. Basing the measure on what is actually spent – which is all that the data allow – overstates the degree to which a health system achieves a fair distribution of the financing burden.

The measure also says nothing about how a family obtains the cash

to pay out of pocket for health care (or for some forms of prepayment such as "health cards" or vouchers). Households much of whose income is in kind rather than cash may forego health care because they cannot obtain the cash when needed, and the data will show only that they did not spend. Without further analysis there is no way to distinguish illiquidity from all the other reasons why a health need did not eventuate in expenditure. A less serious but sometimes still consequential liquidity problem arises when a household has to pay out of pocket for care, and then wait for reimbursement from an insurer. This need to finance care temporarily arises for populations wealthy

enough to have formal – usually private – insurance.

Finally, and most important, fair financing means only equity in how the financial burden of supporting a health system is shared. It says nothing about whether the *utilization* of health services is fair, which is an equally crucial issue in the overall fairness of the system. Fair financing is concerned with the principle of *from each according to ability*, but not with the principle of *to each according to need*. Unfairness in use relative to need shows up in inequalities in health status, because service utilization ought to reduce such inequalities so far as they are amenable to intervention.

payment in low income countries is commonly too small a share of the total to offset the regressive and very unequal impact of out-of-pocket spending. What is worse, in many countries there is *no* offsetting effect because prepayment via taxes is also regressive. In those cases the poor thus suffer twice – all of them have to pay an unfair share whether or not they use health services, and then some of them have also to pay an even more unfair contribution out of pocket. These are the strongest findings to emerge from the analysis of financing; their implications are developed further in Chapter 5. Box 2.3 discusses four other features of this way of measuring fairness in financing.

Much of the analytical effort behind this report went into developing more and better information about expenditure on health and constructing national health accounts. As described further in Chapter 6, knowledge of where resources are coming from, through what channels they flow and how they are used, is crucial to better stewardship of the system. Annex Table 8 presents the estimates of total health spending, its separation into private and public sources, the distinction between tax-financed and social security health spending in the public sector, and that between insurance and out-of-pocket spending in the private sector, and the overall distinction between prepayment and out-of-pocket spending that helps determine how fairly health systems are paid for. These data, besides being of direct interest, have been used to check the estimates of household expenditure discussed above and to estimate values for indicators that are strongly related to spending.

Whatever the sources and distribution of finance, the level of resources devoted to health is an input into the system, not an outcome: it is what makes the outcomes possible, and against which the system's achievements should be evaluated. The next two sections take up the question of how best to do this, first by developing an overall measure of attainment and then by relating that achievement to resource use, as a measure of performance.

Box 2.4 Weighting the achievements that go into overall attainment

To derive a set of weights for the different achievements that compose overall attainment, WHO conducted a survey of 1006 respondents from 125 countries, half from among its own staff. The questions were designed to elicit not only views about how important each goal is relative to the others (for example, responsiveness compared to health status), but also opinions about what kind of inequality matters most. The responses were checked for consistency and bias, and yielded nearly identical values in each of many different groups – poorer versus richer countries, men versus women, WHO staff versus other respondents. The final weights are shown in the table.

As expected, health is regarded as the most important of the objectives, clearly the primary or defining goal of a system. But fully half of the concern for health is a concern for equality, not simply for a high average. Taking "health" apart into two goals emphasizes the great value of fairness, and not only of goodness. This is fully consistent with WHO's concentration on the poor, the least healthy, the worst-off in society. Equal weights also result from the survey for the overall level and for distribution or equality where responsiveness is concerned. In total, how the system treats people in non-health aspects is as important as either health level or health

equality. And fairness in how health is paid for, which is not a major traditional concern of WHO or the ministries of health it deals with and supports, receives the relatively large weight of one-fourth, equal to that for responsiveness. Both in this case and in that of responsiveness, the weight assigned by respondents probably reflects the direct or intrinsic importance of the objective, and also the indirect or instrumental contribution it makes to achieving good health; it is difficult to separate these two aspects. There is clear agreement that a well-functioning health system should do much more than simply promote the best possible level of overall health.

The exercise of weighting the five objectives also provides values for the relative importance of goodness and fairness. Together, the *levels* of health and of responsiveness receive a weight of three-eighths of the total. The three distributional measures, which together describe the *equity* of the system, account for the remaining five-eighths. Countries which have achieved only rather short life expectancies and cannot adequately meet their peoples' expectations for prompt attention or amenities may nonetheless be regarded as having health systems which perform well with respect to fairness on one or more dimensions.

Health (disability-adjusted life expectancy)	
Total	50%
Overall or average	25%
Distribution or equality	25%
Responsiveness	
Total	25%
Overall or average	12.5%
Distribution or equality	12.5%
Fair financial contribution	
Distribution or equality	25%

OVERALL ATTAINMENT: GOODNESS AND FAIRNESS COMBINED

To the extent that a health system achieves a long disability-adjusted life expectancy, or a high level of responsiveness (or a high degree of equality in either or both), or a fair distribution of the financing burden, it can be said to perform well with respect to that objective. Since a system can do well on one or more dimensions and poorly on others, comparison across countries or through time requires that the five goals be summed into a single overall measure. There is no natural scale on which to add together years of life, responsiveness scores, and measures of inequality or fairness, so combining the measures of achievement means assigning a weight or relative importance to each one. Box 2.4 describes the procedure and the results.

Applying these weights to the achievements described in Annex Tables 5, 6 and 7 yields an overall attainment score for each health system. These scores are presented in Annex Table 9, together with an estimate of the uncertainty around each value, derived from the uncertainties for the components. Because rich countries generally enjoy good health, and because high incomes allow for large health expenditures which are also predominantly prepaid and often largely public, the ranking by overall attainment is closely related to income and health spending. However, the large weight given to distributional goals explains why, for example, Japan outranks the United States and why Chile, Colombia and Cuba outrank all other Latin American countries. It is not surprising that, with three Asian exceptions, the 30 worst-off countries are all in Africa.

PERFORMANCE: GETTING RESULTS FROM RESOURCES

The overall indicator of attainment, like the five specific achievements which compose it, is an absolute measure. It says how well a country has done in reaching the different goals, but it says nothing about how that outcome compares to what might have been achieved with the resources available in the country. It is *achievement relative to resources* that is the critical measure of a health system's performance.

Thus if Sweden enjoys better health than Uganda – life expectancy is almost exactly twice as long – that is in large part because it spends exactly 35 times as much per capita on its health system. But Pakistan spends almost precisely the same amount per person as Uganda, out of an income per person that is close to Uganda's, and yet it has a life expectancy almost 25 years higher. This is the crucial comparison: why are health outcomes in Pakistan so much better, for the same expenditure? And it is health expenditure that matters, not the country's total income, because one society may choose to spend less of a given income on health than another. Each health system should be judged according to the resources actually at its disposal, not according to other resources which in principle could have been devoted to health but were used for something else.

Health outcomes have often been assessed in relation to inputs such as the number of doctors or hospital beds per unit of population. This approach indicates what these inputs *actually* produce, but it tells little about the health system's *potential* – what it could do if it used the same level of financial resources to produce and deploy different numbers and combinations of professionals, buildings, equipment and consumables. In these comparisons, the right measure of resources is money, since that is used to buy all the real inputs.

To assess relative performance requires a scale, one end of which establishes an upper limit or "frontier", corresponding to *the most that could be expected of a health system*. This frontier – derived using information from many countries but with a specific value for each country – represents the level of attainment which a health system might achieve, but which no country surpasses. At the other extreme, a lower boundary needs to be defined for *the least that could be demanded of the health system* (17). With this scale it is possible to see how much of this potential has been realized. In other words, comparing actual attainment with potential shows how far from its own frontier of maximal performance is each country's health system.

WHO has estimated two relations between outcomes and health system resources. One estimate relates resources only to average health status (disability-adjusted life expectancy, DALE), which makes it somewhat comparable to many previous analyses of performance in health. The other relates resources to the overall attainment measure based on all five objectives. The same value of total resources is used for a country in both cases, because there is no way to identify expenditure as being directed to producing health services, determining responsiveness or making the financing more or less fair. The same is true of resources used to improve the distribution of health or responsiveness, rather than the average level.

Each frontier is a function of one other variable besides health system expenditure. That is the average years of schooling in the adult population, which is a measure of human

---

Box 2.5 Estimating the best to be expected and the least to be demanded

WHO's estimates of the upper and lower bounds of health system performance differ in two important ways from most analyses of what health systems actually achieve. The first is that a "frontier" is meaningful only if no country can lie beyond it, although at least one must lie on it. The frontier or upper limit is therefore estimated by a statistical technique which allows for errors in one direction only, minimizing the distances between the frontier and the calculated performance values. (The lower bound is estimated by the conventional technique of allowing errors in either direction.) The second is that the object is not to *explain* what each country or health system has attained, so much as to form an estimate of what should be possible. The degree of explanation could be increased by introducing many more variables. If tropical countries show systematically lower achievement in health, because of the effects of many diseases concentrated near the equator, a variable indicating

tropical location would raise the explanatory or predictive power. Similarly, if outcomes are worse with respect to equality in ethnically diverse countries, a variable reflecting that heterogeneity would explain the outcomes observed.

The difficulty with the attempt to explain as much as possible is that it leads to a different frontier, according to every additional variable. There would be one for tropical countries and another for colder climates; one for ethnically mixed countries and another for those with more uniform populations; and so on. If performance were measured relative to the frontier for each type of country, almost every health system might look about equally efficient in the use of resources, because less would be expected of some than of others. Every additional explanation would be the equivalent of a reason for not doing better. This is particularly true of explanations related to individual diseases: AIDS and malaria are major causes of health loss in many sub-Saharan African countries, but to include

their effects in the estimation of the frontier means judging those countries only according to how well they control all *other* diseases, as though nothing could be done about AIDS and malaria. This is the reason for estimating the frontier according to nothing but expenditure and human capital, which is a general measure of society's capacity for many kinds of performance, including performance of the health system.

The measures of attainment draw on data referring to the past several years, to make the estimates more robust and less susceptible to anomalous values in any one year. The measures of expenditure and human capital are similarly constructed from more than one year's data. Nonetheless, both the outcomes and the factors that determine potential performance are meant to describe the current situation of countries. They do not take into account how past decisions and use of resources may have limited what a system can actually achieve today – which could also be a rea-

son for poor performance – nor do they say how quickly a poorly performing system might be expected to improve and come closer to the frontier.

This way of estimating what is feasible bypasses two particularly complex issues which are well illustrated by control of tobacco-related mortality and disability. One is that many actions taken by health systems produce results only after a number of years, so that resources used today are not closely related to outcomes today. If a health system somehow persuaded all smokers to quit and no one to take up the habit, it would be many years before there was no more tobacco-induced disease burden.[1] The other is that no health system could reasonably be expected to bring smoking prevalence down to zero any time soon, no matter how hard it tried. Determining how to evaluate progress rather than only a health system's current performance is one of many challenges for future effort.

[1] Jha P, Chaloupka F, eds. *Tobacco control policies in developing countries*. Oxford, Oxford University Press for the World Bank and the World Health Organization, 2000.

capital and therefore of the long-run potential, if not the current or actual, state of development of the country. It is a proxy for most of the factors outside the health system that contribute to health status, and probably also to the degree of responsiveness and to how health is financed. Box 2.5 explains how the upper and lower limits are estimated and how they should be interpreted.

Since the estimation is based entirely on country data rather than a model of what is ideal or feasible, and since there are upper limits to all the achievements, the frontier rises rapidly with additional resources when spending is low, and then rises more and more slowly as expenditure reaches the levels typical of rich countries. A health system can move *towards* the frontier by improving performance, that is by achieving more with the same resources. It can move *along* the frontier by spending more or less on health and reaching a different level of attainment but the same degree of performance. The entire frontier can also move *outward*, as new knowledge makes it possible to achieve better health or other outcomes, for given health system resources and a given level of human capital. Most of the enormous improvement in health over the last century and a half, described in Chapter 1, is due to such an expansion or outward movement of what it is possible to achieve.

If there were no health system in the modern sense, people would still be born, live and die; life expectancy would be much less than now, but it would not be zero. There would be no expenditure on health and hence no question of how fairly the financial burden was distributed. Similarly, there would be no responsiveness. So the minimum level of achievement would involve only health status, and in the absence of information about inequalities, only the average level of health. In the measure of overall attainment the values for the other four objectives, including all those related to inequality, would be set at zero. To estimate this minimum, WHO has used information from a limited number of countries *circa* 1900, relating life expectancy – with no adjustment for disability – to estimates of income. The situation at the turn of the last century is taken as the starting point for the great advances made possible by increased knowledge, investment and resources devoted to health. Some of the changes have the effect of raising the minimum – the eradication of smallpox is the best example. The emergence of HIV/AIDS and of tobacco-related disease have the opposite effect, making it harder than it was in 1900 to achieve a given level of health.

The question for any health system today is, given the country's human capital and the resources devoted to its health system, how close has it come to the most that could be asked of it? Relating outcomes in this way to the estimated minimum and maximum attainments and to the use of economic resources defines the overall indicator of system *performance*: to perform well means to move away from the minimum attainment and come close to the maximum. In economic terms, performance is a measure of efficiency: an efficient health system achieves much, relative to the resources at its disposal. In contrast, an inefficient system is wasteful of resources, even if it achieves high levels of health, responsiveness and fairness. That is, it could be expected to do still better, because countries spending less do comparably well or countries spending a little more achieve much better outcomes.

Annex Table 10 presents two indicators of health system performance. The first is based only on the average health status in disability-adjusted life expectancy (DALE) presented in Annex Table 5, comparing the frontier for that objective alone to a country's resource use and human capital. In this case, the upper and lower bounds between which performance lies are strictly comparable, and the measure can be compared to other estimates of what determines health outcomes. As with the measures of attainment, these values carry estimates of uncertainty. Figure 2.6 shows the estimated distribution of performance for all countries with respect to DALE. Higher health expenditure is associated with better health outcomes, even when performance is judged relative to expenditure rather than absolutely. Very poor countries evidently suffer from other handicaps than low spending and low educational attainment. The few countries where spending is below $10 per person per year seldom appear to achieve more than 75% of the life expectancy that should be possible, whereas most countries spending more than $1000 achieve at least 75% of the possible. Higher spending is also associated with less variation in performance. Disturbingly large variations in life expectancy relative to spending and education occur at low and middle levels of expenditure where there is the greatest need to understand and reduce differences in achievement. A large part of the explanation is the HIV/AIDS epidemic: the 25 worst-off countries are all African nations suffering from a severe burden of AIDS. (Box 2.5 explains why the epidemic was not taken into account in defining the frontier of the possible.)

The second indicator in Annex Table 10 is based on the overall attainment measure presented in Annex Table 9 and assesses performance relative to the frontier defined for all five elements of achievement. The intervals around these values are much larger than for DALE alone because of the uncertainty surrounding the other components. These components also account for some considerable changes in the ranking, but the best performing systems still seem to be those of relatively rich countries and the worst off are predominantly poor and in Africa. Figure 2.7 presents the distribution of overall performance, which shows somewhat less variation than Figure 2.6: countries that perform poorly with respect to health alone sometimes compensate for this by doing better in responsiveness or financing or in dealing with health inequality. Nonetheless the rankings of the two performance measures are rather closely associated, with a small number of countries that do much better by one measure than by the other.

The belief that the system should be accountable for the level and distribution of attainment on the goals of health, responsiveness and fair financing, all relative to health

Figure 2.6 Performance on level of health (disability-adjusted life expectancy) relative to health expenditure per capita, 191 Member States, 1999

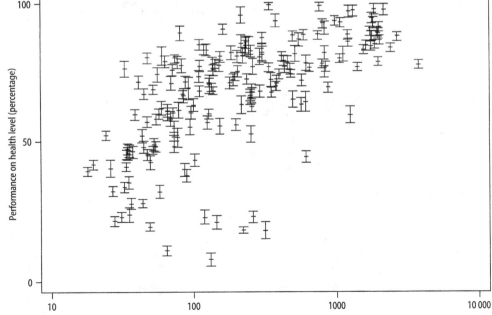

Health expenditure per capita, 1997 international dollars

expenditure, will remain central in WHO's work to support health systems development over the coming years. From this issue, each year's *World health report* will contain more complete and better measures of countries' achievements, and WHO will support countries to strengthen local skills to analyse and improve health system attainment and performance.

IMPROVING PERFORMANCE: FOUR KEY FUNCTIONS

Policy to improve performance requires information on the principal factors which explain it. Knowledge of the determinants of health system *performance*, as distinct from understanding of what determines health *status*, remains very limited. This report focuses on a few universal functions which health systems perform, as indicated in Figure 2.1 above, asking what it means for those functions to be discharged well or poorly and suggesting how they are associated with differences in achievement among countries. This helps to look at the health system overall, rather than building up from the component sub-systems, organizations or programmes, as is more common in evaluations of performance *(18)*.

The service provision function is the most familiar, and in fact the entire health system is often identified with just service delivery. The classification here emphasizes that providing services is something the system *does*; it is not what the system *is*. Much of what is included in the financing function occurs outside what is usually considered to be the health system, as a process which happens to collect revenues and put them at the system's disposal. Treating fairness in financial contribution as one of the intrinsic goals of the system requires viewing the function partly as another of the tasks that the system *does*, rather than pas-

Figure 2.7 Overall health system performance (all attainments) relative to health expenditure per capita, 191 Member States, 1997

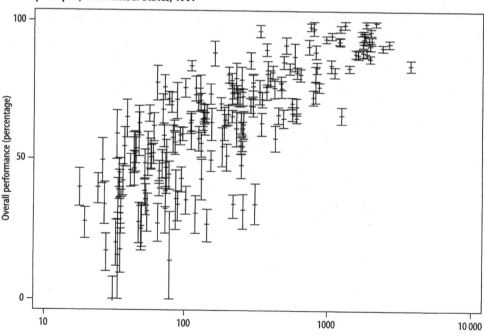

Health expenditure per capita, 1997 international dollars

sively receiving money from somewhere else. It is the system which collects some of the funds directly, pools all that are pooled except for general taxation, and purchases goods and services. This means the system is at least partly accountable to society for how resources are raised and combined, and not only for how they are ultimately used.

Every health system makes some investments in creating resources, but these also are sometimes regarded as coming from outside the system itself. In the short run, the system can only use the resources created in the past, and often can do little to change even how they are employed. But in the long run, investment also is something the system does – and precisely because investments are long-lived, it has a responsibility to invest wisely. Relating achievements to total system expenditure may show that a system is performing badly precisely because what can be obtained from today's resources is needlessly limited by how resources were invested yesterday and the day before.

The fourth function is called *stewardship*, because the concept is well described by the dictionary definition: *the careful and responsible management of something entrusted to one's care (19)*. People entrust both their bodies and their money to the health system, which has a responsibility to protect the former and use the latter wisely and well. The government is particularly called on to play the role of a steward, because it spends revenues that people are required to pay through taxes and social insurance, and because it makes many of the rules that are followed in private and voluntary transactions. It also owns facilities on trust from the citizens. Private insurers and practitioners, however, perform this function in only a slightly restricted degree, and part of the state's task as the overall steward or trustee of the system is to see to it that private organizations and actors also act carefully and responsibly. A large part of stewardship consists of regulation, whether undertaken by the government or by private bodies which regulate their members, often under general rules determined by government. But the concept embraces more than just regulation, and when properly conducted has a pervasive influence on all the workings of the system.

These functions are identifiable in widely differing health system structures *(20, 1)*. At one extreme is a system in which functions are substantially combined in a single organization which raises, pools and allocates funds to a fairly monolithic group of service providers who are its own employees. The Norwegian health system resembles this type of structure, as did the British National Health Service prior to 1990. A system may instead have a high degree of "vertical" segmentation. Separate organizations such as the ministry of health, social security funds, the armed forces, charitable organizations, or private insurers may pay their own providers, raise and allocate funds and provide services, for non-overlapping populations. The health systems of much of Latin America bear some resemblance to this model, although patients often get care from two or more of the vertically separate organizations. A system could also have "horizontal" integration of each function – one organization performing it – but a different organization for each function. No system quite corresponds to this, because there is never a single bloc of providers, unless they are part of a fully integrated system. However, some systems such as that of Chile separate collection and pooling for a large share of resources, and employ a large number of providers under a single organization. At the opposite extreme from a monolithic organization is a system with separate institutions raising funds and paying providers under pluralistic provision arrangements in which few providers "belong" to the financing institution. The Colombian system, following the reforms introduced since 1993, looks somewhat like the latter.

Chapters 3, 4, 5 and 6 concentrate in turn on key characteristics of each of the four functions – service delivery, investment, financing and stewardship – and on some factors affecting performance, examining patterns in countries at different income levels. The financing function obviously is most important for the goal of fairness in paying for the system, but how it is carried out also affects health outcomes and even has some effect on responsiveness. The service delivery function is most tied to health outcomes, but also matters greatly for responsiveness. And stewardship affects everything.

REFERENCES

1. **Murray CJL, Frenk J.** *A WHO framework for health system performance assessment.* Geneva, World Health Organization, 1999 (GPE Discussion Paper No. 6).

2. **Roemer MI.** *National health systems of the world.* New York, Oxford University Press, 1991.

3. **Centers for Disease Prevention and Control, Centro Latino-Americano de Investigación en Sistemas de Salud, and Pan American Health Organization.** *Public health in the Americas.* Washington, DC, Pan American Health Organization, 1999 (unpublished document).

4. *World development report 1993 – Investing in health.* Washington, DC, The World Bank, 1993.

5. **Acheson D et al.** *Independent inquiry into inequalities in health.* London, The Stationery Office, 1998.

6. **Gilson L, Alilio M, Heggenhougen K.** Community satisfaction with primary health care services: an evaluation undertaken in the Morogoro region of Tanzania. *Social Science and Medicine,* 1994, **39**(6): 767–780.

7. **Bassett MT, Bijlmakers L, Sanders DM.** Professionalism, patient satisfaction and quality of health care: experience during Zimbabwe's structural adjustment programme. *Social Science and Medicine,* 1997, **45**(12): 1845–1852.

8. **Hurst J.** Challenges to health systems in OECD countries. *Bulletin of the World Health Organization,* 2000, **78**(6) (in press).

9. **Donelan K et al.** The cost of health system change: public discontent in five nations. *Health Affairs,* 1999, **18**(3): 206–216.

10. **King S.** Vaccination policies: individual rights v. community health. *British Medical Journal,* 1999, **319**: 1448–1449.

11. **de Silva A.** *A framework for measuring responsiveness.* Geneva, World Health Organization, Global Programme on Evidence for Health Policy, 1999 (unpublished paper).

12. **Fabricant S, Kamara C, Mills A.** Why the poor pay more: household curative expenditures in rural Sierra Leone. *International Journal of Health Planning and Management,* 1999, **14**: 179–199.

13. **Nolan B, Turbat V.** *Cost recovery in public health services in sub-Saharan Africa.* Washington, DC, Economic Development Institute of The World Bank, 1995.

14. **Bennett S, Creese A, Monasch R.** Health insurance schemes for people outside formal sector employment. Geneva, World Health Organization, 1998 (Current Concerns, ARA paper No. 16, document WHO/ARA/CC/98.1).

15. **Friedman M.** *Theory of the consumption function.* Princeton, NJ, Princeton University Press, 1957.

16. **Bevan A.** *In place of fear.* London, Heinemann, 1952.

17. **Donabedian A, Wheeler JRC, Wyszewianski L.** Quality, cost, and health: an integrative model. *Medical Care,* 1982, **20**: 975–992.

18. **Cumper GE.** *The evaluation of national health systems.* Oxford, Oxford University Press, 1991.

19. *Meriam Webster's deluxe dictionary.* Pleasantville, New York/Montreal, Reader's Digest, 1998.

20. **Murray CJL, Kreuser J, Whang W.** Cost-effectiveness analysis and policy choices: investing in health systems. *Bulletin of the World Health Organization,* 1994, **72**(4): 663–674.

CHAPTER THREE

Health Services: Well Chosen, Well Organized?

Health services aim to protect or improve health. Whether they do so effectively depends on which services are provided and how they are organized. Resources should be used for interventions that are known to be effective, in accordance with national or local priorities. Because resources are limited, there will always be some form of rationing but prices should not be the chief way to determine who gets what care. Both hierarchical bureaucracies and fragmented, unregulated markets have serious flaws as ways to organize services: flexible integration of autonomous or semi-autonomous health care providers can mitigate the problems.

3

HEALTH SERVICES:

WELL CHOSEN, WELL ORGANIZED?

ORGANIZATIONAL FAILINGS

*J*ust as the principal objective of a health system is to improve people's health, the chief function the system needs to perform is to deliver health services. The other functions matter partly because they contribute to service provision. It is therefore a major failing of the system when effective and affordable health interventions do not reach the populations that would benefit from them. Sometimes this happens because the providers have inadequate skills, or because of a lack of drugs and equipment: these are the consequence of failures of training and investment, as discussed in Chapter 4, or of purchasing, as discussed here and in Chapter 5. Sometimes services are not delivered to potential beneficiaries because of price barriers: this is the result of a failure to finance the services fairly, as discussed in Chapter 5. But often a failure of service delivery is due to dysfunctional organization of the health system, even when the needed inputs exist and financial support is adequate and fairly distributed. Such an organizational failing can result from the wrong arrangements among different parties involved in service delivery, which in turn creates perverse incentives and leads to mistaken choices about what services to provide, to whom to deliver them, or how to ration when it is not possible to meet everyone's needs or wants. This chapter considers how to choose which services to provide, how to organize provision and how to assure the right incentives for providers.

The complexities of organizing service provision are illustrated by the following example, which is not at all unusual. A poor young woman walks to a rural government health post with her sick baby. There is no doctor at the post, and there are no drugs. But a nurse gives the mother an oral rehydration kit and explains how to use it. She tells the mother to come back in a couple of days if the baby's diarrhoea continues. The nurse sees only half a dozen patients that day. Meanwhile, at the outpatient clinic of a community hospital about an hour's drive away, several hundred patients are waiting to be seen. Some are given cursory examinations by the doctors there and are able to obtain any prescribed drugs at the hospital dispensary. When the outpatient clinic closes, even though it is still early in the day, patients who have not been seen are asked to return the next day, without being given appointments. Some of the doctors then hurry off to work in a private "nursing home" or clinic to supplement their salaries.

The doctors' low pay and the absence of more qualified staff and drugs at the health post might be shrugged off as the consequences of spending too little. But a lack of resources cannot be blamed for the maldistribution of those resources between the health post and the hospital, the low productivity of the nurse, the under-utilization of the hospital when its clinic closes early, the failure to have some doctors on duty over a longer interval, and the waste of people's time in waiting and then having to return another day because there is no system of appointments. These problems reflect failures of priority and of organization, both in initial investments and training and then in service delivery or the lack thereof. If the story has a happy ending for the mother and baby, it is only because the child was lucky to have diarrhoea and not malaria or some other condition the nurse could not recognize or could not treat, or requiring care which the mother would have to pay for out of pocket. Getting even limited care for free may also be the reason the mother goes to a public facility rather than to one of the private pharmacies or traditional healers, patronized by large numbers of people.

This chapter looks at how to set priorities for which services health systems should provide, and at the choices and mechanisms involved in rationing so as to make priorities effective. It then considers the organizational factors that help to make sure that the right services reach people at the right time.

PEOPLE AT THE CENTRE OF HEALTH SERVICES

The story of the mother and baby illustrates another fact about health systems: service delivery is where people meet most directly, as providers and users of interventions. But people play more than those two roles, as Figure 3.1 indicates. At the centre of service delivery is the patient, in the case of clinical interventions, or the affected population, in the case of non-personal public health services. People are also consumers, because they behave in ways that influence their health, including their choices about seeking and utilizing health care. The consumer may be the patient, or someone such as a mother acting on his

Figure 3.1 The multiple roles of people in health systems

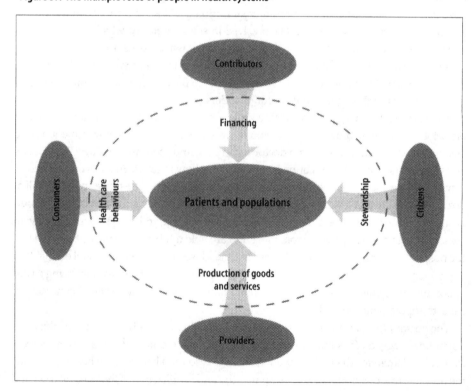

or her behalf, or simply a person making choices about diet, lifestyle and other factors that affect health.

Sometimes the roles of consumer, patient and provider are all combined into one person and one moment, as happens when a woman gives birth with little or no assistance. Every minute, thousands of women across the world are giving birth. In countries where the attendance by trained staff is low (9% in Nepal, 8% in Bangladesh and Ethiopia, 5% in Equatorial Guinea, 4% in Gabon and Mauritania, 2% in Somalia), births usually take place in the presence of lay birth attendants or family members. Even when the delivery is by caesarian section with a trained provider, each woman must still actively participate in birth and the postpartum recovery.

Often the choices people make, particularly about seeking care, are influenced by the responsiveness of the system as described in Chapter 2. Utilization does not depend only on the consumer's perception of need or of the likelihood of benefiting from a service. Although marked differences exist between societies, the basic tenets of ethical provider–patient relations usually include similar elements of consent, confidentiality, discretion, veracity and fidelity *(1)*. Calling the elements of dignity, autonomy and confidentiality that go into responsiveness "respect for persons" underscores the importance of people, and not simply patients, as the recipients of health services.

People also play the role of contributors to financing the system. Millions of poor people pay for all of the services they receive at the time they are ill. In health systems with fairer contribution arrangements, people who are not sick contribute most to financing the health system, through taxes or health insurance contributions, so that the contributor may or may not be the patient or the consumer. Finally, as citizens – and particularly as officials whose job it is to represent citizens and protect their interests – people participate in the system as stewards. In the same way that all four functions have to be carried out in order for the system to perform well, people have to play all these roles in order for the potential benefits to reach the patients and populations at the centre.

People act as providers, consumers, contributors and stewards of the health system during their adult working lives. In contrast, they can assume the role of patients at any time from before birth right up to death. The need to deliver services for people at all ages greatly complicates the choice of what services to emphasize and how to organize them, because people are exposed to different risks at different ages, and priority to any particular intervention is at least in part also a priority for a particular age group. These differences are what make a demographic transition – lower mortality and longer life – into an epidemiological transition – a change in the relative importance of different threats to health, particularly a shift from communicable to noncommunicable diseases.

Besides the variation with age, there are marked differences in disease patterns among regions, countries and specific population groups. For example, in Africa infectious diseases account for nearly 70% of the disease burden, as Annex Table 4 shows. In Europe, they account for less than 20%. The poor suffer more from infectious diseases than the rich *(2)*, but over the next 20 years even the poor will be vulnerable to cardiovascular and cerebrovascular diseases linked to tobacco use *(3)*. It may seem natural to focus health system choices on the causes that account for a large share of the disease burden, either because they affect large populations or because they cause substantial health loss for each victim.

However, all that health systems can actually *do* is to deliver specific services or interventions. Even if a first choice is made to concentrate on one or more particular diseases, it is still necessary to decide what to do – that is, which specific interventions to emphasize. The number of interventions available greatly exceeds the number of diseases, and the appropriate strategy for disease control may depend on just one intervention or on a combination of several activities. To make matters more complicated, a given intervention may be effective against more than one disease or cause, because it works on a common risk factor or symptom. This is especially true of diagnostic activities: taking blood samples, or using X-rays or other imaging techniques may be appropriate for a great variety of problems. Thus, emphasizing an intervention, or investing in the inputs necessary for providing it, does not automatically focus effort on just one disease. Setting priorities also involves deciding what a particular intervention should be used for.

The range of diagnostic approaches and medical and surgical interventions for many conditions is extensive and likely to expand significantly over the coming decades. This means that services need to be designed and implemented so as to allow for innovation and adaptation to new health challenges and interventions, all the while responding to the needs of people who differ in age, income, habits and health risks. No health system can meet all those needs, even in rich countries. So either there must be conscious choices of what services should have priority, or the services actually delivered may bear little relation to any reasonable criterion of what is most important.

CHOOSING INTERVENTIONS: GETTING THE MOST HEALTH FROM RESOURCES

The ancient Greeks believed that *Asclepios,* the god of medicine, had two daughters. One, *Hygieia,* was responsible for prevention, while the other, *Panacea,* was responsible for cure *(4).* While some preventive activities are applied to specific individuals – immunization is the clearest example – the distinction between prevention and cure or treatment corresponds closely to the difference between public health interventions directed to entire populations and clinical interventions directed to individuals. Since there is usually demand for the latter but there may not be any demand for the former, one of the principal tasks in choosing which services should have priority is that of balancing public health and clinical activities *(5).*

To require the health system to obtain the greatest possible level of health from the resources devoted to it, is to ask that it be as cost-effective as it can be. This is the basis for emphasizing those interventions that give the most value for money, and giving less priority to those that, much as they may help individuals, contribute little per dollar spent to the improvement of the population's health. It is the implicit basis of the measure of performance with respect to disability-adjusted life expectancy presented in Chapter 2 and Annex Table 10. So far as the level of health is concerned, the allocative efficiency of the health system could be enhanced by moving resources from cost-ineffective interventions to cost-effective ones *(6).* The potential gains from doing this are sometimes enormous, because the existing pattern of interventions includes some which cost a great deal and produce few additional years of life. For example, a set of 185 publicly-funded interventions in the United States cost about $21.4 billion per year, for an estimated saving of 592 000 years of life (considering only premature deaths prevented). Re-allocating those funds to the most cost-effective interventions could save an additional 638 000 life years if all potential beneficiaries were reached. At the level of specific services, the cost per year of life saved can be as low as $236 for screening and treating newborns with sickle-cell anaemia or as high as $5.4 million for radionuclide emission control *(7).* In poor countries all the absolute numbers will be smaller, but the ratio between more and less cost-effective actions may still be very large.

Combining calculations of the cost with measures of the effectiveness of interventions and using them to determine priorities is a very recent development. Early work using such techniques in developing countries looked mainly at the cost-effectiveness of specific disease control programmes *(8–13)*. This type of work expanded following publication of the *World development report* by the World Bank in 1993 *(14)* and subsequent work by WHO *(15)*. Table 3.1 provides examples of interventions that, if implemented well, can substantially reduce the burden of disease, especially among the poor, and do so at a reasonable cost relative to results. Services can also be classified by their importance in the burden of disease of particular age and sex groups, and their cost-effectiveness for those groups *(14)*.

Ideally, services with these virtues will also be inexpensive, so that they can be applied to large beneficiary populations and still imply reasonable total expenditures. However, there is no guarantee that low cost per life saved or healthy life year gained will mean low cost per person: some cost-effective interventions can be very expensive, with great variation

Table 3.1 Interventions with a large potential impact on health outcomes

Examples of interventions	Main contents of interventions
Treatment of tuberculosis	Directly observed treatment schedule (DOTS): administration of standardized short-course chemotherapy to all confirmed sputum smear positive cases of TB under supervision in the initial (2–3 months) phase
Maternal health and safe motherhood interventions	Family planning, prenatal and delivery care, clean and safe delivery by trained birth attendant, postpartum care, and essential obstetric care for high risk pregnancies and complications
Family planning	Information and education; availability and correct use of contraceptives
School health interventions	Health education and nutrition interventions, including anti-helminthic treatment, micronutrient supplementation and school meals
Integrated management of childhood illness	Case management of acute respiratory infections, diarrhoea, malaria, measles and malnutrition; immunization, feeding/breastfeeding counselling, micronutrient and iron supplementation, anti-helminthic treatment
HIV/AIDS prevention	Targeted information for sex workers, mass education awareness, counselling, screening, mass treatment for sexually transmitted diseases, safe blood supply
Treatment of sexually transmitted diseases	Case management using syndrome diagnosis and standard treatment algorithm
Immunization (EPI Plus)	BCG at birth; OPV at birth, 6, 10, 14 weeks; DPT at 6, 10, 14 weeks; HepB at birth, 6 and 9 months (optional); measles at 9 months; TT for women of child-bearing age
Malaria	Case management (early assessment and prompt treatment) and selected preventive measures (e.g. impregnated bed nets)
Tobacco control	Tobacco tax, information, nicotine replacement, legal action
Noncommunicable diseases and injuries	Selected early screening and secondary prevention

between one health service and another, for the same disease. This is clear in the case of malaria, where two interventions that are about equally cost-effective – chloroquine prophylaxis and two annual rounds of insecticide spraying – differ enormously in how much they would cost to apply to all the affected population of a low income African country *(16)*. Cost differences are even greater for interventions against an infection.

The reverse is also true: health interventions can be cost-ineffective even when they do not cost very much and are intended to benefit large numbers of people. For example, many service providers continue to rely on antibiotics to treat viral illnesses, even though this is known to be ineffective. Even in rich countries, there is a need to ensure that the main output of health services remains focused on effective and affordable public health and clinical interventions. In low income countries, where the full range and cost of possible interventions significantly outstrip available resources, such wasteful practices deprive other patients of critical treatment.

Cost-effectiveness analysis, then, is essential for identifying the services that will produce the most health gain from available resources, but it has to be applied to individual interventions, not broadly against disease or causes. This requirement means that a large set of interventions needs to be evaluated. For all but the richest societies, the cost and time required for such an evaluation may be prohibitive. Moreover, such analysis, as currently practised, often fails to identify existing misallocation of resources because it focuses on the evaluation of new technologies and ignores the existing distribution of productive assets and activities *(6)*.

Intervention costs can also vary greatly from one country, context, and intervention mode to another *(17)*. A naive generalization could lead to serious mistakes in planning and implementing otherwise effective interventions. Even if they cover a relatively small number of interventions, studies in individual countries or populations are needed to avoid such errors. In Guinea, for example, 40 interventions have been studied. These were chosen partly on the basis of more general studies elsewhere, but with detailed local information to confirm what would really be most appropriate in that country *(18)*.

Variations in cost and results among interventions are particularly relevant when a combination of several interventions may be suitable against a particular disease. To take the case of malaria again, at low levels of health expenditure in a country with a high burden of the disease, case management and prophylaxis for pregnant women would be very cost-effective and affordable *(16)*. With more resources available, impregnated mosquito nets could be added – they would prevent more cases but cost more per unit of health benefit gained. A single estimate of cost-effectiveness of malaria control could lead to the wrong conclusion that malaria control is not affordable, for example if the estimate for a low income country is based on a programme combining all technically feasible options. In general, the most cost-effective combination of services depends on the resources available. That relation does not, of course, determine the appropriate level of expenditure on malaria control, which depends on what the country can afford, given its other health problems and priorities. In particular, there is no presumption that it should spend only the amount consistent with one or more of the cheapest interventions. Spending more and using a mixed strategy might yield much greater health gains.

Misuse of cost-effectiveness analysis could also lead to a serious underestimate of the actual cost of control if the estimate were based on the costs and effectiveness of a single type of intervention but multiple interventions were used. Many factors may alter the actual cost-effectiveness of a given intervention programme during implementation. These include: the availability, mix and quality of inputs (especially trained personnel, drugs, equipment and consumables); local prices, especially labour costs; implementation capacity; underlying organizational structures and incentives; and the supporting institutional framework *(17, 19)*.

All these obstacles imply that even on the sole criterion of cost-effectiveness, analysis of a health system's potential for getting more health from what it spends needs to begin with the current capacities, activities and outcomes, and consider what steps can be taken *from that starting point* to add, modify or eliminate services. This is likely to have profound implications for investment if little can be changed simply by re-directing the existing staff, facilities and equipment *(20)*.

CHOOSING INTERVENTIONS: WHAT ELSE MATTERS?

Cost-effectiveness by itself is relevant for achieving the best overall health, but not necessarily for the second health goal, that of reducing inequality. Populations with worse than average health may respond less well to an intervention, or cost more to reach or to treat, so that a concern for distribution implies a willingness to sacrifice some overall health gains for other criteria. More generally, cost-effectiveness is only one of at least nine criteria that a health system may be asked to respect. A health system ought to protect people from financial risk, to be consistent with the goal of fair financial contribution. This means that the cost matters, and not only its relation to health results, whether money is public or private. A health system should strive for both horizontal and vertical equity – treating alike all those who face the same health need, and treating preferentially those with the greatest needs – to be consistent with the goal of reducing health inequalities. And it should assure not only that the healthy subsidize the sick, as any prepayment arrangement will do in part, but also that the burden of financing is fairly shared by having the better-off subsidize the less well-off. This generally requires spending public funds in favour of the poor.

Figure 3.2 Questions to ask in deciding what interventions to finance and provide

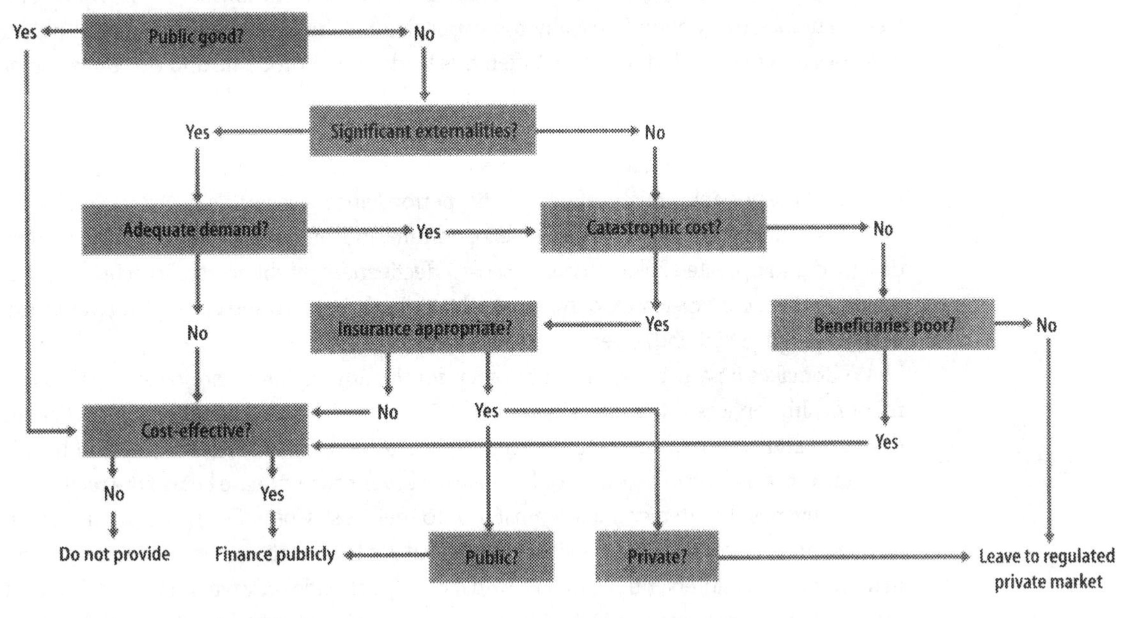

Source: Adapted from Musgrove P. Public spending on health care: how are different criteria related? *Health Policy*, 1999, 47(3): 207–223.

Public money is also the principal, if not the only significant way to pay for public goods, interventions which private markets will not offer because buyers cannot appropriate all the benefits, and non-buyers cannot be excluded. The same is true for partly public goods with large externalities – that is, spillovers of benefits to non-users. Private demand for such services will generally be inadequate. Interventions of this sort are most important in communicable disease control, where treating one case may prevent many others, and especially where it is the environment, rather than identifiable individuals, that is treated. Analysts and decision-makers also correctly argue that resource allocation decisions affecting the entire health system must take into account social concerns, such as a priority for the seriously ill and for promoting the well-being of future generations. Figure 3.2 summarizes the choices for spending public or publicly mandated funds, showing how the different criteria should be considered sequentially and how they can be used to determine whether an intervention is worth buying or not. This way of setting priorities reinforces the emphasis on the two goals of health outcomes and financial fairness. It also emphasizes the importance of public health activities, by starting with interventions that are public or quasi-public goods.

Ignoring these other criteria and using only disease burden and cost-effectiveness as a method for determining priorities can lead to a "race for the bottom of the barrel" among advocates of different interventions, each trying to prove that their programme achieves a greater benefit or costs less than other programmes, sometimes without considering the full range of complicating factors. This often leads to underestimates of the real cost of programmes and their subsequent failure during implementation because of resource shortages.

Too narrow an approach also ignores the important role that the public sector should be playing in protecting the poor and addressing insurance market failure – the tendency of insurance to exclude precisely those people who need it most, because they are at greater than usual risk of ill-health. Many families will be faced at some time with a health problem of low frequency for which there is an effective but high cost intervention. Those who can afford it will turn to the private sector for the needed care. But without some form of organized insurance this option is usually too expensive for the poor who will turn to public hospitals as a place of last recourse. Often this leads to inappropriate and excessive use of hospital care, and it undermines the financing function that health systems should be playing.

Actual health systems always deliver services that correspond to a variety of criteria. The frontier of the possible which defines relative performance reflects this fact, since it is based on actual outcomes relative to health expenditure and human capital. A health system designed and operated solely to pursue cost-effectiveness might be able to achieve much longer average life expectancy or more equality or both, but it would correspond much less to what people want and expect.

What makes it particularly difficult to set priorities among interventions and beneficiaries of health services is that the different criteria are not always compatible. In particular, efficiency and equity can easily be in conflict, because the costs of treating a given health problem differ among individuals, or because the severity of a disease bears little relation to the effectiveness of interventions against it or to their cost. Cost-effectiveness is never the *only* justification for spending public resources, but it *is* the test that must be met most often in deciding which interventions to buy. And it can be set aside only when costs are low and the beneficiaries are not poor, so that they can make their own judgements about the value of a particular purchase and the market can be left to supply it; or when protection from catastrophic cost is the overriding consideration and prepayment can protect against that risk. Determining the priorities for a health system is an exercise that draws on a variety of technical, ethical and political criteria and is always subject to modification as a result of experience in implementation, the reaction of the public, and the inertia of financing and investment *(21)*.

CHOOSING INTERVENTIONS: WHAT MUST BE KNOWN?

Setting priorities realistically requires a great deal of information, starting with epidemiological data. Major progress has been made recently in understanding global health and disease patterns *(14, 15, 22)*, including analysis of risk factors which influence several diseases at once. The most significant of such risk factors are malnutrition in children, and poor water and sanitation practices. Other major risk factors include unsafe sex, alcohol, indoor pollution, tobacco, occupational hazards, hypertension and physical inactivity. The public health services in a given country should attempt to deal with such preventable risk factors, taking account of local contexts. For example, the origins of malnutrition vary greatly from one country to another and from one region to another. In sub-Saharan Africa and south Asia, the problem is often a combination of micronutrient deficiency and absolute shortage of calories. In central and eastern Europe, malnutrition is often "poor calories" rather than a "lack of calories" – a diet too high in fat and refined starch. Public health activities will therefore vary, depending on local risk factors and diseases conditions.

Although there are good data on national patterns of risk and disease today, few countries break this information down sub-nationally by income level, sex or vulnerable groups, such as the handicapped, minority ethnic populations, and the frail elderly. Even fewer countries have information on the health-seeking behaviour of those groups or their utilization of health care facilities. Without such information, the effectiveness of interventions is difficult to assess, as the same intervention may have very different effects when applied to different populations.

Governments need to know how to influence the health-seeking behaviour of target groups in need of care. For example, intergroup variations in under-5 mortality are particularly large in Brazil, Nicaragua, and the Philippines, whereas in Ghana, Pakistan, and Viet Nam these differences are much smaller. This shows the need for a greater emphasis on equity in providing health services in the former countries *(23)*. And there are often significant differences in the utilization of preventive and clinical medical attention from one intervention to another, in the same country. In Peru, differences between the rich and poor are far greater with respect to attended deliveries than with respect to immunization *(24)*, largely because of the much higher cost of deliveries.

A key recommendation for policy-makers is to collect and combine data on risk factors, health conditions and interventions with data from household and facilities surveys, focus groups and other qualitative methods, and academic studies, since global and national aggregate data may not reflect local needs. Public health and clinical services should be customized to respond to the latter, and should allow for innovative adaptation during implementation. While gathering and analysing such data is more difficult in the very poorest countries which need this type of analysis the most, the methods are becoming routine and more easily used even at low incomes *(25)*.

The following steps will make health systems more likely to produce effective interventions at an affordable cost, especially for needy populations.

- First, there should be an ongoing detailed assessment of underlying risk factors, disease burden, and utilization patterns of the target populations.
- Second, global information on the cost and effectiveness of interventions, as well as intervention strategies and practice patterns, should be adapted to local prices and local contexts.
- Third, all countries need explicit policies to ration interventions and to ensure that limited resources are spent in identified high priority areas. How to achieve this is taken up next. Few countries have clinical protocols that can be used to standardize practice patterns and match known priority interventions with needs. Fewer still have the means to enforce such guidelines in privately financed provision.
- Finally, none of these steps will matter unless the quality of service delivery is assured.

ENFORCING PRIORITIES BY RATIONING CARE

Stating priorities is one thing: actually delivering the supposedly most valuable services at the expense of other services is another thing. Markets solve this problem through rationing by price, which means that who gets what goods and services depends not only on how much those goods and services are valued by people, but on who has the means to buy them. Priorities are not set by anyone but emerge from the play of the market. As indicated, this is almost the worst possible way to determine who gets which health services. Every health system therefore confronts the question of what other means to use, when resources are inadequate to needs or wants.

In low-income countries, the difficulties involved in setting priorities and rationing services are extreme. The HIV/AIDS epidemic kills over two million people in Africa every year – more than 10 times the number that perish in wars and armed conflict during the same period. The health services of many low income countries in south Asia and sub-Saharan Africa have been burdened in recent years by this epidemic. In this case, health systems are faced with a long-term problem. Difficult choices have to be made on how resources should be allocated to cover AIDS prevention campaigns, and care for people with AIDS, while maintaining other essential health services. This problem is chronic, and quite different from the need to ration non-urgent care when the system is temporarily burdened by a short-lived epidemic of disease or the results of a natural or man-made disaster. Then emergency services get priority, elective procedures are delayed, and the system concentrates on the epidemic until it is sufficiently under control that business as usual can be resumed.

The most common chronic approach to rationing care is to impose strict expenditure controls that do not try to target any specific disease group or broad category of interventions but simply limit budgetary obligations to affordable levels. This technique has been most commonly used in health systems with global budget financing and leaves it to the budget-holder to ration care. It has been used in the pre-1990 British National Health Service and the ministries of health of many low income countries. Other cost-containment techniques are now being used with varying degrees of success in many European Union countries and some developing countries (26).

The major disadvantage of this approach is that, in low income countries, it usually leads to a degradation of overall standards and quality of care. If resources are in the hands of the better-off, there may be a failure to target vulnerable groups. The available budget is usually captured by the politically strongest providers, such as specialists and hospitals, rather than being used according to the needs of the population. Thus, in many low income countries, an approach based solely on expenditure control leads to the exclusion of large segments of the population from access to organized care.

A second approach is to ration explicitly, following priorities which were set according to some predetermined criteria, as discussed above. This approach, first introduced in the mid-1980s, has now been partially implemented in the Netherlands, New Zealand, Norway, Sweden and Oregon (USA) (27). All use a combination of social, political and cost-effectiveness criteria. Since 1993, several developing countries have tried to introduce intervention packages, variously described as including "essential" or "basic" or "core" interventions that are affordable within each country context (28). Mexico was the first country to design and adopt such a package (29). Bangladesh, Colombia and Zambia have also begun implementation.

The explicit priorities established through this process are a major improvement over the traditional passive cost-containment approach. One serious disadvantage is that in real life, providers are faced with demand for services that are not included in the defined benefit package. They usually react to this demand in one of two ways – by cross-subsidizing the excluded activities through the budget received to pay for the defined benefit package; or by charging extra for the additional services. The first leads to a financing shortfall for the defined benefit package. The second leads to increases in out-of-pocket expenditure and erosion in financial protection. Attempts to curtail such behaviour by providers have been largely unsuccessful.

Another problem is that there are "limits to rationality" (30), particularly if rationality is identified purely with cost-effectiveness. Politicians, providers and the public care about all the criteria discussed above, and may be very sceptical of the estimates underlying allocative choices. The success of explicit priority setting depends on the acceptance and support of providers and consumers.

Even within the set of services financed by prepayment, and particularly those financed by public or publicly mandated funds, there is no clearly best way to ration care. Figure 3.3 illustrates four simplified approaches, based on a combination of what services cost per individual treated or affected, and how frequently the service is likely to be needed. In general, very costly services are seldom needed, while there is much more frequent need for a variety of interventions with intermediate costs. The upper curve in each panel of the figure shows what the demand for different services might look like in the absence of any form of rationing – that is, if every need were expressed as a demand and there were no price or other barriers to obtaining care. That represents the most that the health system might want or try to deliver.

One way to limit what is actually delivered is to exclude all or most of the rare but very expensive services – to cut off the right-hand tail of the distribution of needs. This is relatively common in private insurance, either by explicit exclusion of services or by risk selection of potential clients so as to reduce the likelihood of those services. This may be, but need not be, consistent with cost-effectiveness, and it is almost a necessary form of rationing in systems with very limited resources. But it maximizes people's exposure to financial risk if the intervention can be had by paying out of pocket, or to catastrophic health losses if the service is simply not available at all.

The opposite approach is to exclude common but very inexpensive services from prepayment schemes and in effect require that they be paid out of pocket – that is, to cut off the left-hand end of the distribution. This is likely to save administrative costs, but may or may not represent substantial overall cost saving. As a general rule, prices should not be the main instrument of rationing, and low prices paid by the non-poor present a relatively minor problem. The difficulty with this approach is clear: it exposes the poor to risks that would be acceptable for the non-poor, and so worsens inequality in financial contribution. Rationing may need to be differently conducted for the poor than for the rest of the population, if prices are to play any role.

A health system could also try to ration all services in the same proportion, giving everyone who needs it the same likelihood of obtaining care independently of its cost or of how many other people need the same intervention. There is little to be said for this way of delivering less care than people need, since it does not respect any of the criteria discussed above. At best it represents an attempt to spread the frustration of not obtaining care more or less equally, but that does not even correspond to equality of responsiveness. It may be the response of a system under pressure and with no clear guidance as to the relative importance of different services.

The last panel of Figure 3.3 corresponds to explicit priority setting, so that rationing is much more severe for some services than for others. Only if this happens are nominal priorities really being enforced so as to affect service delivery. And only if the priorities are chosen according to some appropriate criteria can rationing, however it is enforced, actually contribute to better health system performance.

Figure 3.3 Different ways of rationing health interventions according to cost and frequency of need

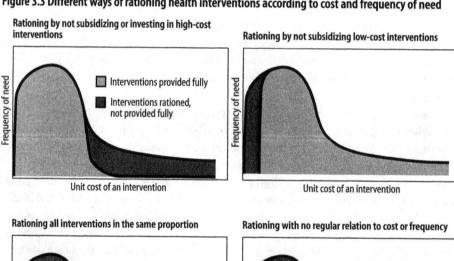

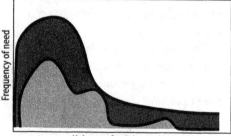

AFTER CHOOSING PRIORITIES:
SERVICE ORGANIZATION AND PROVIDER INCENTIVES

Priority setting is generally considered a public sector exercise, particularly concerning the proper use of public or publicly mandated expenditure. It does not matter for this purpose whether the delivery of services is public or private, nor how providers are paid. What matters is that by contracting with private providers or reimbursing them through public insurance, the government can assure that its priorities are respected even where it does not provide the services. In the sphere of private, voluntary financing of services there generally are no explicit priorities: that part of the health system responds to demands rather than to needs. It is important to take into consideration the impact of out-of-pocket spending on the poor due to increased demand in the private sector for interventions that are not in the public package. But some priorities can nonetheless be enforced through regulation, as for example by requiring all private insurance policies to include a package of essential services or by limiting the degree to which private providers or insurers can select patients or clients on the basis of risk. These are among the tasks of stewardship discussed in Chapter 6. More generally, since it is ultimately providers who do or do not deliver the priority services, rationing requires "careful governance of the agents" who act for patients and assess their competing health needs *(31)*.

Given a list of priorities, and given one or more mechanisms for rationing care, the way services are actually delivered – who benefits from which interventions, how efficiently they are provided, how responsive the system is – can still differ markedly from one health system to another. These differences reflect the fact that while providers may be urged or enjoined to deliver particular services, and public budgets and regulations are designed to reinforce those choices, there is still a variable latitude for providers themselves to decide whom to treat, for what, and how. Just how much latitude providers should have is one of the crucial questions for a health system. The outcome depends on organizational and institutional characteristics, which together determine some of the fundamental incentives to which providers respond.

The relationship between organizations, institutions, and interventions parallels that between the players, the rules and the objects of a game. *Organizations* are the players – for example, individual providers, hospitals, clinics, pharmacies, and public health programmes. *Institutions* are the rules (formal rules and informal customs) – the socially shared constraints that shape human interactions, along with the mechanisms by which these rules are enforced. The key institutions that affect the service delivery system include rules relating to stewardship (governance, information dissemination, coordination, and regulation) and purchasing. *Interventions*, in the sense of services or activities as described above, are the objects of the game and include clinical treatment, public health measures, and health-promoting intersectoral actions *(32)*. *Incentives* are all the rewards and punishments that providers face as a consequence of the organizations in which they work, the institutions under which they operate and the specific interventions they provide.

Both among and within countries there are marked differences in all these features, reflecting the complexity of the production process for health interventions and the variations in culture and tradition. The characteristics that exert the most powerful influence on clinical and public health services are the organizational structures or forms, the service delivery configurations, the organizational incentive regimes, and the linkages among services. As emphasized in Chapter 1, health services deal with an asset – the human body – that is very different from those that other economic activities deal with. Nonetheless there are some aspects of how health services are produced that do not differ greatly from the production of other services. Evidence of the importance of these factors is slowly growing as a result of progress made in applying systems analysis and organizational theory to health services (33–35).

ORGANIZATIONAL FORMS

Health services can be organized in three fundamentally different ways – via hierarchical bureaucracies, through long-term contractual arrangements under some degree of non-market control, and as direct, short-term market-based interactions between patients and providers (36). These arrangements are independent of whether ownership is public or private. For example, the ownership of services that are organized as hierarchies can be public, as in the extensive network of public health, hospital, and ambulatory clinics that are part of the Turkish Ministry of Health service delivery system and that of many other countries. But they can also be private, as in a United States health management organization like Kaiser Permanente. Such private entities often suffer from many of the same bureaucratic rigidities as public ones. Likewise although market-based interaction between providers and patients is most common in the private sector, short-term market exchanges in the form of user fees are pervasive in the public sector in many low income countries.

India provides examples of all three organizational forms. The services delivered by government are hierarchical, with providers who are employed directly. At the other extreme are direct, market-based, non-contractual interactions between the population and providers. These include both private providers *per se* and informal fee charging in public facilities: 80% of total health care spending takes place in this domain. In between are several forms of contractual arrangement. One type comprises long-term contracts between the public sector and nongovernmental providers (both non-profit and for-profit). This arrangement is used predominantly for treating patients suffering from cataract and, by increasing the number of providers that are financed publicly, has allowed for a large expansion of surgery to prevent blindness, particularly among the poor. Another contractual arrangement characterizes private insurance, which may or may not be publicly regulated. The client has one kind of relation with an insurer, which in turn has a different relation – one that may or may not be contractual – with providers.

Each of these ways to organize health services has its strengths and weaknesses in various contexts and when applied to different types of population-based and clinical services. When a strongly coordinated approach is needed, as was the case for example during the postwar (late 1990s) reconstruction of the health service in Bosnia and Herzegovina or during an outbreak of cholera, hierarchical controls are better. Largely inspired by experiences such as the British National Health Service and the difficulty of addressing health problems through markets alone, many low and middle income countries have, over the past 50 years, established state-funded health care systems with services produced by a vertically integrated public bureaucracy. This has led to improved access to health care for millions of people and underpinned many successful public health programmes.

But hierarchical bureaucracies also have some serious shortcomings when it comes to the provision of health services. These shortcomings have become more apparent in recent years (37, 38). Bureaucracies are vulnerable to capture by the vested interests of the bureaucrats and providers who work in them. They are often not as effective in downsizing or reorienting priorities as they are in expanding capacity and adding services. And they are often associated with many of the same shortcomings as private markets in terms of abuse of monopoly power (such as the collection of rents in the form of informal charges) and information asymmetry. Over time, many of the hierarchical service delivery systems have become excessively rigid, with inefficient processes producing low-quality care that is unresponsive to the needs and expectations of the populations and individuals that they serve. This has been the motive for many recent reform efforts, as described in Chapter 1.

Where there is a call for innovation and flexibility to respond to specific needs, as in the development of new drugs and equipment, markets are better. But direct market interactions between patients and providers in the health sector have the major disadvantage of exposing individuals to the financial risks of illness unless the financial resources are adequately pooled. And it is difficult or impossible to assure that such transactions respect any priorities among interventions and patients that the health system is trying to implement.

Because of the disadvantages of both rigid hierarchies and out-of-pocket payment in the health sector, countries throughout the world are today experimenting with long-term contracts to achieve the combined advantages of greater flexibility and scope for innovation while maintaining overall control over strategic objectives and financial protection. There is already some analysis of experiments with contracting for service provision in low and middle income countries (39), and much effort has also gone into drawing lessons from the better documented instances, particularly in the United Kingdom, which may also be relevant elsewhere (40).

SERVICE DELIVERY CONFIGURATIONS

Health services, like many other forms of production, can be implemented in more dispersed or more concentrated configurations, or in hybrid arrangements that combine some concentrated with some dispersed elements (41). Dispersed service configurations are usual for activities which do not benefit from economies of scale – unit costs are no lower for large than for small production units – such as primary care, including the integrated management of childhood illness; pharmacies; dental offices; field-based implementation of public health programmes; counselling; social work; and community and home-based care. Such ambulatory services usually involve a fairly broad range of activities of varying degrees of complexity, such as the management of common clinical and nonclinical activities by individuals or small teams of people.

Dispersed, competitive production by small producing units works well wherever markets are a satisfactory way to organize output. It is less successful in health, for all the reasons that markets work more poorly for health care. However, attempts to offset market failings by integrating such dispersed activities into a hierarchical bureaucratic structure have almost always run into problems of staff motivation and accountability. Close supervision is difficult to implement, while excessive control is detrimental. A more successful approach has been to establish a contractual relationship that relies on professional reputation, and a strong sense of commitment and responsibility. Such contractual relationships have a long history of success in countries such as Denmark and Norway, and have recently been tried successfully in Croatia, the Czech Republic, and Hungary.

Concentrated service configurations are common for activities such as hospital care, central public health laboratories, and health education facilities, which do benefit from economies of scale – lower costs with larger size – and scope – lower costs from undertaking a variety of activities (42, 43). These interventions are highly specialized and expensive, and require large teams of people with a wide range of skills. Some require continuous observation (for surgical treatment and care), and highly controlled sterile conditions (for surgical and burns units). Accountability can usually be enforced through direct observation of outputs or outcome. Most personnel can be employed as regular or part-time staff, rather than under the contractual relationships that appear to be better for dispersed activities. Countries have been more successful in integrating these services into hierarchical public bureaucracies but pay the price of the disadvantages of this organizational form.

There is both an upper and a lower efficiency boundary for concentrated service configurations. At the upper end, the large 1000 to 2000 bed hospitals and huge public health laboratories in central and eastern Europe were characterized by over-specialization, low productivity and low quality of care *(44)*. At the lower end, there are also considerable efficiency and quality problems when facilities that perform specialized care are too small. Cottage or district-level hospitals with 20 to 50 beds are common in many low and middle income countries, such as Ethiopia, Morocco, and Turkey, especially in rural regions and in the private sector *(45)*. Often they have low bed-occupancy rates and the staff do not see a sufficient volume of patients to maintain the clinical skills needed to treat rarer conditions. They may deal well with more common conditions, but then they must be integrated into a referral system that can treat more difficult or unusual ailments.

Hybrid service configurations fall somewhere between these two extremes. Many of the activities with a large potential impact on outcomes (shown in Table 3.1) are implemented in this form. Programmes to control infectious diseases such as malaria, tuberculosis and HIV/AIDS benefit from the planned coordination of some of their strategic elements at the national level. Yet their implementation can sometimes be more effective when carried out under contractual relationships with local providers than when implemented as vertical programmes isolated from other ambulatory services. For example, the implementation of the integrated management of childhood illness in Egypt requires close national coordination of activities such as immunization, malaria control and iron supplementation, but implementation would be impossible without local providers with the broad range of skills needed, for example, to treat acute respiratory infections, diarrhoea, and childhood illnesses.

This latter example highlights a key challenge in health service delivery. That is, to balance the need for broad policy oversight with sufficient flexibility so that managers and providers can innovate and adapt policies to local needs and contexts in a dynamic way. Population-based and clinical health services that can be refashioned through negotiation and adapted during implementation at the discretion of agencies and their staff are more responsive to the health needs and non-health expectations of the population than those that are implemented through rigid centralized bureaucracies *(46–49)*. This is consistent with the relations between responsiveness and service characteristics described in Chapter 2. But this approach may lead to outcomes quite different from those intended at the outset. The more focused managers and staff are in pursuing a clear mandate, the more likely it is that broader policy objectives will be achieved without having to resort to rigid hierarchical structures for control *(50)*.

ALIGNING INCENTIVES

Service providers need flexibility, not for arbitrary purposes, but so that they can respond to well-defined incentives – that is, so the incentives defined by organizational and institutional arrangements can be effective instead of being frustrated by rigidities. The growing awareness of the structural nature of problems in hierarchical service delivery systems has led policy-makers in many countries to examine the incentive environment of organizations and alter the distribution of decision-making control, revenue rights, and financial risk among the different participants, as analysed in *The world health report 1999 (16)*.

There is a wide range of ways to change the organizational incentive regime of health services. In many Latin American countries, including Argentina and Brazil, decentralization has led to a shift in decision-making control and often revenue rights and responsibilities from central to lower levels of government. The devolution of central control to provinces in Sri Lanka is another form of decentralization. The creation of semi-autonomous hospitals in Indonesia shifted decision-making and control even further down the line to the level of facilities. In Hungary, during the early 1990s, general practitioners were transformed from civil servants into semi-autonomous practitioners on contract with local governments and the newly created National Health Insurance Fund.

In each of these examples, there is a change in one or more organizational incentives that exerts a powerful influence on how the organizational unit in question behaves, be it a province, region, district, or individual provider unit such as a hospital or ambulatory clinic *(51)*. Figure 3.4 shows the relation between the organizational forms discussed earlier and the following five incentives.

- The degree of *autonomy* (decision rights) that the organization has *vis-à-vis* its owners, policy-based purchasers such as insurance funds, the government, and consumers. Critical decision rights include control over input mix and level, outputs and scope of activities, financial management, clinical and nonclinical administration, strategic management and market strategy (where appropriate).
- The degree of *accountability*. As decision rights are delegated to the organization, the ability of governments to assert direct accountability (through the hierarchy) is diminished. When autonomy increases, accountability must be secured by shifting from hierarchical supervision to reliance on monitoring, regulations, and the economic incentives embedded in contracts.
- The degree of *market exposure* or revenues that are earned in a competitive way rather than through a direct budget allocation. Market participation need not imply out-of-pocket financing; it is preferable for provider organizations to compete for prepaid revenues. When governments bail out organizations that run deficits or are indebted as a result of weak technical performance, they undermine the impact of market exposure.
- The degree of *financial responsibility* for losses and rights to profit (retained earnings and the proceeds from the sale of capital). This determines the financial incentive for managers and staff to economize. Under increased autonomy they, rather than the public purse, become the "residual claimant" on revenue flows, but such claims must be clearly spelled out and regulated.
- The degree of *unfunded mandates*. Where the share of total revenues earned through markets is significant, organizations are at financial risk because of the unrecoverable costs associated with requirements for which no funds are provided, such as care for the poor or very sick. Organizational reforms that increase autonomy should therefore be accompanied by complementary reforms in health financing to protect the poor. Chapter 5 discusses some recent examples in Latin America.

How far countries can safely go in pushing service provision away from hierarchical control and towards an incentive environment (the right of the spectrum in Figure 3.4) depends on the nature of the services and the capacity to create accountability for public objectives through indirect mechanisms such as regulation and contracting. There is no single blueprint for a successful service delivery system. But countries such as Canada *(52)* that have succeeded in creating a more coherent framework for these three organizational characteristics perform better than countries such as the United States (53) where there are many conflicting signals because market incentives are very strong in some places and more tightly controlled in others.

The coherence of organizational incentives is especially important in the hospital sector because of the central role of these organizations in service provision. Countries that have introduced consistent objectives and that have aligned the five organizational incentives appear to have been more successful than countries that have ended up with conflicting objectives and incentives regimes. For example, in Singapore, the public hospitals have been given considerable autonomy over management decisions ranging from procurement to personnel (54). Accountability is now enforced through contracts rather than hierarchical controls. The hospitals compete with each other for patients and can keep any surpluses they generate through savings. And there is an explicit subsidy scheme for low income groups, although cross-subsidies are still needed to cover some unfunded mandates. Follow-up assessments indicate that the reforms have succeeded in improving responsiveness to patients and efficiency in resource management, while protecting poor patients against opportunistic behaviour by hospitals trying to increase their revenues. In Indonesia, the degree of autonomy is much less but the various incentives are nevertheless more balanced than in New Zealand and the United Kingdom where there has been less policy coherence across the five organizational incentives (39, 55, 56). Hospitals are without question the most complex organizations involved in service delivery, and their role has been undergoing rapid change as new procedures shift the balance between inpatient and ambulatory care and as financial pressures have increased (57). How to organize hospital services and how to integrate them with other providers is perhaps the hardest question a service delivery system faces.

Figure 3.4 Different internal incentives in three organizational structures

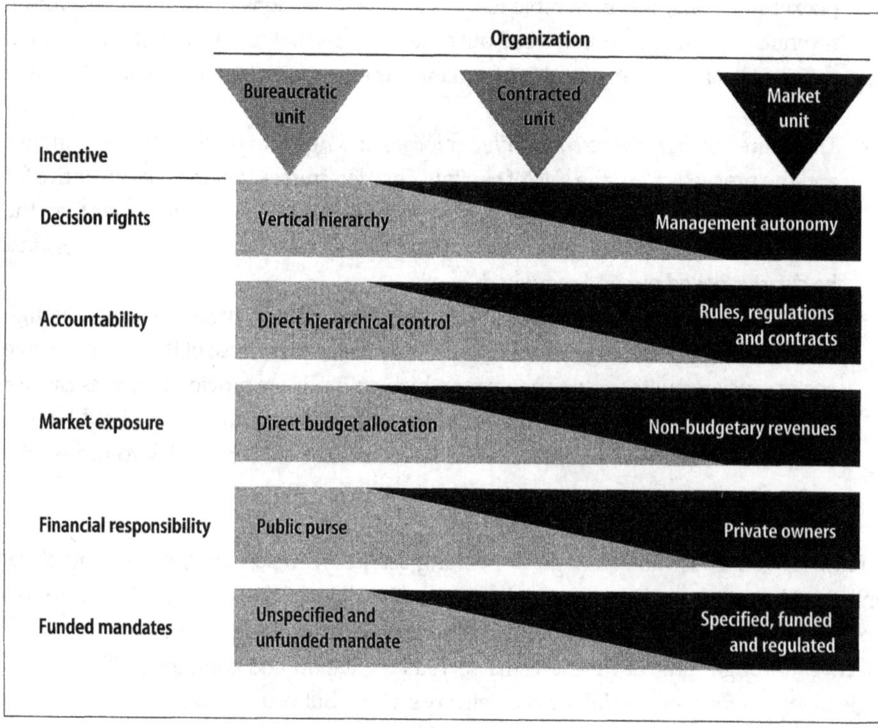

One way that many countries have tried to increase market exposure of hospitals is to "outsource" or "unbundle" some hospital activities. Experience so far in this area has been mixed. For example, there has been some success in outsourcing the maintenance of medical equipment in Thailand, management services in South Africa, and routine custodial, dietary, and laundry services in Bombay. Most of these activities benefit from the efficiency gains that can be provided by external suppliers that specialize in a given service. But with few exceptions, outsourcing is much more difficult with clinical services because of loss of strategic control over part of the production process, cost shifting, and difficulties in monitoring the quality of the outputs *(58)*.

Many public health interventions, such as malaria control programmes, nutrition programmes in Senegal, and reproductive health programmes in Bangladesh, are now carried out through long-term contracts with nongovernmental providers rather than rigid vertical programmes under a central hierarchical bureaucracy. And there has been a marked increase in the autonomy and privatization of general practitioners, dentists, pharmacists and other ambulatory health care workers in central and eastern Europe, with both good and bad consequences.

As in the case of hospitals, ambulatory services that are made autonomous perform better when there are minimal conflicts between the objectives and organizational incentive regimes. Table 3.2 provides some examples of organizational incentives for ambulatory

Table 3.2 Examples of organizational incentives for ambulatory care

Organization affected	Country examples
Local or district teams that manage several clinical facilities and public health services Includes district level ministry of health offices and municipal councils. Changes in organizational incentives are often modest and mostly related to decision rights over budget and staff. Financial risk remains limited. Actual degree of market exposure may be greater than intended when user fees are significant.	**Finland:** municipalities own and manage health centres, employ staff, raise taxes and set fees. **Philippines:** decentralization of responsibility for primary health care (and other social services) to local governments in 1993. Assets, staff and budgets transferred to local level. Ministry of Health (MoH) set up community health care associations along with each local government unit. Health workers now report to local government, not to MoH. Supervision by MoH has become more difficult. **Zambia:** the Central Board of Health (CBoH), the executive arm of the MoH, now contracts through annual district plans with independent district health boards/ district teams. Districts have gained greater control over their non-salary recurrent budget. But staff are mostly still employed by the civil service. This is changing as new graduates are hired by districts and unskilled staff are recruited locally. Accountability to CBoH is retained through sanctions if agreed performance targets are not met. Income from user fees is retained by facilities.
Individual facilities	**Belarus:** polyclinics now receive their own budget and can retain a proportion of their earnings from user fees. **Burkina Faso:** community-managed health centres established under the Bamako Initiative comprise one-third of public facilities and manage user fees (up to 10% of recurrent budget) for drugs mainly. Staff management is formally centralized. There are no clear accountability lines between community boards and health centre staff. **Mali:** independent health centres are not-for-profit cooperative establishments owned, financed and managed by community associations. These health centres recruit their own staff. Few are as yet financially independent in practice.
General practitioners	**Croatia:** previously centrally employed, salaried ambulatory care physicians. Now they are independent contractors.

care. Tensions often occur when decision rights are not extended to managers (for example, when political pressure makes it impossible to dismiss staff), when accountability mechanisms are neither built into long-term contracts nor enforced through market discipline, and when the providers are not allowed to retain their surpluses or made responsible for their losses. The latter undermines the incentive to economize.

There is still considerable debate about whether long-term contracts with private providers create better incentives than similar contracts with public providers. Which incentives are most appropriate may depend on which goals have priority. The global trend is to try to avoid the inefficiencies and unresponsiveness that occur when a hierarchy becomes too rigid, while avoiding the opposite extreme of unregulated markets. The latter almost always undermine financial protection and may interfere with the strategic coordination needed to provide effective care.

INTEGRATION OF PROVISION

As organizational units like hospitals or clinics become more autonomous, the service delivery system is at risk of becoming fragmented. Fragmentation may occur among similar provider configurations (hospitals, ambulatory clinics, or public health programmes) or between different levels of care. Such fragmentation has negative consequences for both the efficiency and the equity of the referral system unless explicit policies are introduced to ensure some sort of integration among the resulting semi-autonomous service delivery units.

When health services become fragmented, allocative efficiency suffers. For example, nonclinical health facilities designed to provide public health services in Poland and Hungary often engage in secondary prevention and a wide range of basic care because they are not adequately linked to ambulatory care networks. The university hospitals that have recently been made autonomous in Malaysia provide a wide range of inpatient and outpatient care for conditions that could have been treated effectively at lower levels in a community setting. The newly autonomous general practitioners in the Czech Republic have been quick to buy a large quantity of expensive equipment that is rarely used *(59)*.

When organizational changes among providers cause fragmentation, disillusionment with a market-oriented system can lead to some vertical and horizontal reintegration, with more hierarchical control. Armenia, Hungary, New Zealand and the United Kingdom have recently experimented with such steps. Both the market model and the hierarchical model present problems; it is important not to forget the shortcomings of the centrally planned models that were apparent in countries as diverse as Costa Rica, Sri Lanka, Sweden, the United Kingdom and the former Soviet Union (59).

One way to preserve the virtues of autonomy for providers without fragmentation is via "virtual integration" instead of traditional vertical integration. Under vertical integration, a clinic takes orders from a hospital or a government department, limiting its responses to local needs. Virtual integration means using modern communication systems to share information quickly and without cumbersome controls. This is particularly valuable for referrals, and can include nongovernmental providers hard to incorporate under hierarchical schemes. Bangladesh and Ghana are experimenting with this innovation.

Even in the United States, vertical integration under health maintenance organizations (HMOs) is being eclipsed by virtual integration between the provider network HMOs, other provider groups, and a globalized insurance industry. Vertical integration between production and distribution units is now being viewed as a coordination mechanism of last resort, and is used mainly when contractual alternatives are not available *(60)*.

Efforts at virtual integration face three common problems, related to decentralization, separating purchasers from providers, and user charges. In many countries, there has recently been an increased enthusiasm for decentralization as a means of attaining a wide variety of policy and political goals in health as in other areas. The explicit objective of decentralization is often to improve responsiveness and incentive structures by transferring ownership, responsibility and accountability to lower levels of the public sector. This is usually done through a shift in ownership from the central government to local levels of the public sector – states or provinces, regions, districts, local communities, and individual publicly owned facilities.

A common difficulty with such reforms has been that the internal structural problems of the hospitals, clinics and public health facilities do not disappear during the transfer. In Uganda, decentralization did not close the financing gap experienced by many health facilities. In Sri Lanka, decentralization exposed weak management capacity but failed to address it. In Ghana, the unfunded social obligations were passed on to lower levels of government which did not have the financial capacity to absorb this responsibility because the proposed social insurance reforms had stalled. In many cases, central governments reassert control in a heavy-handed fashion when local governments deal with politically sensitive issues in a way that does not accord with the views of the national government on how such issues should be treated.

Where there is a split between purchasers and providers, similar tensions often arise. In Hungary and also in New Zealand there has been conflict between purchasing agencies situated in different branches of the government and still responsible for stewardship (such as ministries of health and finance) and the owners of the contracted providers (such as municipalities and local governments). In Hungary, constitutional powers were given to a self-governing National Health Insurance Fund that was controlled by the labour unions during the early 1990s. For about eight years, until the abolition of this arrangement in 1998, there was an open conflict between the Ministry of Finance and the Health Insurance Fund over fiscal policy and expenditure control. Providers were often not paid on time.

Finally, the introduction of user fees creates tensions between policy-based and prepaid purchasing and market-driven purchases of services by individual consumers. This has been especially true in many of the central Asian republics and in countries affected by the east Asia crisis, where the revenues channelled through policy-based purchasing have experienced a dramatic drop in recent years. This can undermine national policies on priority setting and cost containment, and as discussed in Chapter 2, it makes financing much less fair. The issue of how to organize purchasing as an integral part of the financing function is treated at more length in Chapter 5.

In order to attain the goals of good health, responsiveness and fair financial contribution, health systems need to determine some priorities and to find mechanisms that lead providers to implement them. This is not an easy task, because of two sources of complexity. Priorities should reflect a variety of criteria that are sometimes in conflict, and that requires a great deal of information that most health systems simply do not now have available. And to make priorities effective requires a mixture of rationing mechanisms, organizational structures, institutional arrangements and incentives for providers that must above all be consistent with one another and with the goals of the system.

REFERENCES

1. **Beauchamp TL, Childress JF.** *Principles of biomedical ethics, 3rd ed.* Oxford, Oxford University Press, 1989.

2. **Gwatkin DR, Guillot M.** *The burden of disease among the global poor: current situation, future trends, and implications for strategy.* Washington, DC, and Geneva, The World Bank and the Global Forum for Health Research, 1999.

3. **Jha P, Chaloupka FJ, eds.** *Tobacco control policies in developing countries.* Oxford, Oxford University Press, 2000.

4. **Loudon IS, ed.** *Western medicine: an illustrated history.* Oxford, Oxford University Press, 1997.

5. **McKee M.** For debate – does health care save lives? *Croatian Medical Journal,* 1999, **40**(2): 123–128.

6. **Murray CJL et al.** *Development of WHO guidelines on generalized cost-effectiveness analysis.* Geneva, World Health Organization, 1999 (GPE Discussion Paper No. 4).

7. **Tengs TO.** *Dying too soon: how cost-effectiveness analysis can save lives.* Irvine, California, University of California, National Center for Policy Analysis, 1997 (Policy Report No. 204).

8. **Barnum H, Tarantola D, Setiady I.** Cost-effectiveness of an immunization programme in Indonesia. *Bulletin of the World Health Organization,* 1980, **58**(3): 499–503.

9. **Barnum H.** Cost savings from alternative treatments for tuberculosis. *Social Science and Medicine,* 1986, **23**(9): 847–850.

10. **Prescott N, de Ferranti D.** The analysis and assessment of health programs. *Social Science and Medicine,* 1985, **20**(12): 1235-1240.

11. **Mills A.** Economic evaluation of health programmes: application of the principles in developing countries. *World Health Statistics Quarterly,* 1985, **38**(4): 368–382.

12. **Mills A.** Survey and examples of economic evaluation of health programmes in developing countries. *World Health Statistics Quarterly,* 1985, **38**(4): 402–431.

13. **Lee M, Mills A, eds.** *Health economics in developing countries.* Oxford, Oxford University Press, 1984.

14. *World development report 1993 – Investing in health.* Washington, DC, The World Bank, 1993.

15. **Murray CJL, Lopez AD, eds.** *The global burden of disease: a comprehensive assessment of mortality and disability from diseases, injuries and risk factors in 1990 and projected to 2020.* Cambridge, MA, Harvard School of Public Health on behalf of the World Health Organization and The World Bank, 1996 (Global Burden of Disease and Injury Series, Vol. I).

16. *The world health report 1999 – Making a difference.* Geneva, World Health Organization, 1999.

17. **Hammer J.** *Economic analysis for health projects.* Washington, DC, The World Bank, 1996 (Policy Research Working Papers, No. 1611).

18. **Jha P, Bangoura O, Ranson K.** The cost-effectiveness of forty health interventions in Guinea. *Health Policy and Planning,* 1998, **13**: 249–262.

19. **Peabody J et al.** *Policy and health: implications for development in Asia.* Cambridge, Cambridge University Press, 1999.

20. **Murray CJL, Kreuser J, Whang W.** Cost-effectiveness analysis and policy choices: investing in health systems. In: Murray CJL, Lopez A. *Global comparative assessments in the health sector: disease burden, expenditures and intervention packages.* Geneva, World Health Organization, 1994.

21. **Bobadilla JL.** Investigación sobre la determinación de prioridades en materia de salud [Inquiry into the determination of priorities in health]. In: Frenk J, ed. *Observatorio de salud.* Chapter 11. Mexico, Fundación Mexicana para la Salud, 1997 (in Spanish).

22. **Murray CJL, Lopez AD.** *Global health statistics.* Cambridge, MA, Harvard School of Public Health on behalf of the World Health Organization and The World Bank, 1996 (Global Burden of Disease and Injury Series, Vol. II).

23. **Wagstaff A.** *Inequalities in child mortality in the developing world. How large are they? How can they be reduced?* Washington, DC, The World Bank, 1999 (HNP Discussion Paper).

24. **Cotlear D.** *Peru: improving health care financing for the poor.* Washington, DC, The World Bank, 1999 (Country Studies).

25. **Wagstaff A.** *HNP module of Poverty Reduction Strategy Paper (PRSP) toolkit.* Washington, DC, The World Bank, 2000.

26. **Missialos E, Grand JL, eds.** *Health care and cost containment in the European Union.* Aldershot, Ashgate, 1999.

27. **Ham C.** Corporatization of UK hospitals. In: Preker AS, Harding A, eds. *Innovations in service delivery: the corporatization of hospitals.* Baltimore, Johns Hopkins University Press for The World Bank, 2000 (in press).

28. Bobadilla JL et al. Design, content and financing of an essential national package of health services. *Bulletin of the World Health Organization*, 1994, **72**(4): 653–662.

29. Bobadilla JL et al. *El paquete universal de servicio esenciales de salud [Universal package of essential health services]*. Economía y salud, documentos para el análisis y la convergencia. Mexico, Fundación Mexicana para la Salud, 1994 (in Spanish).

30. Robinson R. Limits to rationality: economics, economists and priority setting. *Health Policy*, 1999, **49**: 13–26.

31. Maynard A. Rationing health care: an exploration. *Health Policy*, 1999, **49**: 5–11.

32. Berryman SE et al. *Assessing institutional capabilities*. Washington, DC, The World Bank, 1997 (World Bank Working Paper).

33. Wilson JQ. *Bureaucracy: what government agencies do and why they do it*. New York, Basic Books, 1989.

34. Schmalensee R, Willing RD. *Handbook of industrial organization, Vols I and II*. Amsterdam, Elsevier Science, 1989.

35. Williamson O. *The economic institutions of capitalism: firms, markets and relational contracting*. New York, Free Press, 1985.

36. Williamson OE. Comparative economic organization: the analysis of discrete structural alternatives. *Administrative Science Quarterly*, 1991, **36(2)**: 269–296

37. Barr N, ed. *Labor markets and social policy in Central and Eastern Europe*. Oxford, Oxford University Press for The World Bank,1994.

38. World Bank. *World development report 1996 – From plan to market*. New York, Oxford University Press, 1996: 123–132

39. Lieberman S. Corporatization of Indonesia hospitals. In: Preker AS, Harding A, eds. *Innovations in service delivery: the corporatization of hospitals*. Baltimore, Johns Hopkins University Press for The World Bank, 2000 (in press).

40. Palmer N. *The theory and evidence of contracting for primary care services: lessons for low and middle income countries*. London, London School of Hygiene and Tropical Medicine, 1999 (unpublished paper).

41. Gregory R. Accountability, responsibility, and corruption: managing the 'public production process'. In: Boston J, ed. *The state under contract*. Wellington, New Zealand, Bridget Williams Books, 1995.

42. Panzar J, Willing R. *Economies of scale and economies of scope in multi-output production*. Murray Hill, NJ, Bell Laboratories, 1975 (Economic Discussion Paper No. 33).

43. Teece DJ. Economies of scope and the scope of the enterprise. *Bell Journal of Economic Behavior and Organization*, 1980, **1**: 223–247.

44. Ho T. Hospital restructuring in the European and Central Asian Regions. In: McKee M et al, eds. *The appropriate role of the hospital*. Copenhagen, World Health Organization Regional Office for Europe, 2000 (in press).

45. Barnum H, Kutzin J. *Public hospitals in developing countries: resource use, cost and financing*. Baltimore, Johns Hopkins University Press, 1993.

46. Lipsky M. *Street-level bureaucracy*. New York, Russell Sage, 1980.

47. Tarimo E. *Towards a healthy district: organizing and managing district health systems based on primary health care*. Geneva, World Health Organization, 1991.

48. Conyers D, Cassels A, Janovsky K. *Decentralization and health systems change: a framework for analysis*. Geneva, World Health Organization, 1993 (document WHO/SHS/NHP/93.2).

49. Janovsky K, Travis P. *Decentralization and health systems change: case study summaries*. Geneva, World Health Organization, 1998.

50. Pressman J, Wildavsky A. *Implementation*. Berkeley, University of California Press, 1973.

51. Harding A, Preker AS. Conceptual framework for organizational reform of hospitals. In: Preker AS, Harding A, eds. *Innovations in health service delivery: corporatization in the hospital sector*. Baltimore, Johns Hopkins University Press, 2000 (in press).

52. Evans B. General revenues financing: a comparison of US and Canada. In: Figueras J et al, eds. *Funding health care and long-term care: options in Europe*. Copenhagen, World Health Organization Regional Office for Europe, 2000 (in press).

53. Robinson JC. *The corporate practice of medicine: competition and innovation in health care*. Berkeley, University of California Press, 1999.

54. Phua K. Corporatization of hospitals in Singapore. In: Preker AS, Harding A, eds. *Innovations in health service delivery: corporatization in the hospital sector*. Baltimore, Johns Hopkins University Press, 2000 (in press).

55. Scott G. Corporatization in New Zealand hospitals. In: Preker AS, Harding A, eds. *Innovations in health service delivery: corporatization in the hospital sector*. Baltimore, Johns Hopkins University Press, 2000 (in press).

56. **Ham C.** Priority setting in health care: learning from international experience. *Health Policy*, 1997, **42**(1): 49–66.

57. **McKee M, Healy J.** *The role of the hospital in a changing environment.* European Observatory on Health Care Systems and London School of Hygiene and Tropical Medicine, 1999 (unpublished paper).

58. **Mills A.** Contractual relationship between government and the commercial private sector in developing countries. In: Bennett S, McPake B, Mills A. *Private health providers in developing countries: serving the public interest.* London, Zed Books, 1997.

59. **Preker AS, Feachem RGA.** *Market mechanisms and the health sector in Central and Eastern Europe.* Washington, DC, The World Bank, 1996 (Technical Paper No. 293).

60. **Klein B, Crawford RG, Alchian AA.** Vertical integration, appropriable rents, and the competitive contracting process. *Journal of Law and Economics*, 1978, **21**: 297–326.

CHAPTER FOUR

What Resources are Needed?

Providing health care efficiently requires financial resources to be properly balanced among the many inputs used to deliver health services. Large numbers of physicians, nurses and other staff are useless without adequately built, equipped and supplied facilities. Available resources should be allocated both to investments in new skills, facilities and equipment, and to maintenance of the existing infrastructure. Moreover, these delicate balances must be maintained both over time and across different geographical areas. In practice, imbalances between investment and recurrent expenditures and among the different categories of inputs are frequent, and create barriers to satisfactory performance. New investment choices must be made carefully to reduce the risk of future imbalances, and the existing mix of inputs needs to be monitored on a regular basis. Clear policy guidance and incentives for purchasers and providers are necessary if they are to adopt efficient practices in response to health needs and expectations.

4

WHAT RESOURCES

ARE NEEDED?

BALANCING THE MIX OF RESOURCES

*T*he provision of health care involves putting together a considerable number of resource inputs to deliver an extraordinary array of different service outputs. Few, if any, manufacturing processes match the variety and rate of change of production possibilities in health. Figure 4.1 identifies three principal health system inputs: human resources, physical capital, and consumables. It also shows how the financial resources to purchase these inputs are of both a capital investment and a recurrent character. As in other industries, investment decisions in health are critical because they are generally irreversible: they commit large amounts of money to places and activities which are difficult, even impossible, to cancel, close or scale down.

The fact that some investment decisions lie outside the authority of the ministry of health makes the achievement of overall balance even more difficult. For example, the

Figure 4.1 Health system inputs: from financial resources to health interventions

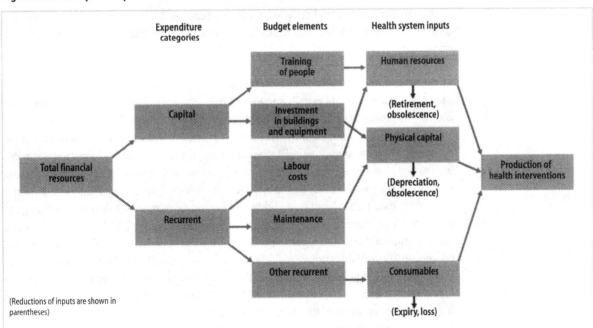

training of doctors often comes under the ministry of education, and there may be private investment in facilities and equipment.

Capital is the existing stock of productive assets. Trained health workers and mobile clinics, as well as fixed assets, are part of the capital stock of the health system. Investment is any addition to this stock of capital, such as more pharmacists or additional vehicles. The typical productive lifetime of different investments will vary from as little as 1–2 years for certain equipment to 25–30 years or more for buildings and some kinds of professionals.

Technological progress influences the economic lifetime of a piece of capital: old investments quickly become outdated as new and improved technologies emerge. The way in which assets are managed also affects their lifetime. With proper handling and maintenance, buildings and vehicles lose their value more slowly. Without care and maintenance, health capital deteriorates rapidly. The planning of maintenance also needs to take the physical environment into account. For example, bad roads reduce the average lifetime of vehicles; so the planning of maintenance, operation and replacement of vehicles should allow for this.

Human capital can be treated conceptually in the same way as physical capital, with education and training as the key investment tools to adjust the human capital stock and determine the available knowledge and skills (1). Unlike material capital, knowledge does not deteriorate with use. But, like equipment, old skills become obsolete with the advent of new technologies, and human capital needs to be maintained too. Continuing education and on-the-job training are required to keep existing skills in line with technological progress and new knowledge. Human capital is also lost through retirement and death of individuals.

Investment also refers, in a broader sense, to any new programme, activity or project. Capital investment costs are all those costs that occur only once (to start up the activity), while the recurrent costs refer to the long-term financial commitment that usually follows from such an investment. If the available medical technology is seen as "capital", and research and development as the investment tool to expand the technology frontier and develop new ideas, these concepts may also be applied to diagnostic equipment, medicines and the like.

Investment is the critical activity for adjusting capital stock and creating new and productive assets. Such adjustments typically occur gradually over time. Thus, the current physical infrastructure of hospital buildings and facilities in many countries is the product of an evolution that has taken many years. Among OECD countries, expenditures for investment in buildings and equipment are typically not more than 5% of total annual health care expenditures and are usually somewhat lower than they were 15 or 20 years ago: cost control has been enforced partly by controlling additions to capital.

In low income countries, however, there is greater variation. Investment levels can be substantially higher than the OECD figures, especially when physical infrastructure is being created or restored with the help of donor agencies. Countries such as Burkina Faso, Cambodia, Kenya, Mali and Mozambique report capital expenditures of between 40% and 50% of the total public health care budget in one or more years (2). A large percentage of the remaining recurrent budget usually pays for health care staff. This means that only a small fraction of the total budget is spent on the maintenance of physical and human capital and on consumable inputs, including pharmaceuticals. The balance between investments and other expenditures is more critical in low income countries as there is little room for mistakes. In general, however, very little is known about health investments in low income countries, even in the public sector. For the private sector, the available national health accounts estimates often have no data, or present implausibly high ratios of investment to total spending, maintained over many years. Not to know how much is being invested, and in what kinds of inputs, makes it nearly impossible to relate capital decisions to recurrent costs or assure that capital is not wasted or allowed to drain off funds needed for other inputs.

Even less data are available on the size of annual investments in education and training. These investment costs include medical and nursing schools, on-the-job training in different forms, and clinical research. Many players are involved and investments are often neither controlled by a single ministry nor guided by a common purpose. There is reason to believe that the sum of investments in human capital is far greater than investment in physical capital, at least in high income countries. As is the case for investment in physical capital, additions to human capital usually occur slowly over time. The training of a specialist, for example, can take 10 years or more of studies in medical school and on-the-job training. New investments in human capital also have long-term consequences, similar to investments in physical capital. The creation of a cadre of health workers with new skills, for example, will require a long-term investment in new curricula for basic and continuing education as well as a long-term commitment to paying their salaries.

HUMAN RESOURCES ARE VITAL

Human resources, the different kinds of clinical and non-clinical staff who make each individual and public health intervention happen, are the most important of the health system's inputs. The performance of health care systems depends ultimately on the knowledge, skills and motivation of the people responsible for delivering services.

Furthermore, the human resources bill is usually the biggest single item in the recurrent budget for health. In many countries, two-thirds or more of the total recurrent expenditures reflect labour costs. But people would not be able to deliver services effectively without physical capital – hospitals and equipment – and consumables such as medicines, which play an important role in raising the productivity of human resources. Not only is a workable balance between overall health capital formation and recurrent activities needed, but the three input categories shown in Figure 4.1 should also be in equilibrium.

What treatment alternatives should be used for a certain illness or medical condition? Should services be offered at hospitals or primary care facilities? What is the level of skills and knowledge required to deliver this set of services? These questions have one thing in common. They are concerned with the degree of flexibility that exists in delivering health services, i.e. the possibility of substitution between one type of input and another, or the substitution of one form of care for another, all the while maintaining a constant level and quality of output. From a societal point of view, such positive substitution to achieve cost-effective delivery of services should be encouraged. A balanced combination of the different resource inputs will depend on identified health needs, social priorities and people's expectations.

Health systems are labour intensive and require qualified and experienced staff to function well. In addition to a balance between health workers and physical resources, there needs to be a balance between the different types of health promoters and care-givers. It would be an obvious waste of money to recruit physicians to carry out the simplest tasks. As a particular health system input is increased, the value added by each additional unit of input tends to fall *(3)*. For example, where there are too few physicians, the arrival of another physician will have a positive effect on health care; but where there are already too many physicians, an additional physician is more likely to increase costs than improve care.

Some ways of dealing with imbalances among health care providers are outlined in Box 4.1.

A health system can have plentiful human resources, with excellent knowledge and skills, but still face impending crisis if future health needs, priorities and available resources are not taken into account. For example, where the education and training for junior doctors and nurses functions poorly, or where senior staff lack adequate time and resources to update their knowledge and skills, future shortfalls can be expected. Similarly, a health system with a skewed age distribution among staff towards the point of retirement poses a real problem. Thus, a health care system must balance investments in human capital to cover future needs as well as present demands. Some of the most critical and complex input problems relate to human resources (see Box 4.2).

Without functioning facilities, diagnostic equipment, and medicines, it does not matter if the knowledge, skills and staff levels are high. The delivery of services will still be poor. A lack of complementary inputs will also have a negative impact on staff motivation, a factor that influences the capacity of human resources. Motivation, however, depends not only on working conditions. Financial incentives and compensation, i.e. income and other benefits, are also important, as are the overall management of staff and the possibilities for professional advancement.

Inadequate pay and benefits together with poor working conditions – ranging from work in conflict zones to inadequate facilities and shortages of essential medicines and consumables – are frequently mentioned in less developed countries as the most pressing problems facing the health care workforce *(4)*. In some countries, for example Bangladesh and Egypt, a clear majority of all publicly employed physicians see private paying patients to supplement income from their regular jobs. In Kazakhstan, "informal payments" are estimated to add 30% to the national health care bill *(5)*. Possibilities for doctors to work privately in public institutions are being offered in some countries to neutralize an ongoing brain drain of qualified staff from the public sector. This strategy is considered successful in Bahrain, but experiences from Ghana and Nepal show that such incentives can lead to the diversion of scarce resources from public services and can induce professionals to engage in independent private practice *(6)*.

People, as thinking creatures, are very different from machines and human capital cannot be managed in the same way as physical capital. First of all, human resources, and in

---

Box 4.1 Substitution among human resources

A large number of countries face an overall shortage of physicians. Other countries that are following a long-term strategy to shift resources to primary care find that they have too many specialists and too few general practitioners. Many are dealing with the problems by substituting among various health care-givers.

*Reorientation of specialist physi-*cians. While limiting admissions to specialist training and changing internship programmes is a long-term strategy to balance the professional distribution of physicians, the reorientation of specialists into family practice is a short-run substitution strategy being used, for example, in central and eastern Europe.

Substitution for other health professionals. The training of a physician may cost three times more than that of a nurse.[1] As a result, training of more nurses as well as other health professionals may be a cost-effective substitute for physicians. In Botswana, training of more nurse practitioners and pharmacists has offset the lack of physicians in some areas.[2]

Introduction of new cadres. Ensuring a closer match between skills and function may demand the creation of new cadres. In Nepal, an educational programme allowed health assistants and other health workers in rural areas to train for higher professional postings.[3]

[1] *World development report 1993 – Investing in health.* New York, Oxford University Press for The World Bank, 1993.
[2] Egger D, Lipson D, Adams O. *Achieving the right balance: the role of policy-making processes in managing human resources for health problems.* Geneva, World Health Organization, 2000 (Issues in health services delivery, Discussion paper No. 2, document WHO/EIP/OSD/2000.2).
[3] Hicks V, Adams O. *The effects of economic and policy incentives on provider practice. Summary of country case studies using the WHO framework.* Geneva, World Health Organization, 2000 (Issues in health services delivery, Discussion paper No. 5, document WHO/EIP/OSD/2000.8 (in press)).

particular physicians, determine the use of other available inputs. An oversupply of physicians will almost certainly mean an oversupply of the kind of services that physicians provide. The high density of private physicians working in urban areas of many middle income countries, such as Thailand, usually correlates with frequent use of expensive equipment and laboratory testing, and with more services of sometimes doubtful value being provided to the urban population. In Egypt, the high ratio of physicians – for every occupied bed in Egypt there are two physicians – combined with extensive self-medication explain the very high use of drugs. According to estimates, the poorest households in Egypt spend over 5% of their income on drugs alone (2).

Incentives and management related to human resources have an indirect impact on the use of other resources as well. For example, many payment systems provide physicians and providers with incentives to use more or less medical equipment, laboratory testing and medicines. In Bangladesh, physicians get 30–40% of the laboratory charges for each referral generated, creating a clear interest to expand the volume of such services (2). In both China and Japan, many physicians derive part of their income from the sale of drugs which they prescribe. In many countries, the use of branded drugs instead of generics is still common, and this can to a large extent be blamed on the incentives offered to physicians and pharmacists by pharmaceutical producers. Lack of the skills needed to assess technology and control quality is an additional factor causing imbalances among resources.

Another difference between human and physical capital, which affects how people are managed, is that physicians, nurses and other health workers are not motivated only by present working conditions, income and management. They are also influenced by what they believe those conditions will be in the future, based on past experiences, views expressed by others and current trends. If qualified staff believe that future payment, benefits and working conditions will deteriorate, their job-related decisions and motivation will reflect that belief. This "shadow of the future" can easily result in a continuing negative spiral towards lower motivation and performance.

A first step to prevent such a development is to find a sustainable balance among the different types of resources and between investment and recurrent costs. Perhaps the most

---

Box 4.2 Human resources problems in service delivery

Numerical imbalances. A recent study of human resources in 18 low and middle income countries, one or more in each of the WHO regions, indicates that most countries experience varying degrees of shortages in qualified health personnel. In sub-Saharan Africa in particular, the limited training capacity and low pay for qualified health workers causes severe problems in service delivery. Elsewhere, for example in Egypt, oversupply is a problem. Generally, shortages and oversupply are defined relative to countries in the same region and at similar levels of development. Oversupply, thus, may be absolute, as is the case for specialist physicians in many countries of eastern Europe and central Asia, or relative to geographical location.

Training and skill mix imbalances. Health care workers are often unqualified for the tasks they perform because of a shortage of training opportunities, as in many African countries, or a mismatch between available skills and the needs and priorities of the health care system, as in eastern Europe and central Asia. The number of physicians and other health personnel with a certain type of training or qualification, however, tells only part of the story. Neither formal training nor professional affiliation necessarily equates with skill in dealing with specific problems.

Distribution imbalances. Almost all countries have some urban/rural imbalances among their human resources and face problems in meeting the needs of specific groups such as poor or handicapped people or ethnic minorities. It is almost universally true that providers tend to concentrate in urban areas. In Cambodia, 85% of the population live in rural areas, but only 13% of the government health workers work there. In Angola, 65% live in rural areas, but 85% of health professionals work in urban areas. In Nepal, only 20% of rural physician posts are filled, compared to 96% in urban areas.

Failure of past public policy approaches. Although progress has been made in recent years to develop national policies and plans for human resources for health, they are not fully implemented in most countries. Moreover, very few countries monitor and evaluate the progress and impact of policy implementation.

important part of such a balance is to ensure that there are individual incentives to invest in human capital in the form of improved earnings, career opportunities and working conditions. Indeed, many low and middle income countries have increased pay or benefits as a key strategy for developing human resources and improving delivery of services to meet health needs and priorities (7). Public sector pay in Uganda rose by 900% (in nominal terms) between 1990 and 1999, which represents a doubling in real terms (8).

In general there are no easy answers in the area of human resources development. Left unmanaged, human skills markets take years, even decades, to respond to market signals.

And, unlike physical capital, human resources cannot be scrapped when their skills are no longer needed or obsolete; even laying off public sector health workers is often so difficult that it can only be achieved as part of a broader policy to reform the civil service.

Public intervention to produce the required balance is thus essential to reduce waste and accelerate adjustment. Some successful experiences are summarized below but many problems remain (7).

Utilization levels, mix and distribution. The relative prices of different skill categories should guide decisions about their most efficient mix, where labour markets are functioning. There are no absolute norms regarding the right ratio of physicians or nurses to population; rules of thumb are often used. Generally, shortages or oversupply are assessed on the basis of need and priorities combined with comparisons with neighbouring countries or those at a similar level of development. Such assessment requires sound data about available human resources and their geographical and professional distribution: such information is often lacking. In Guinea-Bissau, 700 "ghost" workers were removed from the payroll of the Ministry of Finance, following an inventory of the health care workforce. Cambodia's 1993 survey of health workers revealed a poorly distributed and largely unregistered workforce, with widely differing competencies (2).

Three types of human resource strategy have been pursued with some success:

- making more efficient use of available personnel through better geographical distribution;
- greater use of multiskilled personnel where appropriate;
- ensuring a closer match between skills and functions.

The latter strategy responds to a widespread problem. Formal training of health workers, particularly for more highly skilled staff, too seldom reflects the actual tasks being performed. This is both wasteful and demoralizing.

Some success has been recorded with mandatory service and multiple incentives (financial, professional, educational, etc.) to make otherwise unattractive technical or geographical areas more appealing, as has been done in Canada and the Scandinavian countries to deploy staff in their northern regions. Countries such as Fiji, Oman and Saudi Arabia have successfully recruited foreign workers to fill critical gaps, as an interim strategy. This strategy can, however, create other difficulties and tensions. Oman at present has a policy to recruit primarily a domestic workforce, as the pool of potential medical students has increased.

Intake training and continuing education. A clear case can be made for strong public sector involvement in training and in monitoring the quality of continuing education to stimulate the development of human resources in targeted areas. New public health schools have recently been established in Hungary and Jamaica to meet needs for professionals with skills in epidemiology, statistics, management and health education. They aim to integrate initial formal training, subsequent continuing education, and actual service provision.

This has two potential benefits. It ensures that training has strong practical foundations, and it continually exposes service providers to new thinking and development. In countries with large rural populations several strategies have been used to recruit staff to rural areas. Examples are intake of medical students from rural areas and training in the locations where physicians will later practise.

A related problem concerns the brain drain of trained staff from low income countries to wealthier countries or from the public sector to the private sector within a country. The more successful trainees often emigrate, tempted by higher standards of practice and living abroad. Many Jamaican nurses have migrated to the United States. Physicians migrate from Egypt and India to other countries in the Middle East and to the USA and Europe. Inadequate pay and benefits rank as the most serious problem confronting the public sector health workforce in many countries, with growing formal and informal private practice as a consequence. Service contracts that require a certain number of years in public service, especially when the training is state sponsored, have been implemented in the Philippines and the United Republic of Tanzania, and are common in Latin America but there are attendant difficulties. The staff concerned are usually junior, placements are short term and unpopular, mentoring arrangements are seldom adequate, and overall geographical imbalance is little affected. Globalization has led to greater mobility of staff and opportunity for overseas training, and students who qualify abroad may wish to stay in the country where they were trained.

ADJUSTING TO ADVANCES IN KNOWLEDGE AND TECHNOLOGY

Growth in the available knowledge or advances in technology – such as new drugs or diagnostic equipment – can substantially increase the capacity of human resources to solve health problems, and thereby improve the performance of a health care system. New knowledge is also a challenge to each country's existing input balance, as relative prices change and the efficient mix of resources alters (9). In the past few decades, revolutionary advances in medicine and technology have shifted the boundaries between hospitals, primary health care, and community care (10). Corresponding resource shifts in health systems have been much slower to emerge.

Antibiotic drugs provide one example of new knowledge affecting cost structures. Since their introduction in the 1940s, patients suffering from a bacterial infection have most often been cared for at home or at outpatient clinics rather than in special hospitals, significantly reducing costs and improving outcomes. The recent growth of unregulated self-treatment and the increasing incidence of drug-resistant bacteria have compromised some of these gains. There is now a need for active stewardship to regulate the quality of diagnosis, prescribing and compliance. Vaccines have similarly altered the strategy and costs of tackling epidemic diseases such as measles and poliomyelitis, and new vaccines will continue to necessitate re-thinking to ensure an efficient mix of inputs in national health strategy.

All countries – rich as well as poor – need to find and maintain a reasonable balance between inputs. The choices involved in finding this balance, however, vary depending on the amount of total resources available. In a poor country, the possibilities of investing in modern medical technologies or paying for modern medicines are very limited. Moving from the use of essential drugs to new and expensive drugs for cardiovascular diseases would mean an enormous opportunity loss in terms of health outcome for a poor country. This difference in opportunities across countries also has an impact on the optimal balance between resources (see Box 4.3).

Some input prices are determined locally; others are set in international markets. In most countries, prices for human resources (incomes for physicians, nurses and other health care personnel) are determined nationally, and the general income level for each country or region will be an important determinant. Prices for such items as patented drugs and medical equipment, on the other hand, are determined in a global market. Although differences in income levels across countries will induce manufacturers and distributors of medicines and equipment to differentiate prices somewhat, stewards of individual country health systems are far less able to influence these prices than the prices of human resources. International stewardship is needed to represent the interests of consumers in low income countries that face heavy burdens of infectious and parasitic diseases. This type of stewardship, led by agencies such as WHO and the World Bank, will assume increasing importance as globalization of the economy continues and free trade agreements are implemented.

PUBLIC AND PRIVATE PRODUCTION OF RESOURCES

With the exception of skilled human resources, most inputs used for health services are produced in the private sector, with varying degrees of public stewardship over the level and mix of production, distribution, and quality. For example, local markets successfully produce most consumables and unskilled labour. Government intervention is needed mainly to ensure that quality and safety standards are met, that reliable information is available about the products, and that a fair competitive environment exists.

Other inputs, such as manufactured pharmaceuticals and specialized medical equipment, often face barriers to entry into the market in the form of patents and licensing requirements, manufacturing standards, large initial investment costs, expensive research, and long development periods. This gives the manufacturers of these inputs considerable market power to abuse by manipulating prices and demand. Strong policy measures are therefore needed, such as anti-trust legislation, limited formularies, generic drug policies, bulk purchasing, and formal technology assessments *(11–13)*. Furthermore, by procuring

---

Box 4.3 A widening gap in technology use?

A vast quantity of valuable medical technologies and innovative clinical methods have been developed over the past decades and many more are on the way. Unfortunately, the new possibilities are not open to all because of the lack of available income in some countries. Diseases that are treated effectively in rich countries by professional staff using modern technology are handled by unskilled staff or informally at home in less developed countries. Moreover, some of these diseases are more prevalent in the poorest countries.

Medicines are now available for *HIV/AIDS* that can, at a huge cost, at least postpone further development of the disease. But treatment patterns and resource inputs for HIV/AIDS currently follow different paths in different countries. In poor countries, HIV/AIDS is still a disease without treatment alternatives. The sick are mainly taken care of informally at home or in institutions with predominantly unskilled staff. South Africa has improved the availability of HIV treatment by obliging insurers to cover its cost for members of insurance schemes.

Malaria transmission can be prevented by means of house spraying, insecticide-treated nets, chloroquine prophylaxis, and so on, but such measures are not always available to the people who need them most. Several different projects to develop a malaria vaccine are under way.[1] A breakthrough in this research would present a tremendous opportunity to improve quality of life and prevent death. Such a technological breakthrough would also demand a new mix of resources, but only for those countries that could afford the new vaccine.

For *tuberculosis*, the incidence of bacterial resistance to first-line drugs is increasing. It is of major concern, for example, in the Russian Federation. Lack of effective medical treatment and improper use of medicines continue to create obstacles to dealing with this escalating problem.[2]

[1] *The world health report 1999 – Making a difference.* Geneva, World Health Organization, 1999.
[2] *Global tuberculosis control: WHO report 2000.* Geneva, World Health Organization, 2000 (document WHO/CDS/TB/2000.275).

medicines and medical technologies on the international market, countries can ensure that local producers remain competitive *(14, 15)*.

Publicly subsidized production of consumables, pharmaceuticals and medical equipment often leads to low quality, lack of innovation, outmoded technology, inefficient production modalities and distribution delays. The most striking example of this occurred in the former Soviet Union. Most countries that have followed this model have quickly fallen behind in productivity and production technology. Many Western firms that entered the pharmaceutical and medical equipment market in central and eastern Europe during the early 1990s found it cheaper and easier to build new factories than to convert and modernize the old capital stock *(16–18)*.

Decisions on physical capital, such as hospitals and other large facilities, require more public attention. Ambulatory clinics, laboratories, pharmacies, cottage hospitals, and other small clinical facilities often have small capital requirements, and private providers may be able to finance these themselves or through small personal loans in parallel to public investments. In the case of large hospitals, most countries have in the past relied heavily on public investments. Investment decisions in this area have consequences that may last for 30–40 years or more. Once built, hospitals are politically difficult to close. The need for strong public policies, however, does not necessarily mean the public financing of the entire capital stock. Increasingly, many countries are looking to the private sector to support investments in their health system even when the resulting facilities will not have for-profit objectives, and the running costs will be publicly financed *(19)*. Chapter 6 illustrates some pitfalls of developing joint venture investments, and the different skills required for compe-

---

Box 4.4 The Global Alliance for Vaccines and Immunization (GAVI)

Every year, nearly three million children die from diseases that could be prevented with currently available vaccines, yet nearly 30 million of the 130 million children born every year are not receiving vaccinations of any kind. The great majority of unreached children – 25 million – live in countries that have less than US$ 1000 per capita GNP.

The Global Alliance for Vaccines and Immunization (GAVI) is a coalition of public and private interests that was formed in 1999 to ensure that every child is protected against vaccine-preventable diseases. GAVI partners include national governments, the Bill and Melinda Gates Children's Vaccine Program, the International Federation of Pharmaceutical Manufacturers Associations (IFPMA), research and technical health institutions, the Rockefeller Foundation, UNICEF, the World Bank Group, and WHO.

GAVI is seeking to close the growing gap of vaccine availability between industrialized and developing countries. Beyond the six basic vaccines of the Expanded Programme on Immunization (against poliomyelitis, diphtheria, whooping cough, tetanus, measles and tuberculosis), newer vaccines, such as those for hepatitis B, *Haemophilus influenzae* type b (Hib), and yellow fever are now widely used in industrialized countries. A major priority is to see that all countries of the world achieve at least 80% immunization coverage by 2005. Based on current assumptions of vaccine delivery costs it is estimated that an additional $226 million annually are needed to reach this level of coverage in the poorest countries with the traditional EPI vaccines; to cover the same number of children with the newer vaccines, according to the guidelines adopted at GAVI's first board meeting, would require an additional $352 million.

At the second meeting of the GAVI board, held during the World Economic Forum in Davos in February 2000, the GAVI partners discussed policies for attaining the 80% immunization objective and announced a multimillion-dollar global fund for children's vaccines. Governments, businesses, private philanthropists, and international organizations are working together to manage these resources so as to provide the protection of immunization to children in all countries, under the campaign title of "The Children's Challenge". Members of GAVI argue that protecting the world's children against preventable diseases is not only a moral imperative but an essential cornerstone of a healthy, stable global society.

All countries with incomes of less than $1000 per capita GNP (74 countries worldwide, with the majority in Africa) have been invited to express their interest in collaborating with GAVI in this campaign.

Nearly 50 countries, from all WHO regions, have already provided details of their immunization activities and needs. Resources from the fund will primarily be used to purchase vaccines for hepatitis B, *Haemophilus influenzae* type b (Hib), and yellow fever, and safe injection materials.

It is envisaged that GAVI partners at the country level will collaborate with national governments to help close the gaps identified in the country proposals other than those directly related to the provision of vaccines. By placing more of the responsibility for providing the necessary information and commitment on the countries themselves, the GAVI partners are hoping that resulting efforts will be more country-driven and therefore more sustainable.

tent stewardship of such developments. With regard to the training of specialized labour and the generation of knowledge, the story is similar. There is a need for strong public involvement in setting the policy agenda and ensuring adequate regulation, but private capital can be mobilized to support investments in both training and research activities.

The dominant force underlying the 20th-century revolution in health services has been the new global knowledge made possible by research and development. Chapter 1 echoes *The world health report 1999* in arguing that today's health systems have a clear responsibility to provide the knowledge for the health systems of tomorrow *(20)*. Investment in knowledge which can be used by all has a special merit (see Box 4.4). Although most research and development is, and should be, financed through private capital, there should be public involvement in supporting such endeavours and directing them towards areas of greatest need. Attempts to directly manage the dynamics of research and development from the top, however, often fail. Experience suggests that indirect approaches and providing the research community with appropriate incentives will be more successful. Once again, imaginative international stewardship may make a vital difference.

THE LEGACY OF PAST INVESTMENTS

Past investments in the poorest countries in the world have focused on the accumulation of physical infrastructure. Such programmes have often been supported by multilateral and bilateral donor agencies in the hope that they would lead to improved performance and that the countries themselves would be able to collect sufficient public money to cover recurrent costs *(21)*. In reality, resources to maintain and operate both physical and human capital have often been insufficient. Health facilities are unable to function well because of poor maintenance and shortages of essential drugs and supplies. Vehicles are often immobile for lack of repair and maintenance. For example, in Ghana at one point in 1992, 70% of Ministry of Health vehicles were reported immobile, pending repair at government workshops. Reorganization of maintenance and repair arrangements and budget practice led to rapid improvement, but Ghana's recent experience is widespread. Even in places where vehicles are mobile, fuel is often a scarce resource. These are just some examples of imbalances that all lead to reduced performance, a shorter lifespan of the physical infrastructure and low staff morale. In terms of physical capital, the situation is often irreversible. The cost of renovating is higher than the cost of building anew.

Lack of necessary skills, poor cost information systems, rigid budgeting systems, and fragmentation of tasks – such as separation of responsibility for investment from operating budgets – are further reasons behind input imbalances. If information on needed quantities is not available, it is difficult to estimate reasonable budget levels for inputs such as consumables and fuel for transportation. If providers are then responsible for holding each of these budget lines, serious barriers are created to delivering health services effectively. Shortages of essential production inputs too frequently coexist with unused funds in over-compartmentalized health budgets.

Chapter 6 considers the recent development of formal partnerships, such as sector-wide approaches (SWAPs), between government and groups of donors. On the capital investment front, donors could do much better. External agencies have contributed to unbalanced input mixes by focusing on highly visible investments without adequate consideration of compatibility with other investments (for example, with respect to spare parts), or recurrent costs. Political success in health system investment is seldom the ally of long-term sustainability. There are often incentives in less developed countries for decision-makers to accept donor support irrespective of the long-term consequences on the balance among existing resources or between investments and recurrent costs. For example, Sri Lanka accepted a donor contribution of a 1000-bed hospital: to operate it took needed resources away from many other activities. Competing agendas among donors have led to further fragmentation in responsibility and short-term thinking *(22)*.

HEALTH CARE RESOURCE PROFILES

Large differences in the mix of resources used by high and low income countries can partly be explained by differences in relative prices. A full system of national health accounts offers the most complete information on health system inputs and their prices, as discussed below. In a poor country, unskilled human resources will be relatively cheap, whereas medical technology, facilities and highly qualified staff will be expensive. As a result, a large percentage of the total public budget is often allocated to investment. Once staff have been paid from the recurrent budget, there will be little left to spend on equipment, medicines, consumables and maintenance of facilities. This is evidence that there are simply too many staff, often reflecting the training of staff relative to population norms or need-based planning, rather than in accordance with resource-based planning. Drug consumption in low income countries – often high in relative terms – is to a large extent financed privately by consumers through out-of-pocket payment. In a more developed country, spending on consumables will be much higher in absolute numbers, but still low in relative terms due to the fact that human resources will be more expensive. But even for countries with comparable income levels there are sometimes wide differences in country-specific resource profiles.

Figure 4.2 shows resource profiles for four high income countries: Denmark, Sweden, the United Kingdom, and the United States *(23)*. Each country's input level, on each of eight inputs, is expressed as a percentage of the highest value for that indicator in the group: the figures do not show "best performance" in the sense of Chapter 2 but simply compare input levels.

The United States is at or close to the maximum on every input. On expenditure and technology it is at the maximum of this group of countries. Sweden has the largest stock of human resources and beds and, with Denmark, the highest drug spending. The United Kingdom is within the boundary set by this group on every input: it is particularly far from the maximum on expenditure per capita and technology (magnetic resonance imaging (MRI) and computerized tomography (CT) scanners). However, in terms of beds and drugs the UK is comparable to the rest of the group and higher than the USA.

This simple comparison between countries shows clear differences in terms of input mix. The differences can in part be explained by past conditions of competition and payment methods among US hospitals, which have focused more on quality than on price and cost-effectiveness. Relative price differences also play a role. The 'medical arms race' in Sweden and particularly in the UK has been more restrained under global budgets. This also means that the US health system (and ultimately US tax-payers and health insurance payers) pays a larger share of the global costs involved in bringing new medical technologies and medicines to the market. Trend data (not in the diagrams) show that, with respect to MRI and CT scanners, both Sweden and the UK are catching up with levels in the United States. This supports the view that the US health system is an early adopter of new medical technology. The relative price of physicians and nurses in Sweden is low compared to that in the United States, and the different input mixes illustrate a degree of substitutability between human resources and other health inputs.

Figure 4.3 shows similar resource profiles for Egypt, Mexico, South Africa and Thailand. These four middle income countries spend substantially less on all types of health care resources than the group of high income countries. As is the case for the group of high income countries, there are considerable contrasts in the mix of resources and these differences do not seem to be due primarily to differences in income or prices.

South Africa is at the maximum of the group for expenditure, nurses, beds and MRI scanners, while it is furthest from the maximum for drugs and physicians (with Thailand). Egypt has the lowest total health expenditure per capita within the group, but the highest ratio of physicians and the second highest level of drug consumption. Both physicians and drugs in Egypt are mostly paid for directly by patients out of pocket. Some 80% of physicians' income is estimated to come from private practice, and households finance close to 60% of total drug costs through direct payments *(2)*. Doubts have been raised about skill

Figure 4.2 Health systems input mix: comparison of four high income countries, around 1997

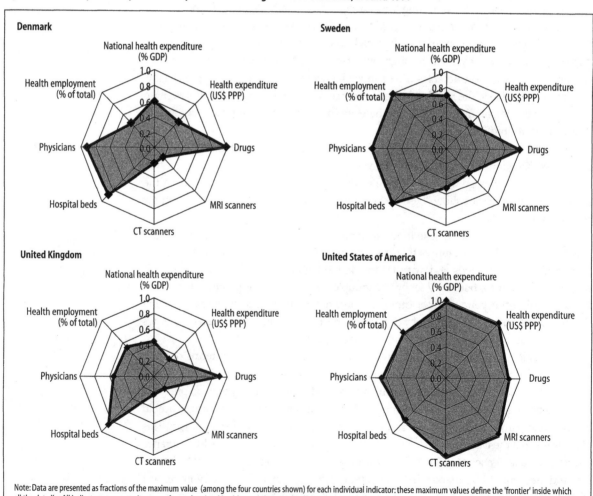

Note: Data are presented as fractions of the maximum value (among the four countries shown) for each individual indicator: these maximum values define the 'frontier' inside which all the data lie. All indicators are per capita except for total national health expenditure and health employment.
PPP= purchasing power parity. MRI = magnetic resonance imaging. CT= computerized tomography.
Source: OECD health database 2000.

levels of physicians. There is extensive use of branded as opposed to generic drugs. In part this pattern of drug use is explained by little knowledge and poor perception of generic drugs by consumers, combined with extensive self-medication. Irrational prescribing by physicians and dispensing by pharmacists of expensive drugs are other important explanatory factors.

Mexico has a high ratio of physicians and, together with Thailand, the lowest ratio of nurses within the group. It is estimated that about 15% of all physicians in Mexico are either inactive, underemployed or unemployed *(2)*. Despite this evidence of surplus, there are a large number of unfilled posts in rural areas. In contrast, Thailand and South Africa have a low ratio of physicians. Indeed, Thailand's health authorities estimate that at least another 10 000 physicians are needed *(2)*. The ratios of physicians to nurses show great contrasts: in South Africa nurses greatly outnumber physicians, possibly due to greater international mobility of doctors, but in Egypt and Mexico the proportions are reversed.

The distribution of available resources between urban and rural areas is a major problem in all four middle income countries but is not illustrated by the figure, which presents

Figure 4.3 Health systems input mix: comparison of four middle income countries, around 1997

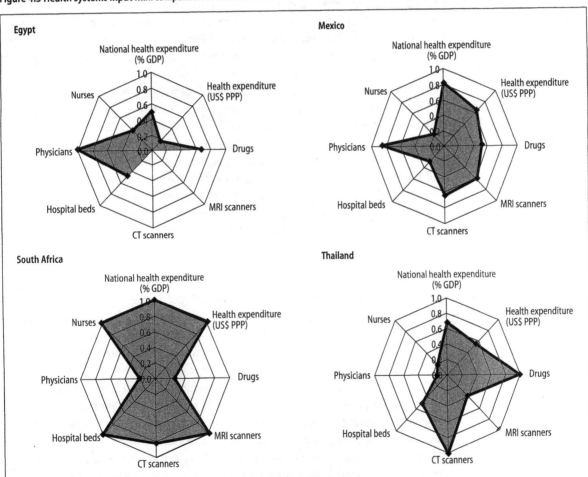

Note: Data are presented as fractions of the maximum value (among the four countries shown) for each individual indicator: these maximum values define the 'frontier' inside which all the data lie. All indicators are per capita except for total national health expenditure.
PPP= purchasing power parity. MRI = magnetic resonance imaging. CT= computerized tomography.
Source: WHO health system profiles database, WHO national health accounts estimates, and personal communications from WHO and ministry of health staff.

only averages. Physicians mostly work where health status levels are highest. The distribution of resources across ethnic groups is a particular problem in South Africa. In Thailand, most of the high technology equipment is concentrated in urban hospitals, whereas the use of technology at the primary care level is scarce. Most of the about 900 physicians produced annually in Thailand remain in urban areas, and shortages of qualified staff in rural areas are expected to persist.

CHANGING INVESTMENT PATTERNS

Experience points to political difficulties in changing existing investment patterns and resource profiles. Every euro, bhat or kwacha spent on health service delivery or investment is income to someone and therefore creates a vested interest *(24)*. If the income is large, this "someone" will lobby for more resources and resist changes that do not match his or her particular interests. Such lobbying and resistance come from both the medical industry and from labour groups. Attempts to reform systems for paying providers are often highly controversial, as are changes in medical school admissions or educational programmes. Lobbying also comes from interest groups and politicians. Health care investments usually attract popular support and it can be difficult to rearrange investments in favour of a new balance. This will often be the case even if large imbalances exist compared to social priorities. Vested interests and lobbying related to the distribution of cost and benefits are important factors in the inertia that has to be overcome in order to change the existing capital structure and mix of resource inputs.

The predominant investment emphasis in the health system over past decades has been on hospitals and specialist care. In addition to the other forces opposing primary health care, discussed in Chapter 1, investment decisions played a part. The allocation of investment capital to hospital buildings is not the main reason. More importantly, the focus on specialist care entailed investments in the employment and training of human resources to staff hospitals. The focus on hospital care led to a rapid accumulation of beds. In high income countries, the accumulation of beds was accompanied and driven by rapid technological change, resulting in a greater intensity of care and increasing costs. Population ageing, and the accompanying higher health systems utilization rates by elderly people, maintained this upward pressure on bed supply.

In less developed countries the accumulation of beds has been accompanied by much slower technological change and slower cost increases, but also by less intensity of care, inadequate maintenance of facilities and lower quality of services because of a lack of funding for recurrent costs *(24)*. In many middle and low income countries, occupancy rates at public hospitals have been low. In Mexico, for example, occupancy rates at Ministry of Health hospitals have been 50% on average, because of inadequate staffing and maintenance, with consequent inefficient use of existing resources *(25)*.

During the 1990s, many countries started to reduce the size of their hospital sector and many small hospitals, in particular, were closed or used for other purposes (see Box 4.5). Reflecting technical progress and lower costs in ambulatory care, the number of beds has declined and the average length of stay has been reduced. Closure of small hospitals and emergency wards and a declining number of beds mean that new strategies will have to be developed to respond to fluctuating demand, with greater integration among providers, transport of patients, pooling of resources and information as key components.

With fluctuating demand, there is a need for some surplus capacity to absorb changes in demand. The influenza epidemic that swept across Europe in 1999–2000 revealed that surplus bed-capacity to deal with sudden changes in health need is limited in many countries, for example in the UK *(26)*. In other industries (electricity supply, public transport) temporary surges in demand can be met through peak-load pricing. As discussed more fully in Chapter 3, rationing by price is not an acceptable allocation mechanism in the health system. Excess demand that cannot be repressed by higher prices must be accommodated by other means of rationing – postponing non-emergency care, transferring patients, shortening inpatient stays and so on.

In countries with a hierarchical planning structure, resource allocation and investment planning is often incremental. Last year's budget is often the starting point for next year's planning. Ongoing activities are usually not questioned: this greatly reduces the country's scope for shifting to a more cost-effective overall allocation of inputs. The planning process can be described as a game in which ministries that deliver services (such as ministries of health) call for increased resources, while the guardians of the treasury try to maintain expenditure at its previous level *(27)*. This approach is attractive because of its simplicity but it demands growing budgets. If budgets are declining, departments should really scrutinize the full range of ongoing programmes and activities, prioritizing activities for possible cutting or elimination. Public bureaucracies typically try to maintain the status quo by cutting costs across the board without changing overall priorities, and without taking special account of the need to protect targeted geographical areas or sub-groups of the population.

Agencies will try, for as long as possible, to maintain what they judge to be critical expenditure such as salaries and cut down on expenditure that does not immediately damage health system performance *(22)*. Planned investments are delayed and ongoing constructions are left incomplete. In the hope that financial crises are short-lived, health systems may decrease their spending on long-term investments in human and physical capital and even on recurrent costs for maintenance, medicines and other consumables. This will eventually constrain severely the capacity of human capital and health system performance. Investments, by their nature, tend to be more volatile than recurrent expenditures: they occur in discrete chunks and then require smaller but regular operating expenditures. Short-

---

Box 4.5 Investment in hospitals in countries of the former Soviet Union prior to policy reform

The majority of health care resources in the former Soviet Union were controlled from the top by ministries of health. Central government managed investments and the consequent accumulation of resources in physical and human capital. The structure of service delivery was determined by such norms as beds or physicians per thousand inhabitants. The result was high hospital capacity.

In the early 1990s the bed ratio for most of the former Soviet Union was considerably higher than that in many western European countries. The number of physicians per capita, most of them allocated to the hospital sector, was also high in comparison with many western countries. Indications of inefficiency were given by long lengths of stay and moderate occupancy rates, especially in small hospitals. The effectiveness of hospital services was also influenced adversely by the poor quality of facilities and medical equipment. Many of the small district hospitals had no more than 4–5 m^2 per bed, and some of the smallest hospitals had no radiology services, and inadequate heating or water.

For example, a 1989 survey found that 20% of Russian hospitals did not have piped hot water, 3% did not even have piped cold water, and 17% lacked adequate sanitation facilities. The survey also found that every seventh hospital and polyclinic needed basic reconstruction. A similar survey of facilities in 1988 found substantial underinvestment in maintenance of polyclinics and hospitals, with 19% of polyclinics and 23% of hospitals rated as either being in a "disastrous" condition or requiring full reconstruction.

In the 1990s, reductions in the number and use of hospitals were an essential part of reforms. A combination of overcapacity and poor quality of physical resources had become a major distortion in the input mix of these countries. Where facilities were not closed, or used as nursing homes or for other functions, they were upgraded and used more effectively in the referral system. In many cases, however, changes have been modest because of political difficulties in transferring resources from one use to another.

Source: Anell A, Barnum H. The allocation of capital and health sector reform. In: Saltman RB, Figueras J, Sakellarides C, eds. *Critical challenges for health care reform in Europe.* Buckingham, UK, Open University Press, 1998 (State of Health Series).

term postponement or cutting of investment may be an appropriate response to a crisis, but it requires an overall picture of capital and recurrent resources as well as a likely time horizon for the crisis. Without these, ad hoc chopping of planned investments will create imbalances and inefficiency.

THE WAY FORWARD

Clear symptoms of imbalances between resources include poor performance, deteriorating facilities, and low working morale among staff. Often, skilled human capital moves to the private sector or to wealthier regions. Physical capital deteriorates in a more visible way. The patient turns to the private sector in search of better quality care.

Whatever a country's income level, there exist efficient ways to allocate health system inputs that will allow the health system to function at its best. The efficient mix will vary over time and across countries, depending on relative prices among inputs, country specific health needs and social priorities. In less developed countries, setting priorities will surely be much harder, and the balance between investments and recurrent costs more critical. Health care systems face major challenges when there is a rapid change either in technology or in available financial resources as a result of a turbulent macroeconomic environment. The failure of health care decision-makers to respond to such a shift in conditions will lead to suboptimal health system performance.

For very different reasons, both developed and less developed countries record imbalances between the available inputs. Because of the rapid technological changes in health services, imbalances have been the rule rather than the exception in developed countries. Problems are much more visible in less developed countries, where imbalances have often been caused by lack of management skills and a decline in the available financial resources. Although some imbalances are likely to exist even in well-functioning health systems, much more could be done to correct them rapidly or even prevent them.

A first step is to create a general awareness of the problem by documenting the various resources used and the performance of health systems. Sound data on the existing numbers and distribution of human resources, especially when linked to data on health system performance, can also contribute to the formulation of policies and plans to address problems. Figures 4.2 and 4.3 present fragments of information on inputs. But they do not reveal how input mix affects performance.

National health accounts (NHAs) offer a more comprehensive framework for bringing together data on inputs and for communicating with various stakeholders on future investment policies. NHAs give a broad picture, which enables ministries to lead health care services through reforms and difficult times. When Finland's economy went into crisis with the loss of its export market with the Russian Federation in the early 1990s, health policymakers were able to use their NHA information to restore productivity in the health system.

More appropriate cost information and accounting systems would also make it easier to achieve a balance among inputs, for example by establishing more reliable budget estimates. A general awareness and improved information through NHAs and accounting systems will not result in any change, however, without a parallel and widespread commitment by health care decision-makers to address the fundamental problems.

Such commitment is best supported by a combination of stewardship – oversight and influence – and more scope for decentralized decision-making by purchasers and providers. Central authority over major investment decisions is essential. This does not mean that all such decisions need to be made centrally. But central policy and guidance, through a bidding or certification process, are necessary to ensure overall coordination between public and private investment decisions, and with the recurrent funding capacity of the public sector. The worst mistake is to promote or allow investments when their running costs cannot be met. Central policy on drugs and major technology registration, the development of essential drugs lists and treatment guidelines, quality assurance and bulk tendering will continue to be necessary. Purchasers and providers need incentives and opportunities to challenge the prevailing allocation of inputs in order to discover the best way to respond to health needs, social priorities and expectations. Rigid hierarchical approaches to balancing resources usually result in reactive rather than continuous change; shortages of essential inputs on one hand and unspent funds on the other are likely to be common problems. But decentralized decision-making among providers must be controlled and guided through active purchasing and appropriate payment mechanisms to meet overall priorities. Decentralized decision-making on the details of service and intervention arrangements also requires new strategies for human resources and investments in planning and management skills at all levels.

Without such explicit stewardship of all input sources and monitoring of developments, there will be too much discretion among decentralized units to engage in opportunistic behaviour. Such behaviour, either at central or decentralized levels, will also deter donor agencies from supporting decentralization, for example through sector-wide approaches and common funding pools. It will also be a reason for aid recipients to mistrust attempts to bring about donor coordination (22). Decentralization does not mean a lack of accountability in resource management, nor that central government should opt out of planning and monitoring. It should be designed to increase accountability and should give central government and ministries a new role, focusing on overall regulation and monitoring.

As part of that new role, the impact of new medical technologies should be assessed and regulatory practice developed in consultation with the important stakeholders. Such assessment of new technologies requires documentation on existing practice and use of resources. This further emphasizes the importance of monitoring. For the less developed countries, donor agencies need to take existing and possible imbalances into account when drawing up support strategies. The information base provided by a consistent use of NHAs will provide a good starting point for a common understanding of existing imbalances.

In both rigid hierarchical systems and in decentralized systems without accountability, proper incentives and stewardship, imbalances among resources will be more difficult to correct and prevent. Such imbalances often create huge problems in their own right, but they will also induce further problems by giving wrong signals to the health care labour market and the industry that supports health services. Well-performing, cost-effective health systems that respond to health needs based on explicit priorities will give both the medical industry and medical schools the incentives to invest properly in research and development, in educational programmes and in the physical inputs essential to the production of better health.

REFERENCES

1. **Becker GS.** *Human capital. A theoretical and empirical analysis with special reference to education,* 3rd edition. Chicago, The University of Chicago Press, 1993.

2. WHO health system profiles database.

3. **Folland S, Goodman AC, Stano M.** *The economics of health and health care.* New York, Macmillan Publishing Company, 1993.

4. **Berckmans P.** *Initial evaluation of human resources for health in 40 African countries.* Geneva, World Health Organization, Department of Organization of Health Services Delivery, 1999 (forthcoming document).

5. **Ensor T, Savelyeva L.** Informal payments for health care in the Former Soviet Union: some evidence from Kazakhstan. *Health Policy and Planning,* 1999, **13**(1): 41–49.

6. **Hicks V, Adams O.** *The effects of economic and policy incentives on provider practice. Summary of country case studies using the WHO framework.* Geneva, World Health Organization, 2000 (Issues in health services delivery, Discussion paper No. 5, document WHO/EIP/OSD/2000.8, in press).

7. **Egger D, Lipson D, Adams O.** *Achieving the right balance: the role of policy-making processes in managing human resources for health problems.* Geneva, World Health Organization, 2000 (Issues in health services delivery, Discussion paper No. 2, document WHO/EIP/OSD/2000.2).

8. *Public sector pay reform project, final report.* Ministry of Public Service, Accra, Uganda, 1999, WHO health system profiles database.

9. **Weisbrod BA.** The health care quadrilemma: an essay on technological change, insurance, quality of care, and cost containment. *Journal of Economic Literature,* 1991, **24**: 523–552.

10. *European health care reform. Analysis of current strategies.* Copenhagen, Denmark, World Health Organization, 1997 (European Series No. 72).

11. *Action Programme on Essential Drugs.* Geneva, World Health Organization, 1999.

12. *Public–private roles in the pharmaceutical sector: implications for equitable access and rational use.* Geneva, World Health Organization, 1997 (Health economics and drugs, DAP Series No. 5).

13. **Banta HD, Luce BR.** *Health care technology and its assessment: an international perspective.* Oxford, Oxford University Press, 1993.

14. *Medical equipment procurement manual.* Washington, DC, The World Bank, 1998.

15. *Standard bidding documents: procurement of health sector goods.* Washington, DC, The World Bank, 2000.

16. **Van Gruting CWD ed.** *Medical devices: international perspective, Part VIII – Geographical situations in central and east Europe.* Amsterdam, Elsevier, 1994.

17. **Issakov A, Richter N, Tabakow S.** Health care equipment and clinical engineering in central and eastern Europe. *New World Health,* 1994: 167-171.

18. *Russian Federation medical equipment project.* Washington, DC, The World Bank, 1996 (Report No. 14968-RU).

19. *Private hospital study.* Washington, DC, International Finance Corporation, 1998.

20. *The world health report 1999 – Making a difference.* Geneva, World Health Organization, 1999.

21. **Lee K.** Symptoms, causes and proposed solutions. In: Abel-Smith B, Creese A, eds. *Recurrent costs in the health sector: problems and policy options in three countries.* Geneva, World Health Organization, 1989 (document WHO/SHS/NHP/89.8).

22. **Walt G et al.** Health sector development: from aid coordination to resource management. *Health Policy and Planning,* 1999, **14**(3): 207–218.

23. **Anell A, Willis M.** International comparison of health care resources using resource profiles. *Bulletin of the World Health Organization,* 2000, **78** (in press).

24. **Reinhardt U.** *Accountable health care: is it compatible with social solidarity?* London, The Office of Health Economics, 1997.

25. **Barnum H, Kutzin J.** *Public hospitals in developing countries: resource use, cost and financing.* Baltimore, John Hopkins University Press, 1993.

26. The health service: bedridden. *The Economist,* 15 January 2000: 31–34.

27. **Wildavsky A.** *Budgeting: a comparative theory of budgetary processes.* Boston, Little, Brown & Co., 1975.

CHAPTER FIVE

Who Pays for
Health Systems?

Choices for financing health services have an impact on how fairly the burden of payment is distributed. Can the rich and healthy subsidize the poor and sick? In order to ensure fairness and financial risk protection, there should be a high level of prepayment; risk should be spread (through cross-subsidies from low to high health risk); the poor should be subsidized (through cross-subsidies from high to low income); the fragmentation of pools or funds should be avoided; and there should be strategic purchasing to improve health system outcomes and responsiveness.

5

WHO PAYS FOR HEALTH SYSTEMS?

HOW FINANCING WORKS

*H*ealth care expenditures have risen from 3% of world GDP in 1948 to 7.9% in 1997. This dramatic increase in spending worldwide has prompted societies everywhere to look for health financing arrangements which ensure that people are not denied access to care because they cannot afford it. Providing such access to all citizens has long been a cornerstone of modern health financing systems in many countries. The main function of the health system is to provide health services to the population, and this chapter concentrates on health financing as a key to effective interaction between providers and citizens. It discusses the purpose of health financing, and the links between health financing and service delivery, through purchasing. The factors affecting the performance of health financing are also examined.

The purpose of health financing is to make funding available, as well as to set the right financial incentives for providers, to ensure that all individuals have access to effective public health and personal health care. This means reducing or eliminating the possibility that an individual will be unable to pay for such care, or will be impoverished as a result of trying to do so.

To ensure that individuals have access to health services, three interrelated functions of health system financing are crucial: revenue collection, pooling of resources, and purchasing of interventions. The main challenges are to put in place the necessary technical, organizational and institutional arrangements so that such interactions will protect people financially the fairest way possible, and to set incentives for providers that will motivate them to increase health and improve the responsiveness of the system. The three functions are often integrated in a single organization, and this is currently the case in many health systems in the world. Although this chapter discusses the three functions separately, it does not imply that an attempt should be made to separate them in different organizations. There is, however, an increasing trend to introduce a separation between financing and provision.

Revenue collection is the process by which the health system receives money from households and organizations or companies, as well as from donors. Contributions by donors are discussed in Box 5.1. Health systems have various ways of collecting revenue, such as general taxation, mandated social health insurance contributions (usually salary-related and almost never risk-related), voluntary private health insurance contributions (usually risk-related), out-of-pocket payment and donations. Most high income countries rely heavily

---

Box 5.1 The importance of donor contributions in revenue collection and purchasing in developing countries

Donor contributions, as a source of revenue for the health system, are of key importance for some developing countries. The absolute amounts of such aid have been large in recent years in Angola, Bangladesh, Ecuador, India, Indonesia, Mozambique, Papua New Guinea, the United Republic of Tanzania and several eastern European countries, but in the larger countries aid is usually only a small share of total health spending or even of government expenditure. In contrast, several countries, particularly in Africa, depend on donors for a large share of total expenditure on health. The fraction can be as high as 40% (Uganda in 1993) or even 84% (Gambia in 1994) and exceeds 20% in 1996 or 1997 in Eritrea, Kenya, The Lao People's Democratic Republic and Mali. Bolivia, Nicaragua, the United Republic of Tanzania and Zimbabwe have obtained 10% to 20% of their resources for health from donors in one or more recent years.

Most aid comes in the form of projects, which are separately developed and negotiated between each donor and the national authorities. Although by no means unsuccessful, international cooperation through projects can lead to fragmentation and duplication of effort, particularly when many donors are involved, each focusing on their own geographical or programme priorities. Such an approach forces national authorities to devote significant amounts of time and effort to dealing with donors' priorities and procedures, rather than concentrating on strategic stewardship and health programme implementation. Donors and governments are increasingly seeing the need to move away from a project approach towards wider programme support to long-term strategic development that is integrated into the budgetary process of the country. In this respect, sector-wide approaches have been effective in countries such as Bangladesh, Ghana and Pakistan.[1]

[1] Cassels A, Janovsky K. Better health in developing countries: are sector-wide approaches the way of the future? *The Lancet*, 1998, 352:1777–1779.

---

on either general taxation or mandated social health insurance contributions. In contrast, low income countries depend far more on out-of-pocket financing: in 60% of countries at incomes below $1000 per capita, out-of-pocket spending is 40% or more of the total whereas only 30% of middle and high income countries depend so heavily on this kind of financing (see Table 5.1).

In most social insurance and voluntary private insurance schemes, revenue collection and pooling are integrated in one organization and one purchasing process. For organizations relying mainly on general taxation, such as ministries of health, collecting is done by the ministry of finance and allocation to the ministry of health occurs through the government budgetary process.

Pooling is the accumulation and management of revenues in such a way as to ensure that the risk of having to pay for health care is borne by all the members of the pool and not by each contributor individually. Pooling is traditionally known as the "insurance function" within the health system, whether the insurance is explicit (people knowingly subscribe to a scheme) or implicit (as with tax revenues). Its main purpose is to share the financial risk associated with health interventions for which the need is uncertain. In this way it differs from collecting, which may allow individuals to continue bearing their own risks from their own pockets or savings. When people pay entirely out of pocket, no pooling occurs.

Table 5.1 Estimated out-of-pocket share in health spending by income level, 1997
(number of countries in each income and expenditure class)

Estimated annual per capita income (US$ at exchange rate)	Estimated share in total expenditure on health (%)						
	Under 20	20–29	30–39	40–49	50–59	60 and over	Total
Under 1000	7	10	9	7	11	19	**63**
1000–9999	16	18	23	15	8	8	**88**
10 000 and over	19	7	4	5	0	2	**37**
All income classes	42	35	36	27	19	29	**188**

Source: WHO national health accounts estimates: income unknown for three countries.

For public health activities and even for aspects of personal health care – such as health check-ups – for which there is no uncertainty or the cost is low, funds can go directly from collecting to purchasing. This is an important consideration with regard to the regulation of mandatory pooling schemes, as consumer preferences for insurance packages often focus on interventions of high probability and low cost (relative to the household capacity to pay), although these are best paid for out of current income or through direct public subsidies for the poor.

Pooling reduces uncertainty for both citizens and providers. By increasing and stabilizing demand and the flow of funds, pooling can increase the likelihood that patients will be able to afford services and that a higher volume of services will justify new provider investments.

Purchasing is the process by which pooled funds are paid to providers in order to deliver a specified or unspecified set of health interventions. Purchasing can be performed passively or strategically. Passive purchasing implies following a predetermined budget or simply paying bills when presented. Strategic purchasing involves a continuous search for the best ways to maximize health system performance by deciding which interventions should be purchased, how, and from whom. This means actively choosing interventions in order to achieve the best performance, both for individuals and the population as a whole, by means of selective contracting and incentive schemes. Purchasing uses different instruments for paying providers, including budgeting. Recently, many countries, including Chile *(1, 2)*, Hungary *(3)*, New Zealand *(4, 5)*, and the United Kingdom *(6–8)*, have tried to introduce an active purchasing role within their public health systems.

PREPAYMENT AND COLLECTION

Traditionally, most policy discussions regarding health system financing centre around the impact of public versus private financing on health system performance. Chapter 3 clarifies the central role of public financing in public health. For personal health care, however, it is not the public–private dichotomy that is most important in determining health system performance but the difference between prepayment and out-of-pocket spending. Thus, private financing, particularly in developing countries, is largely synonymous with out-of-pocket spending or with contributions to small, voluntary and often highly fragmented pools. In contrast, public or mandatory private financing (from general taxation or from contributions to social security) is always associated with prepayment and large pools. The way policy-makers organize public financing or influence private financing will affect four key determinants of health system financing performance: the level of prepayment; the degree of spreading of risk; the extent to which the poor are subsidized; and strategic purchasing.

A health system where individuals have to pay out of their own pockets for a substantial part of the cost of health services at the moment of seeking treatment clearly restricts access to only those who can afford it, and is likely to exclude the poorest members of society *(9–12)*. Some important health interventions would not be financed at all if people had to pay for them, as is the case for the public good type of interventions discussed in Chapter 3 *(13)*. Fairness of financial risk protection requires the highest possible degree of separation between contributions and utilization. This is particularly so for interventions that are high cost relative to the household's capacity to pay.

In addition to affording protection against having to pay out of pocket and, as a result, facing barriers to access, prepayment makes it possible to spread the financial risk among members of a pool, as discussed later in the chapter. Individual out-of-pocket financing does not allow the risk to be shared in that way. In other words, as already proposed by *The world health report 1999 (14)*, there has to be prepayment for effective access to high-cost personal care.

The level of prepayment is mainly determined by the predominant revenue collection mechanism in the system. General taxation allows for maximum separation between contributions and utilization, while out-of-pocket payment represents no separation. Why then is the latter so generally used, particularly in developing countries? *(15)*.

The answer is that separation of contributions from utilization requires the agencies responsible for collection to have very strong institutional and organizational capacity. These attributes are lacking in many developing countries. Thus, although the highest possible level of prepayment is desirable, it is usually very difficult to attain in low income settings where institutions are weak. Relying on prepaid arrangements, particularly general taxation, is institutionally very demanding. General taxation, as the main source of health financing, demands an excellent tax or contribution collecting capacity. This is usually associated with a largely formal economy, whereas in developing countries the informal sector is often predominant. While general taxation on average accounts for more than 40% of GDP in OECD countries, it accounts for less than 20% in low income countries.

All other prepayment mechanisms, including social security contributions and voluntary insurance premiums, are easier to collect, as the benefit of participating is linked to actual contributions. In most cases, participation in social insurance schemes is restricted to formal sector workers who contribute through salary deductions at the workplace. This makes it easier for the social security organization to identify them, collect contributions and possibly exclude them from benefits if no contribution is made. Similarly, identification and collection is easier for voluntary health insurance and community pooling arrangements. Nevertheless, such prepayment still requires large organizational and institutional capacity compared to out-of-pocket financing.

In developing countries, therefore, the objective is to create the conditions for revenue collecting mechanisms that will increasingly allow for separation of contributions from utilization. In low income countries, where there are usually high levels of out-of-pocket expenditure on health and where organizational and institutional capacity are too weak to make it viable to rely mainly on general taxation to finance health, this means promoting job-based contribution systems where possible, and facilitating the creation of community or provider-based prepayment schemes. Evidence shows *(16, 17)*, however, that although the latter are an improvement over out-of-pocket financing, they are difficult to sustain and should be considered only as a transition towards higher levels of pooling or as instruments to improve the targeting of public subsidies in health. In middle income countries, with more formal economies, strategies to increase prepayment as well as pooling arrangements include strengthening and expanding mandatory salary-based or risk-based contribution systems, as well as increasing the share of public financing, particularly for the poor.

Although prepayment is a cornerstone of fair health system financing, some direct contribution at the moment of utilization may be required in low income countries or settings to increase revenues where prepayment capacity is inadequate. It can also be required in the form of co-payment for specific interventions with a view to reducing demand. Such an approach should only be used where there is clear evidence of unjustified over-utilization of the specific intervention as a result of prepayment schemes (moral hazard). The use of co-payment has the effect of *rationing* the use of a specific intervention but does not have the effect of *rationalizing* its demand by consumers. When confronted with co-payments, people, particularly the poor, will reduce the amount of services demanded (even to the extent of not demanding a service at all) but will not necessarily be more rational in distinguishing when to demand services or which services they need to demand. Therefore, using user charges indiscriminately will indiscriminately reduce demand, hurting the poor in particular.

Free-of-charge services do not translate automatically into unjustified over-utilization of services. Services that are free of direct charge are in reality not necessarily free or affordable, particularly for the poor, because of other costs associated with seeking health care, such as the cost of medication (when not available free of charge), under-the-table payments, transportation, or time lost from work *(18, 19)*.

Given its potentially negative impact on necessary services, especially for the poor, co-payment should not be chosen as a source of financing except for low-cost relatively predictable needs. Rather, it can be used as an instrument to control over-utilization of specific interventions (when such over-utilization is evident) or to implicitly exclude services from a benefit package when explicit exclusion is not possible. Because of the desirability of separating contributions from utilization, out-of-pocket payment should not be used unless no other alternative is available. All prepaid arrangements are preferable, except for low-cost interventions for which the administrative costs involved in prepayment arrangements might not be worthwhile.

SPREADING RISK AND SUBSIDIZING THE POOR: POOLING OF RESOURCES

Pooling is the main way to spread risks among participants. Even when there is a high degree of separation between contributions and utilization, prepayment alone does not guarantee fair financing if it is on an individual basis only – that is, via medical savings accounts. Individuals would then have limited access to services after their savings were exhausted. It is claimed for medical savings accounts, which have been implemented in Singapore and in the United States, that they reduce moral hazard and give consumers the incentive to buy services more rationally, but while there is evidence of reduced expenditure and of substantial savings among those who receive tax benefits and can afford to save *(20)*, there is no evidence of more rational purchasing. And individual financing fosters fee-for-service payment and makes it harder to regulate the quality of provision *(21)*. People with a high risk of having to use services, such as the sick and the elderly, would be denied access because they could not save enough from their income. On the other hand, the healthy and the young, whose risk is usually low, might prepay for a long time without needing the services for which they had saved. In this case, mechanisms allowing for cross-subsidies from the young and healthy to the sick and old would benefit the former without damaging the latter. Thus, systems as well as people benefit from mechanisms that not only increase the degree of prepayment for health services, but also spread the financial risk among their members.

Although prepayment and pooling are a significant improvement over purely out-of-pocket financing, they do not take questions of income into account. As a result of large pools, society takes advantage of economies of scale, the law of large numbers, and cross-subsidies from low-risk to high-risk individuals. Pooling by itself allows for equalization of contributions among members of the pool regardless of their financial risk associated with service utilization. But it also allows the low-risk poor to subsidize the high-risk rich. Societies interested in equity are not indifferent to who is subsidized by whom. Therefore, health financing, in addition to ensuring cross-subsidies from low to high risk (which will happen in any pool, unless contributions are risk-related), should also ensure that such subsidies are not regressive (see Figure 5.1).

Health systems throughout the world attempt to spread risk and subsidize the poor through various combinations of organizational and technical arrangements *(22)*. Both risk- and income-related cross-subsidies could occur among the members of the same pool, for example in single pool systems such as the Costa Rican social security organization and the national health service in the UK, or via government subsidies to a single or multiple pool arrangement.

In practice, in the majority of health systems, risk and income cross-subsidization occurs via a combination of two approaches: pooling and government subsidy. Cross-subsidization can also occur among members of different pools (in a multiple pool system) via explicit risk and income equalization mechanisms, such as those being used in the social security systems of Argentina *(23)*, Colombia *(24)* and the Netherlands *(25)*. In these countries, the existence of multiple pools allows members of pools to have different risk and income profiles. Without some compensatory mechanisms, such arrangements would offer incentives for pooling organizations to select low risks, and to exclude the poor and the sick.

Even under single pool organizations, decentralization, unless accompanied by equalization mechanisms for resource allocation, may result in significant risk and income differences among decentralized regions. Brazil has introduced compensatory mechanisms in the allocation of revenues from the central government to the states to reduce such differences *(26)*.

Table 5.2 shows four country examples of different arrangements for spreading risk and subsidizing the poor. Some organizational arrangements are less efficient than others in ensuring that these two objectives are achieved, particularly if the arrangements facilitate fragmentation, creating numerous small pools. Collecting, pooling, purchasing and provi-

Figure 5.1 Pooling to redistribute risk, and cross-subsidy for greater equity
(arrows indicate flow of funds)

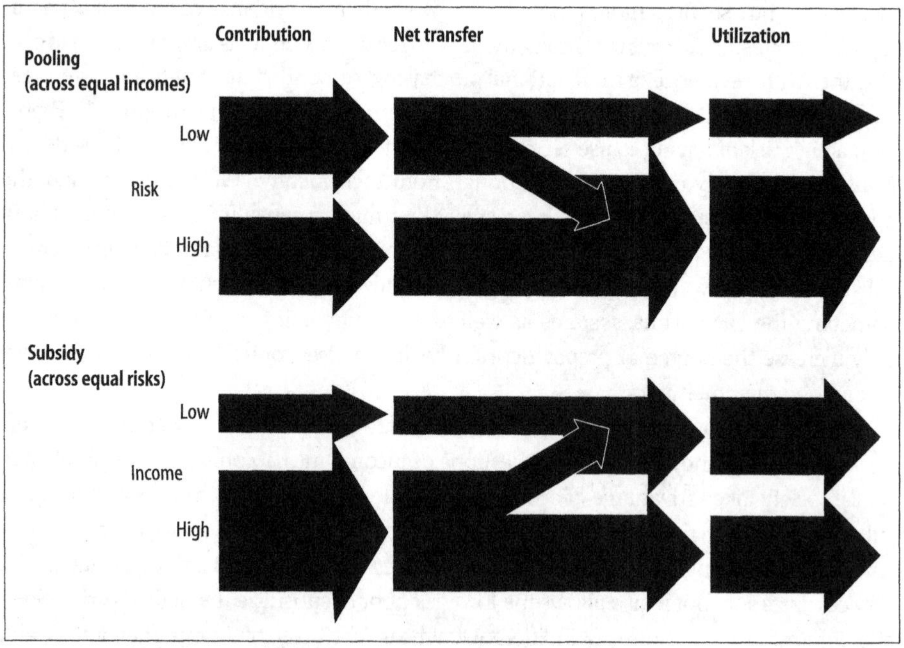

sion imply flows of funds from sources to providers through a variety of organizations, which may perform only one, or several of these tasks. Figure 5.2 illustrates the structure of health system financing in four countries which differ greatly in the degree to which there is formal pooling of funds and purchasing, rather than consumers paying directly to providers without any sharing of risks.

Large pools are better than small ones because they can increase resource availability for health services. The larger the pool, the bigger the share of contributions that can be allocated exclusively to health services. A large pool can take advantage of economies of scale in administration and reduce the level of the contributions required to protect against uncertain needs, while still ensuring that there are sufficient funds to pay for services. Given that needs vary unpredictably, the estimation for an individual could be unaffordably large. By reducing this uncertainty, the pool is able to reduce the amount set aside as a financial reserve to deal with variations in the health expenditure estimates for its members. It can then use the funds released for more and better services.

Fragmentation of the pool – in other words, the existence of too many small organizations involved in revenue collection, pooling and purchasing – damages performance of all three tasks, particularly pooling. In fragmented systems, it is not the number of existing pools and purchasers that matters, but that many of them are too small. In Argentina, prior to the 1996 reforms, there were more than 300 pooling organizations (*Obras Sociales Nacionales*) for formal sector workers and their families, some with no more than 50 000 members. The administrative capacity and financial reserves required to ensure financial viability for the small ones, together with the low wages of their beneficiaries, guaranteed that their benefit packages were very limited. A similar problem occurs with community

Table 5.2 Approaches to spreading risk and subsidizing the poor: country cases

Country	System	Spreading risk	Subsidizing the poor
Colombia	Multiple pools: multiple competing social security organizations, municipal health systems and Ministry of Health.	Intra-pool via non-risk-related contribution and inter-pool via a central risk equalization fund. Mandated minimum benefit package for all members of all pools.	Intra-pool and inter-pool: salary-related contribution plus explicit subsidy paid to the insurer for the poor to join social security; supply side subsidy via the Ministry of Health and municipal systems.
Netherlands	Multiple pools: predominantly private competing social insurance organizations.	Intra-pool via non-risk-related contribution and inter-pool via central risk equalization fund.	Via risk equalization fund, excluding the rich.
Republic of Korea	Two main pools: national health insurance and the Ministry of Health. National health insurance, however, only covers 30% of total health expenditures of any member.	Intra-pool via non-risk-related contribution. Explicit single benefit package for all members.	Salary-related contribution plus supply side subsidy via the Ministry of Health and national health insurance from Ministry of Finance allocations. Public subsidy for insurance for the poor and farmers.
Zambia	Single predominant formal pool: Ministry of Health/Central Board of Health.	Intra-pool, implicit single benefit package for all in the Ministry of Health System and at state level. Financed via general taxes.	Intra-pool via general taxation. Supply side subsidy via the Ministry of Health.

Figure 5.2 Structure of health system financing and provision in four countries

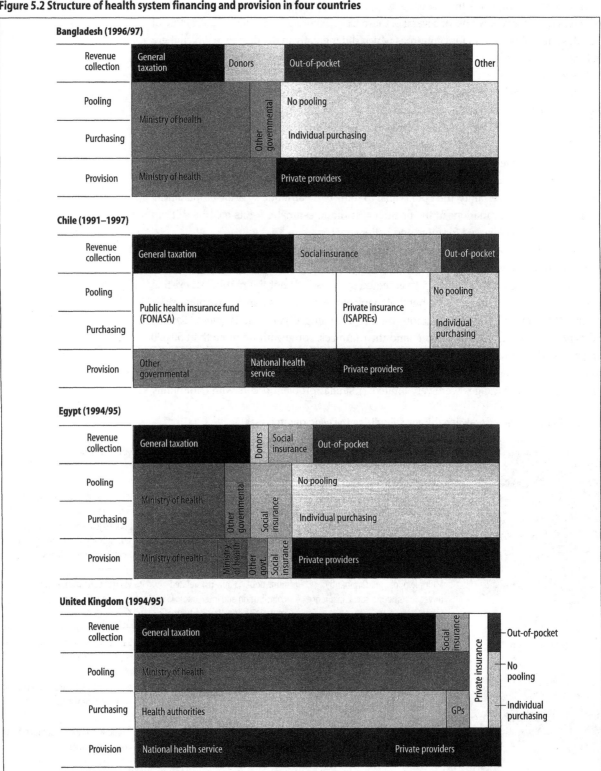

Note: Widths are proportional to estimated flows of funds.
Source: National health accounts estimates.

pooling arrangements in developing countries. Although an improvement over out-of-pocket financing, their size and organizational capacity often threatens their financial sustainability *(16, 17)*. Predominantly out-of-pocket financing represents the highest degree of fragmentation. In such a case, each individual constitutes a pool and thus has to pay for his or her own health services.

Larger is better for pooling and purchasing. But economies of scale show diminishing returns and, beyond a critical size, marginal benefits may be negligible. The argument for large pools is therefore not an argument for single pools when multiple pools can exist without fragmentation, and when their size and financing mechanisms allow for adequate spreading of risk and subsidization of the poor.

Health system policy with regard to pooling needs to focus on creating conditions for the development of the largest possible pooling arrangements. Where a particular country for the moment lacks the organizational and institutional capacity to have a single pool or large pools for all citizens, policy-makers and donors should try to create the enabling conditions for such pools. Meanwhile, policy-makers should promote pooling arrangements whenever possible, as a transitional stage towards the future aggregation of pools. Even small pools or pools for segments of the population are better than pure out-of-pocket financing for all. Opposing or neglecting such arrangements until the capacity exists for the establishment of an effective single pool has two drawbacks. It deprives consumers of improved protection. And it may prevent the state from regulating such initiatives and steering them towards future large or single pool arrangements. Introducing regulations such as community rating (adjusting for the average risk of a group), portable employment-based pooling (insurance that a worker keeps when changing jobs) and equal minimum benefit packages (access to the same services in all pools), in addition to protecting members of the pools, may pave the way for larger pooling in the future.

For low income economies where the formal sector is small, this means promoting pooling at the community level. Communities' lack of trust in local pooling organizations might be a limiting factor, but such initiatives offer an important opportunity for international cooperation whereby donors act as guarantor for the community and help create the necessary organizational and institutional capacity. For middle income developing countries, this means both encouraging the creation of pools and, where possible, either directly establishing a large pool or enacting regulation to specify a minimum size of pool for financial viability, as well as regulating pooling initiatives in a way that will facilitate consolidation in the future.

However, competition among pools is not entirely bad. It can increase the responsiveness of pooling organizations to their members and provide an incentive for innovation. It can also offer incentives for reducing costs (to increase market share and profits), for example through mergers, as in the reform of the quasi-public health insurance organizations (*Obras Sociales*) in Argentina in 1996. Lack of competition meant that the administrators were little concerned about high administrative costs and small benefits for their members, as they had in any case a captive group of contributors. Competition and the resulting mergers, together with explicit subsidies for low-income beneficiaries, have allowed members of small pools to join larger pools and obtain better benefits for the same level of contributions.

Despite its potential benefits, pooling competition poses significant problems to health systems, particularly in selection behaviour by both pooling organizations and consumers. Mandatory participation (that is, all eligible members must join the pooling organization) significantly reduces the scope of selection behaviour but does not totally eliminate the incentives associated with it, particularly under non-risk-related contribution schemes.

Selection behaviour is a potential problem of competition whenever and at whatever organizational level pooling is performed *(27, 28)*. It is particularly a problem for competition under non-risk-related contribution schemes. Either pooling organizations will try to pick the lowest risk consumers (risk selection), who will contribute but not cause expense, or the highest risk consumers will seek coverage more actively than the rest of the population (adverse selection). Pooling competition then becomes a battle for information between consumers (who usually know more about their own risk of requiring health interventions) and the pooling organization (which needs to know more about consumers' risks to ensure long term financial sustainability). This has significant consequences for the administrative costs of pooling organizations. If adverse selection predominates, pooling organizations end up with increasing costs, are obliged to demand increasing contributions, and may eventually face financial default. This applies not only to private health insurance schemes but also to community pooling arrangements. Evidence shows that managing adverse selection is a major challenge for community pooling arrangements *(17)*, which mostly rely on voluntary affiliation. If instead risk selection predominates, as is most likely when there is weak regulation of pooling competition, the poor and the sick will be excluded.

Exclusion from the pool is a problem that should be corrected through a combination of regulation and financial incentives. Regulation may cover such aspects as mandatory participation, non-risk-related contributions or community rating (the same price for a group of members sharing the same geographical area or the same workplace), and prohibition of underwriting (requesting additional information regarding health risks). Financial incentives may include risk compensation mechanisms and subsidies for the poor to join a pool. These approaches reduce the problems of pooling competition but are administratively expensive because of the high transaction costs within the system, associated with moving from hierarchical organizational arrangements for non-competitive pools to a market in pooling *(29, 30)*.

Regulation and incentives should also be directed to avoiding fragmentation of the pool as a result of competition. If organizational and institutional incentives are adequate, large pools are much more efficient than pooling competition. Single national pools, as the largest pools attainable and as non-competing organizations, might be seen as the most efficient way to organize pooling. They avoid fragmentation and all competition problems but also forego the advantages of competition.

In most health financing arrangements, pooling and purchasing are integrated within the same organization. Allocation of funds from pooling to purchasing occurs in the organization through the budgetary process. There are, however, a few instances in the world where attempts have been made to separate the functions and allocate resources from a pooling organization to multiple purchasers through risk adjusted capitation. For example, in Colombia *(31, 32)* and the USA *(33, 34)*, attempts have been made to take advantage of purchasing competition to minimize the pooling competition problems discussed above.

STRATEGIC PURCHASING

Health systems need to ensure that the package of health interventions they provide and finance responds to the criteria discussed in Chapter 3. They also need to ensure that the way interventions are provided helps to improve the system's responsiveness and financial fairness. Strategic purchasing is the way to achieve this.

But, as shown in Chapter 3, the burden of ensuring the effectiveness of health interventions rests mainly on the shoulders of providers. To play their role effectively, providers need adequate inputs and organizational arrangements, as well as coherent incentives, both within and from outside the organization. Purchasing plays a central role in ensuring coherence of external incentives for providers through contracting, budgeting and payment mechanisms.

Strategic purchasing faces three fundamental challenges: What interventions to buy? From whom to buy them? And how to buy them? Size is also important for purchasing organizations. Large purchasers can not only take advantage of economies of scale but also of better bargaining capacity (monopsony power) regarding price, quality and opportunity of services, in dealing with natural monopolies on the provider side.

Strategic purchasing requires a continuous search for the best interventions to purchase, the best providers to purchase from, and the best payment mechanisms and contracting arrangements to pay for such interventions. Identifying the best providers means getting the best deals (for example, fast access for patients to the contracted services). It means establishing strategic alliances for the future development of those providers and for disseminating their best practices to other providers.

The important role of public health and the technical characteristics of what interventions to provide are discussed in Chapter 3. In purchasing personal care, the determination of what interventions to buy takes place at two levels. One level is largely related to stewardship. Here, society determines (most of the time implicitly) the relative weighting of the goals of the system – health, responsiveness, and fair contribution to financing. It does so by determining priorities for the public financing of specific programmes, or via regulation and financial incentives for voluntary or mandated private financing. In the presence of weak stewardship, the relative weighting of health system goals is defined de facto by the purchaser and the market forces. The second level is the purchaser's responsibility. This means that the purchaser is responsible for the day-to-day identification of the interventions to achieve the system goals (as defined at the stewardship level), as well as the determination of co-payment and other financial aspects. It also means that the purchaser has authority for negotiating with providers with regard to the expected quantity, quality, and availability of the interventions to be purchased and provided.

Purchaser organizations also need to define from whom to buy. This definition is crucial in allowing them to avoid becoming involved in the micro-management of providers. In order to set incentives for cost control, an emphasis on preventive care, and maintaining or improving the quality of services, purchasers need to prioritize among *units* of purchasing: that is, whether to buy individual interventions, specified packages of care, all the care for individuals or groups, or all the inputs needed for that care. Each unit of purchasing needs to be of a critical size, and to include a wide enough diversity of individual providers to ensure an appropriate mix of services. Such units make it easier for the purchaser and the provider to agree on a payment mechanism in which the provider shares the risk with the purchaser (that is, the provider is partly responsible for a full range of interventions for a relatively fixed amount of money). The spectrum of risk sharing, from all the risk borne by the purchaser to all of it transferred to providers, is discussed in *The world health report 1999*.

With such units, it is also easier for purchasers to make long-term contracts with providers who would take care of all aspects of necessary health care for groups of members of the pool. If the purchasing unit is too small, the purchaser will have difficulty in agreeing on a risk sharing payment mechanism, because of the potential fragmentation of the pool, and will have to resort to traditional input purchasing or fee-for-service. Such a situation will force the purchaser to focus on short-term isolated interventions, as the absence of a risk sharing agreement will make it difficult to conclude a long-term contract for interventions for groups of the population. This will increase the overall administrative costs in the system relative to the volume of interventions involved.

With regard to how to buy, there are two objectives. The first is to avoid micro-purchasing, that is, such small scale buying of interventions that it constitutes the micro-management of providers. (There are, however, circumstances where micro-purchasing or micro-management may be justified, particularly for high complexity, very expensive and low frequency interventions.) The second is to design and implement effective contractual, budgeting and payment mechanisms. Avoiding micro-purchasing implies focusing the provisioning process on setting the right external incentives and evaluating results. The challenge here is to set purchasing goals that allow providers all necessary discretionary power in the provider–citizen contact, but which leave the purchaser the capacity to influence overall access to personal and non-personal services for members of the pool.

The budgeting and provider payment mechanisms are an essential part of the purchaser–provider interaction. Together with contracting, they establish an environment in which there are incentives for providers to act in accordance with the following four objectives: to prevent health problems of members of the pool; to provide services and solve health problems of members of the pool; to be responsive to people's legitimate expectations; and to contain costs.

No single budgeting or provider payment mechanism can achieve all four objectives simultaneously *(35)*. Table 5.3 summarizes the characteristics of the most common budgeting and payment mechanisms designed to meet those objectives. While line item budgets can be effective in controlling costs, they provide few incentives to achieve the other three objectives. In contrast, while fee-for-service provides strong incentives to deliver services, it also provides incentives that lead to an overall increase in the cost of the system. Therefore, purchasers need to use a combination of payment mechanisms to achieve their objectives. Free choice of provider by consumers increases responsiveness under all payment systems, but particularly under those needing to attract patients to ensure payment by the purchaser (fee-for-service or diagnostic related payment).

Capitation means a fixed payment per beneficiary to a provider responsible for delivering a range of services. It offers potentially strong incentives for prevention and cost control, to the extent that the provider receiving the capitation will benefit from both. If the contract is so short that a particular preventive intervention would have a noticeable effect only beyond the duration of the contract, there will be little or no incentive for prevention.

Table 5.3 Provider payment mechanisms and provider behaviour

Mechanisms \ Provider behaviour	Prevent health problems	Deliver services	Respond to legitimate expectations	Contain costs
Line item budget	+/–	– –	+/–	+++
Global budget	++	– –	+/–	+++
Capitation (with competition)	+++	– –	++	+++
Diagnostic related payment	+/–	++	++	++
Fee-for-service	+/–	+++	+++	– – –

Key: +++ very positive effect; ++ some positive effect; +/– little or no variable effect; – – some negative effect; – – – very negative effect.

Similarly, if the provider is not allowed to benefit from or reinvest the surplus resulting from savings, there is little incentive for cost control beyond that required for the financial sustainability of the provider organization.

Because of its advantages in cost control and prevention, capitation has been introduced in many purchasing organizations in the world. It has been used in the UK national health service with regard to general practitioners and later played a more important role in sharing risk with the introduction of general practitioner fundholding, allowing surpluses to be invested in the fundholder's practice *(6)*. It has also been used for provider networks in Argentina's social security organization for retirees *(23)*, in New Zealand with independent practice associations *(36)*, and in the United States with health maintenance organizations *(37)*. When risk-sharing payment mechanisms are used, depending on the specific terms of the payment mechanism, part of the pooling function of spreading risk among members of the pool may be performed by the provider. Thus, when an integrated pooling/purchasing organization contracts with smaller providers, each provider may also become a pooling organization. There is thus a risk of fragmenting the pool if the provider groups are too small. This has been the main argument for shifting from general practitioner fundholding to larger pools, the primary health care groups, in the UK in 1999.

Supply side provider payment mechanisms, such as line item budgets, focus purchasing efforts on inputs and make it impossible for providers to respond flexibly to external incentives. Too often these are the main resource allocation mechanisms for public providers in developing countries. As a result, providers do not continuously adapt their mix of services. This has been a serious barrier to improving health system efficiency in many developing countries *(38)*. It has also been a major obstacle to the improvement of public–private collaboration in the provision of services *(39)*. Line item budgets are in these respects much worse than global budgets, which also control costs.

What does moving to more flexible resource management at the provider level require? *The world health report 1999* introduced an answer to this question *(14)*: it means reaching more explicit agreements between purchasers and providers regarding services to be provided (performance agreements, quasi-contracts and contracts). Quasi-contractual arrangements refer to non-legally-binding explicit agreements between two parties, in this case between the purchaser and the provider. Resource management also requires the introduction of "money follows the patient" schemes, particularly where policies favouring the free choice of providers are introduced. Doing it well demands significant organizational and institutional capacity, along with propitious political conditions, particularly because of the potential consequences for public providers. Failure to develop such capacity and political conditions before or simultaneously with entering into contracting and demand side financing reforms can have negative consequences to judge from experience in India, Mexico, Papua New Guinea, South Africa, Thailand and Zimbabwe *(40, 41)*. Contracting out clinical services is particularly complex even when limited to non-profit providers such as church hospitals in Ghana, the United Republic of Tanzania and Zimbabwe *(42)*.

In summary, purchasers need to move from supply side payment to demand side provider payment mechanisms, from implicit to explicit contracting, and from fee-for-service to some form of risk sharing payment mechanisms. Contracting, shifting to demand side payment, and introducing risk sharing provider payment mechanisms require a high level of technical, organizational and institutional capacity, as well as significant political leverage because of the likely resistance of providers to bearing more risk and being held more accountable, particularly in the public sector.

ORGANIZATIONAL FORMS

The debate on policy alternatives for health system financing often focuses exclusively on technical aspects, underestimating the importance of organizational and institutional factors. Examples of the results of this approach include the provider payment mechanism reforms designed in the early 1990s in some Latin American countries (Argentina, Chile, Costa Rica, and Nicaragua) *(39)*. These reforms initially underestimated the importance of organizational and institutional effects, assuming that having the right price signals would be sufficient to change provider behaviour. It seems to have been assumed (explicitly or implicitly) that managers of public providers would – mainly by virtue of such new mechanisms as diagnostic-related payments or capitation – understand the price signals, know how to respond and be willing to act accordingly, despite the culture of their organizations. These reforms also underestimated the importance of and difficulties involved in providing managers with a flexible enough legal and administrative environment to make the correct changes. Furthermore, the reforms seem to have assumed that the government would be willing and able to deal with the political problems associated with such flexibility. Experience over the last 10 years shows that these assumptions are not always correct, and that more emphasis on organizational and institutional change is required to make provider payment reforms work.

Characteristics of provider organizations are analysed in Chapter 3. A similar analysis is valid for health financing organizations. Some of the most important factors affecting the performance of health financing organizations and, through it, the financial risk protection provided by the health system are discussed below.

In addition to contributing to the health system via out-of-pocket payment at the moment of demanding services, citizens also contribute to most health systems in the world through various combinations of the following *organizational forms*.

- *Ministry of health*, usually heading a large network of public providers organized as a national health service, relying on general taxation – collected by the ministry of finance – as the main source of revenue, and serving the general population.
- *Social security organization* (single or multiple, competing or not), mostly relying on salary-related contributions, owning provider networks or purchasing from external providers, and serving mostly their own members (usually formal sector workers).
- *Community or provider based pooling organization*, usually comprising a small pooling/purchasing organization relying mostly on voluntary participation.
- *Private health insurance fund* (regulated or unregulated), mostly relying on voluntary contributions (premiums), which may be risk-related but are usually not income-related, and are often contracted by an employer for all a firm's employees.

Providers can play a role as pooling organizations under a non-risk-adjusted capitation payment mechanism, as discussed above. In this scenario, internal incentives for providers coexist with internal incentives for financing organizations, which may impede coherence among incentives.

Each organizational form deals with the technical characteristics of health financing in a particular way. This is particularly evident in comparing private risk-related health insurance with social security. Social security organizations spread risk among the whole pool through non-risk-related contributions. All members of the pool pay a proportion of their salary, regardless of their risk. In contrast, voluntary private health insurance contributions charge the same premium only for the members of a similar risk category in the pool (such as the same sex, age and place of residence). There are multiple categories in private health insurance, and members are charged according to the risk category to which they belong. The social security and risk-related private insurance approaches are contradictory, and their coexistence creates different incentives for consumers. All consumers whose risk category is such that private insurance would charge them less than the amount that they would have to pay under social insurance have the incentive to avoid contributing to social insurance and use private insurance if they are allowed to. High-risk people, however, have the incentive to contribute to social security, loading it with high-risk members and increasing the per capita cost of services for members of the pool. The Chilean case, presented in Box 5.2, is an example of this phenomenon *(43)*, in which contributors can opt out of social security and direct their contributions to private insurers. The contradictory incentives can be controlled only if social insurance is mandatory.

Health financing functions are often integrated in a single organization. For ministries of health (or national health services), however, collecting is usually done by the ministry of finance. Some health systems with multiple social security organizations have introduced central collecting agencies in charge of risk equalization among pools (as in Colombia, Germany, and the Netherlands). Various attempts have been made to separate the pooling

---

Box 5.2 The Chilean health insurance market: when stewardship fails to compensate for pooling competition problems and for imbalances between internal and external incentives

In 1980, Chile implemented a radical reform of the health system. It separated financial administration in the public health sector from public providers and the Ministry of Health, creating the National Health Fund (FONASA), which is financed by a combination of general taxation (for the poor who also are included in the pool) and a 7% payroll tax contribution for formal sector workers. It simultaneously allowed for the introduction of private competing health insurance organizations (ISAPREs). All formal sector workers and their families have to contribute either to FONASA or an ISAPRE. All the rest of the population is covered by FONASA. In contrast with FONASA which charges all members the same 7% payroll tax irrespective of the risk, ISAPREs are allowed to adjust the contribution (with the 7% payroll tax as a minimum contribution) and the benefit package to the risk of the principal and his or her family. These organizational forms reflect opposing rationales. While FONASA is based on salary-related contributions with no exclusions, ISAPREs in practice are based on

risk-related contributions. Apart from the very limited power of the Ministry of Health, no regulatory agency was in a position to regulate ISAPREs until 10 years after they were created. As a result, ISAPREs grew from covering 2% of the population in 1983 to 27% in 1996.

Lack of regulation, weak stewardship (for political reasons), and an explicit policy to channel all cross-subsidies through FONASA only, resulted in severe segmentation of the market. ISAPREs focused on the

Health insurance of formal sector workers, enrolment in FONASA and ISAPREs by income level, Chile, 1994

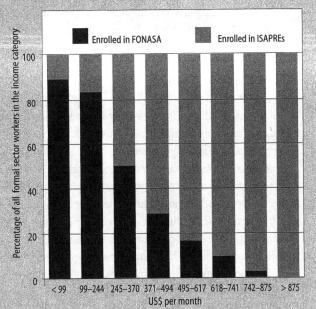

Source: ISAPREs Association and FONASA, 1995.

richest, and risk-selected the healthiest. Only recently has it been possible to introduce regulation to reduce risk selection. Segmentation has determined that while more than 9% of the total Chilean population is older than 60 years of age (generally the highest risk group in the population), that population group represents only about 3% of ISAPRE beneficiaries. At the same time, as shown in the graph, while almost all low income workers are in FONASA, very few are in the ISAPRE system. There is continued debate in Chile over reform of the health insurance system to address this structural problem.

Source: Baeza C, Copetta C. *Análisis conceptual de la necesidad y factibilidad de introducir mecanismos de ajuste de riesgo y portabilidad de los subsidios públicos en el sistema de seguros de salud en Chile. [Conceptual analysis of the necessity and feasibility of introducing mechanisms for risk adjustment and portability of public subsidies in the health insurance system of Chile.]* Santiago, Chile, Centro Latinoamericano de Investigación para Sistemas de Salud (CLAISS) and Fondo de Promoción de Políticas Públicas de la Universidad de Chile, 1999 (in Spanish).

and the purchasing functions (as in Colombia and the United States). The organizational separation of collecting and pooling is less frequent than the separation between purchasing and provision, and it has been less explored. It appears to be less important for setting the right incentives for providers than the separation between purchasing and provision as introduced under managed competition and internal market reforms *(44–47)*.

INCENTIVES

As for provider organizations described in Chapter 3, health financing organizations are subject to internal incentives. Organizational performance depends on the coherence of the following internal incentives.

- The level of *autonomy* or decision rights that the organization has *vis-à-vis* its owner, its overseeing authority or the government. Critical decision rights include setting contribution levels (premiums or payroll tax), co-payment levels, prioritization of interventions to be purchased, designing and negotiating contracts and provider payment mechanisms, selectivity in contracting with providers, and in many cases, freedom to determine investments.
- The degree of *accountability*. As autonomy increases, owners, overseeing authorities or the government require mechanisms to make the organization responsible for the expected results via hierarchical supervision, regulation or financial incentives.
- The degree of *market exposure*, that is, the proportion of revenues earned in a competitive way rather than acquired through a budget allocation. Particularly important for performance is whether governments provide budget supplements for deficits that originate from poor performance.
- The degree of *financial responsibility* for losses, and rights to profits (retained earnings and proceeds from the sale or rental of capital).
- The degree of *unfunded mandates*, that is, the proportion (in terms of revenues allocated) of mandates for which the organization is legally held responsible but for which it is not allowed to charge fees, and for which the organization does not receive any compensatory financial transfer. Such mandates may be to include the very poor or the very sick in the pool, as is usually the case for ministries of health or national health services. There may also be a mandate for the purchaser to pay for emergency care in a life-threatening situation, no matter where the care is provided and whatever the cost.

All prepaid health financing systems in the world are composed of combinations of the four organizational forms described above. It is clear that each organizational form has a different level of exposure to internal incentives. For example, ministry of health or ministry of finance organizations are much more likely to bear unfunded mandates than private insurance funds. Furthermore, because of the differences in market exposure and accountability between such organizations, their responses to unfunded mandates will be significantly different. While ministries of health or finance can respond to unfunded mandates by adjusting the quality or opportunity of interventions or even generating budget deficits, private insurance funds might respond by excluding members who are at a high risk of requiring the services required by the unfunded mandates. To avoid negative equity consequences, particularly under increasing autonomy, regulatory and financial incentives (e.g. risk compensation mechanisms) are necessary to protect the sick and the poor.

Another example of the significant differences in internal incentives concerns to whom each organizational form is accountable. Because ministries of health or finance are accountable to government, external incentives are required to make sure that they are also responsive to consumers. On the other hand, because private health insurance is accountable to owners and consumers, external incentives and regulation are needed to make sure that benefit packages and insurance practices are coherent with national priorities and policies regarding health, financial fairness and responsiveness. Often, as was the case with unregulated private health insurance in Argentina until 1996 *(23)*, private insurance responds to consumer demand by focusing benefit packages on low-cost and high frequency interventions, and excluding very high-cost and low frequency interventions (catastrophic events) which are most appropriately included in pooling arrangements. Regulating minimum benefits for all members, including coverage of catastrophic events by each fund or through re-insurance, is necessary in these circumstances.

Table 5.4 summarizes the level of each internal incentive for each of the four organizational forms.

To increase health system performance, stewardship has a major role to play in health financing. This is because external incentives are needed to compensate for differences in the internal incentives faced by the different health financing organizations.

A set of external incentives (rules and customs) governs the way the different organizational forms interact within the system. The three key external incentives that influence the behaviour of health financing organizations are the rules and customs relating to governance, public policy objectives, and control mechanisms.

- The rules and customs relating to *governance* shape the relationship between organizations and their owners. Ownership (public or private) usually provides the right to make decisions over the use of an asset and the right to the income that remains after all fixed obligations are met. Specification and limitation of these rights is often a major element of regulation.
- The rules and customs related to *public policy objectives* that influence the behaviour of organizations include budget implementation directives (for ministries of health or national health services), criteria for eligibility for public subsidies (for private insurers and community pools), and required auditing procedures.
- The rules and customs relating to *control mechanisms* shape the relationships between organizations and the public authorities, as well as between organizations

Table 5.4 Exposure of different organizational forms to internal incentives

Organizational forms / Internal incentives	Ministries of health or finance	Social security organizations	Community pooling organizations	Private health insurance funds
Decision rights (autonomy)	Limited	Variable but usually high	High	High
Accountability	Government, voters	Board/often government	Owners / consumers	Owners / consumers
Market exposure	None	Variable; high when multiple organizations compete	High	High
Financial responsibility	None or very limited	Low	High	High
Unfunded mandates	High	Low	None or very limited	None or very limited

and consumers. In this context, the public authorities are those involved in areas such as policy-making, regulation and enforcement. The public authorities have a range of instruments at their disposal with which to set external incentives for health financing organizations, ranging from hierarchical command and control (e.g. political or administrative instructions from the government to the ministry of health or national health service) to regulation and financial incentives. These instruments may include rules related to such subjects as the percentage of payroll tax to be devoted to financing social security organizations, the minimum contents of benefit packages, allowed exclusions and pre-existing conditions which must be covered, duration of contracts, commercialization and marketing restrictions, the pricing of private insurance, and the mandatory sending of information to the regulatory agencies.

As for internal incentives, the four organizational forms are subject to different degrees of exposure to the various external incentives. Table 5.5 summarizes the most important differences.

The difference between the external incentives for ministries of health or finance and private health insurance funds is particularly relevant. While hierarchical control influences ministries of health or finance, it has little or no influence on private insurance or community pooling arrangements. The introduction of private competitive health insurance (as an explicit policy option) or the growth of informal community pooling arrangements (or informal health insurance) require stewardship to shift from hierarchical control to using regulations and financial incentives as a means of influencing behaviour. This shift usually represents a significant change in the way control has traditionally worked. It requires an ability to anticipate and implement the necessary legal and administrative changes, and it demands a significant alteration in the skill mix and culture of control organizations.

Evidence from trends in health financing reforms in some eastern European and Latin American countries *(3, 48)* shows the potential negative effects of failure to strengthen control and shift to different external incentive instruments when private competitive health insurance is introduced. Risk selection is almost certain, taking high income low-risk consumers out of the public pools and worsening the financial situation of the latter.

To realize their potential, external and internal incentives should be coherent and aligned to address two fundamental problems increasingly evident in developing countries: the decision-making process being "captured" by other interests; and inefficiencies in supply side financing.

Table 5.5 Exposure of different organizational forms to external incentives

Organizational forms External incentives	Ministries of health or finance	Social security organizations	Community pooling organizations	Private health insurance funds
Governance	Public, low level of decision rights	Public or quasi-public with variable levels of decision rights	Private, high level of decision rights	Private, high level of decision rights
Financing for public policy objectives	High	Variable; government and market	None, except when receiving conditional public subsidies	None, except when receiving conditional public subsidies
Control mechanisms	Hierarchical control	Variable degrees of hierarchical control, regulations and financial incentives	Regulations and possibly financial incentives	Regulations and possibly financial incentives

As internal and external incentives make ministries of health or finance and even single social security organizations focus more on political concerns than on the interests of consumers, these organizations are particularly vulnerable to capture. In other words, decision-making in the pooling or purchasing organization is driven by interests other than health, responsiveness to beneficiaries and financial fairness. Capture may happen as a result of fiscal interests, corporate interests, union interests, political party interests, and so on. There are many examples of systems where social security revenues are used for fiscal purposes (a common problem in Latin America in the past) or where the government, as an employer, simply does not pay its social security dues under tripartite financing arrangements (workers, employers and government all contribute), as in Costa Rica during the 1980s. Strikes by physicians and their effects on salaries in national health services also show the vulnerability of such systems to capture by professional interests and illustrate one danger of large-scale public provision.

How financing affects equity and efficiency

The most important determinant of how fairly a health system is financed, as illustrated in Chapter 2, is the share of prepayment in total spending. Out-of-pocket payment is usually the most regressive way to pay for health, and the way that most exposes people to catastrophic financial risk. How revenues are collected therefore has a great impact on the equity of the system.

But even if nearly any form of prepayment is preferable, on these grounds, to out-of-pocket spending, it also matters greatly how the revenues are combined so as to share risks: how many pools there are, how large they are, whether inclusion is voluntary or mandatory, whether exclusion is allowed, what degree and kind of competition exists among pools, and whether, in the case of competing pools, there are mechanisms to compensate for differences in risk and in capacity to pay. All these features affect the fairness of the system, but they also help determine how efficiently it operates. The argument in favour of a single pool or a small number of pools of adequate size, and against fragmentation, concerns the financial viability of pools, the administrative costs of insurance, the balance between the economies of scale and (when there is little or no competition) the risks of capture and unresponsiveness, and the limitation of risk selection (which is a matter of efficiency as well as equity). Inefficiencies in collecting and pooling revenues reduce both the funds available for investment and for providing services, and people's access to those services that can be financed.

Purchasing, finally, also affects both equity and efficiency, by determining which investments are made and which interventions are bought, and for whom. Revenues may be collected fairly and with minimal waste, and be pooled so as to assure that the healthy help support the sick and the rich help support the poor. The performance of the system will still fall short of its potential if the pooled resources are not used intelligently to purchase the best attainable mixture of actions to improve health and satisfy people's expectations.

REFERENCES

1. **Musgrove P.** Reformas al sector salud en Chile: contexto, logica y posibles caminos [Reforms to the Chilean health sector: context, logic and possible trajectories]. In: Giaconi J, ed. *La salud en el siglo XXI.* Santiago, Chile, Centuro de Estudios Publicos, 1995 (in Spanish).

2. **Oyarzo C, Galleguillos S.** Reforma del Sistema de Salud Chileno: Marco Conceptual de la Propuesta del Fondo Nacional de Salud [Reform of the Chilean health system: conceptual framework of the National Health Fund proposal]. *Cuadernos de Economia,* 1995, **32**(95) (in Spanish).

3. **Preker A et al.** *Health financing systems in transition: trends in Eastern Europe and Central Asia.* Washington, DC, The World Bank, 1999 (World Bank Technical Paper, forthcoming).

4. **New Zealand Ministry of Health.** *Healthy New Zealanders: briefing papers for the Minister of Health 1996.* Wellington, Ministry of Health, 1996.

5. **Hornblow A.** New Zealand's health reforms: a clash of cultures. *British Medical Journal,* 1997, **314:** 1892–1894.

6. **Robinson R, Le Grand J.** *Evaluating the National Health Service reforms.* Oxford, Policy Journals, Transaction Books, 1994.

7. **UK Department of Health.** *Working for patients.* London, HMSO, 1989.

8. **UK Department of Health.** *The new NHS.* London, The Stationery Office, 1998.

9. **Gertler P, van der Gaag J.** *The willingness to pay for medical care: evidence from two developing countries.* Baltimore, MD, The Johns Hopkins University Press, 1990.

10. **Bitran R, McInnes DK.** *The demand for health care in Latin America: lessons from the Dominican Republic and El Salvador.* Washington, DC, Economic Development Institute of The World Bank, 1993.

11. **Lavy V, Quingley JM.** *Willingness to pay for the quality and intensity of medical care by low-income households in Ghana.* Washington, DC, The World Bank, 1993 (Living Standards Measurement Study, Working Paper No. 94).

12. **Nyonator F, Kutzin J.** Health for some? The effects of user fees in the Volta Region of Ghana. *Health Policy and Planning,* 1999, **14**(4): 329–341.

13. **Musgrove P.** *Public and private roles in health: theory and financing patterns.* Washington, DC, The World Bank, 1996 (World Bank Discussion Paper No. 339).

14. *The world health report 1999 – Making a difference.* Geneva, World Health Organization, 1999: 37–43.

15. **Shieber G, Maeda A.** A curmudgeon's guide to financing health care in developing countries. In: *Innovations in health care financing.* Proceedings of a World Bank Conference, Washington, DC, 1997.

16. **Bennett S, Creese A, Monash R.** *Health insurance schemes for people outside formal sector employment.* Geneva, World Health Organization, 1998 (document WHO/ARA/CC/98.1).

17. **ILO.** *Estudio de casos de esquemas de extension de cobertura en salud para el sector informal en America Latina* [*Case studies of schemes for extending health coverage for the informal sector in Latin America*]. Santiago, Chile, Centro Latinoamericano de Investigación para Sistemas de Salud (CLAISS), 1999 (in Spanish).

18. **Newhouse JP, Manning WG, Morris CN.** Some interim results from a controlled trial of cost sharing in health insurance. *New England Journal of Medicine,* 1981, **305:** 1501–1507.

19. **Abel-Smith B, Rawal P.** Can the poor afford 'free' health services? A case study of Tanzania. *Health Policy and Planning,* 1992, **7**(4): 329–341.

20. **Schefler R, Yu W.** Medical savings accounts: a worthy experiment. *European Journal of Public Health,* 1998, **8:** 274–276.

21. **Saltman RB.** Medical savings accounts: a notably uninteresting policy idea. *European Journal of Public Health,* 1998, **8:** 276–278.

22. **Londoño JL, Frenk J.** Structured pluralism: towards an innovative model for health system reform in Latin America. *Health Policy,* 1997, **41**(1): 1–36.

23. **World Bank.** *Argentina, facing the challenge of health insurance reform.* Washington, DC, The World Bank, 1997 (LASHD ESW Report 16402-AR).

24. **Baeza C, Cabezas M.** *Es necesario el ajuste de riesgo en los mercados de seguros de salud en América Latina?* [*Is risk adjustment necessary in health insurance markets in Latin America?*]. Santiago, Chile, Centro Latinoamericano de Investigación para Sistemas de Salud (CLAISS), 1999 (in Spanish).

25. **Van de Ven WP et al.** Risk-adjusted capitation: recent experiences in The Netherlands. *Health Affairs,* 1994, **13**(5): 120–136.

26. **Musgrove P.** *Equitable allocation of ceilings on public investment: a general formula and a Brazilian example in the health sector.* Washington, DC, The World Bank, 1996 (Working Paper No. 69).

27. **Arrow K.** Uncertainty and the welfare economics of medical care. *American Economic Review,* 1963, **53**(5): 941–973.

28. **Feldstein P.** *Health care economics.* New York, Delmar Publisher, 1993.

29. **Coase R.** The nature of the firm. *Economica,* 1937, **4**.

30. **Williamson O.** *The economic institutions of capitalism.* New York, The Free Press, 1985.

31. **Londoño JL.** Estructurando pluralismo en los servicios de salud: la experiencia Columbiana [Structuring pluralism in health services: the Colombian experience]. *Revista de Anàlisis Economico,* 1996, **11**(2) (in Spanish).

32. **Titelman D, Uthoff A.** *The health care market and reform of health system financing.* Santiago, Chile, ECLA, 1999.

33. **Weiner J et al.** Risk-adjusted Medicare capitation rates using ambulatory and inpatient diagnoses. *Health Care Financing Review,* 1996, **17**(3): 77–99.

34. **Actuarial Research Corp.** *Medical capitation rate development.* Annandale, VA, US Department of Commerce, 1996 (National Technical Information, 1996 PB 96214887).

35. **Barnum H, Kutzin J, Saxenian H.** Incentives and provider payment methods. *International Journal of Health Planning and Management,* 1995, **10**: 23–45.

36. **Wilton P, Smith RD.** Primary care reform: a three country comparison of budget holding. *Health Policy,* 1998, **44**(2): 149–166.

37. **Sekhri Feachem N.** Managed care: the US experience. *Bulletin of the World Health Organization,* 2000, **78**(6) (in press).

38. **Preker A, Feachem RGA.** *Market mechanisms and the health sector in Central and Eastern Europe.* Washington, DC, The World Bank, 1995 (Technical Paper No. 293).

39. **Baeza C.** *Taking stock of health sector reform in LAC.* Washington, DC, The World Bank, 1998 (World Bank Technical Discussion Paper, LASHD).

40. **Mills A.** Contractual relationships between governments and the commercial private sector in developing countries. In: Bennett S, McPake B, Mills A, eds. *Private health providers in developing countries: serving the public interest?* London, Zed Books, 1996.

41. **McPake B, Hongoro C.** Contracting out clinical services in Zimbabwe. *Social Science and Medicine,* 1995, **41**(1): 13–24.

42. **Gilson L et al.** Should African governments contract out clinical health services to church providers? In: Bennett S, McPake B, Mills A, eds. *Private health providers in developing countries: serving the public interest?* London, Zed Books, 1996.

43. **Baeza C, Copetta C.** *Análisis conceptual de la necesidad y factibilidad de introducir mecanismos de ajuste de riesgo y portabilidad de los subsidios públicos en el sistema de seguros de salud en Chile [Conceptual analysis of the necessity and feasibility of introducing mechanisms for risk adjustment and portability of public subsidies in the health insurance system of Chile].* Santiago, Chile, Centro Latinoamericano de Investigación para Sistemas de Salud (CLAISS) and Fondo de Promoción de Políticas Públicas de la Universidad de Chile, 1999 (in Spanish).

44. **Enthoven A.** *Reflections on the management of the National Health Service.* London, Nuffield Provincial Hospitals Trust, 1985.

45. **Enthoven A.** Managed competition of alternative delivery systems. *Journal of Health Politics, Policy and Law,* 1988, **13**: 305–321.

46. **Enthoven A.** The history and principles of managed competition. *Health Affairs,* 1993, **12**: 24–48.

47. **Ovretveit J.** *Purchasing for health: a multidisciplinary introduction to the theory and practice of health purchasing.* Buckingham, UK, Open University Press, 1995 (Health Services Management Series).

48. **Baeza C.** *Problemas y desafíos para el sistema de salud chileno en el siglo XXI [Problems and challenges for the Chilean health system in the 21st century].* Santiago, Chile, Centro Latinoamericano de Investigación para Sistemas de Salud (CLAISS), 1999 (Documentos para el Dialogo en Salud No. 3) (in Spanish).

CHAPTER SIX

How is the
Public Interest Protected?

Governments should be the "stewards" of their national resources, maintaining and improving them for the benefit of their populations. In health, this means being ultimately responsible for the careful management of their citizens' well-being. Stewardship in health is the very essence of good government. For every country it means establishing the best and fairest health system possible. The health of the people must always be a national priority: government responsibility for it is continuous and permanent. Ministries of health must take on a large part of the stewardship of health systems.

Health policy and strategies need to cover the private provision of services and private financing, as well as state funding and activities. Only in this way can health systems as a whole be oriented towards achieving goals that are in the public interest. Stewardship encompasses the tasks of defining the vision and direction of health policy, exerting influence through regulation and advocacy, and collecting and using information. At the international level, stewardship means influencing global research and production to meet health goals. It also means providing an evidence base to guide countries' efforts to improve the performance of their health systems.

6

HOW IS THE

PUBLIC INTEREST PROTECTED?

GOVERNMENTS AS STEWARDS OF
HEALTH RESOURCES

Stewardship is the last of the four health systems functions examined in this report, and it is arguably the most important. It ranks above and differs from the others – service delivery, input production, and financing – for one outstanding reason: the ultimate responsibility for the overall performance of a country's health system must always lie with government. Stewardship not only influences the other functions, it makes possible the attainment of each health system goal: improving health, responding to the legitimate expectations of the population, and fairness of contribution. The government must ensure that stewardship percolates through all levels of the health system in order to maximize that attainment.

Stewardship has recently been defined as a "function of a government responsible for the welfare of the population, and concerned about the trust and legitimacy with which its activities are viewed by the citizenry" (1). It requires vision, intelligence and influence, primarily by the health ministry, which must oversee and guide the working and development of the nation's health actions on the government's behalf. Much of this chapter, therefore, addresses the ministry's role.

Some aspects of stewardship in health must be assumed by government as a whole. Affecting the behaviour of health actors in other sectors of the economy, or ensuring the right size and skill mix of the human resources produced for the health system, may be beyond the ministry's reach. The government ought to ensure coherence and consistency across departments and sectors, where necessary by an overall reform of public administration.

Outside of government, stewardship is also a responsibility for purchasers and providers of health services who must ensure that as much health as possible results from their spending. And stewardship in health has an international dimension, relating to external assistance.

But government remains the prime mover. Today in most countries the role of the state in relation to health is changing. People's expectations of health systems are greater than ever before, yet limits exist on what governments can finance and on what services they can deliver. Governments cannot stand still in the face of rising demands. They face complex dilemmas in deciding in which direction to move: they cannot do everything. But in terms of effective stewardship, their key role is one of oversight and trusteeship – to follow the advice of "row less and steer more" (2, 3).

Stewardship has major shortcomings everywhere. This chapter examines some of them, then discusses important stewardship tasks. It considers the main protagonists involved, and strategies for implementing stewardship in different national settings. Finally, it brings together some of the messages from preceding chapters on policy directions for better-functioning health systems.

WHAT IS WRONG WITH STEWARDSHIP TODAY?

"Ministries of health in low and middle income countries have a reputation for being among the most bureaucratic and least effectively managed institutions in the public sector. Designed and initiated in the early 20th century and given wide responsibility for financing and operating extensive public hospital and primary care systems in the post-war period, they became large centralized and hierarchical public bureaucracies, with cumbersome and detailed administrative rules and a permanent staff with secure civil service protections. The ministries were fragmented by many vertical programmes which were often run as virtual fiefdoms, dependent on uncertain international donor funding" *(4)*.

The problems described above are familiar, in greater or lesser degree, in many countries today. The consequences are easy to see, but it is not always easy to see why the problems occur or how to solve them. Often that is because the stewards of health suffer specific visual impairments.

Health ministries often suffer from myopia. Because they are seriously short-sighted, ministries sometimes lose sight of their most important target: the population at large. Patients and consumers may only come into view when rising public dissatisfaction forces them to the ministry's attention. In addition, myopic ministries recognize only the closest actors in the health field, but not necessarily the most important ones, who may be in the middle or far distance.

Ministries deal extensively with a multitude of public sector individuals and organizations providing health services, many of which may be directly funded by the ministry itself. Often, this involvement means intensive professional supervision and guidance. But sometimes just beyond their field of vision lie at least two other groups with a major role to play in the health system: nongovernmental providers, and health actors in sectors other than health.

In their size and potential impact on achieving health goals, these little recognized individuals and organizations may be more important than the public resources directed through the health ministry. Yet information about them may be scant, and a policy approach towards them is often lacking. In Myanmar, Nigeria *(5)*, or Viet Nam, for example, privately financed and provided medical care is three or four times as big, in expenditure terms, as spending on public services. But the many different types of private providers in these countries are barely recognized in legislation and regulation.

Some large health insurance schemes in India currently have no legal status *(6)*. In Europe and the Americas, road traffic accidents rank fourth in the total burden of disease. Yet the main involvement of the health ministry is often as a steward of accident and emergency services, not as a force for prevention. Services funded from public sources are obviously the responsibility of government. But private finance and the provision of *all* health actions clearly need to be within the focus of government as overall steward of the public interest.

Ministries are also myopic in the sense that their vision does not extend far enough into the future. Investment decisions – new buildings, equipment and vehicles – frequently occupy the foreground, while the severe and chronic need to improve the balance between investment and recurrent funding fades into the hazy distance.

Tunnel vision in stewardship takes the form of an exclusive focus on legislation and the issuing of regulations, decrees, and public orders as means of health policy. Explicit, written rules have an important role to play in the performance of the stewardship function. But formulating regulations is relatively easy and inexpensive. It is also often ineffective, with ministries lacking the capacity to monitor compliance: there are seldom enough public health inspectors to visit all food shops and eating places or enough occupational safety inspectors to visit all factories regularly. On the rare occasions when sanctions are invoked they are too mild to discourage illegal practices or to affect widespread disregard of regulations.

Good stewardship needs the support of *several* strategies to influence the behaviour of the different stakeholders in the health system. Among these are a better information base, the ability to build coalitions of support from different groups, and the ability to set incentives, either directly or in organizational design. As authority becomes devolved, delegated and decentralized to a wide range of stakeholders in the health system, the repertoire of stewardship strategies needs to move away from dependence on "command and control" systems towards ensuring a cohesive framework of incentives.

Health ministries sometimes turn a blind eye to the evasion of regulations which they themselves have created or are supposed to implement in the public interest. A widespread example is the condoning of illicit fee collecting by public employees, euphemistically known as "informal charging". A recent study in Bangladesh found that unofficial fee payments were 12 times greater than official payment (7). Paying bribes for treatment in Poland is cited as a common infringement of patients' rights (8). Though such corruption materially benefits a number of health workers, it deters poor people from using services they need, making health financing more unfair, and it distorts overall health priorities.

In turning a blind eye, stewardship is subverted; trusteeship is abandoned and institutional corruption sets in. A blind eye is often turned when the public interest is threatened in other ways. For instance, doctors can remain silent through misplaced professional loyalty in the face of incompetent and unsafe medical practice by colleagues. A 1999 US study commented "whether care is preventive, acute or chronic, it frequently does not meet pro-

---

Box 6.1 Trends in national health policy: from plans to frameworks

National health policy documents have a long history, predating but stimulated by international concern for promoting primary health care. In many centrally planned and developing economies, health policies were part of a national development plan, with a focus on investment needs. Some health policy documents were only a collection of project or programme-specific plans. They ignored the private sector and often took inadequate account of financial realities and people's preferences. Implementation problems were common.

By no means all countries have formal national health policies: France, Switzerland, and the United States do not; Tunisia has no formal single national policy document; the UK produced its first formal document in the 1990s, Portugal in 1998. The lifespan of a policy depends on whether there are fundamental changes to the agenda: India is still using its 1983 plan; Mongolia, in economic transition, revised its 1991 policy in 1996 and again in 1998.

A shift is now occurring towards more inclusive – but less detailed – policy frameworks mapping the direction but not spelling out the operational detail, as in Ghana and Kenya.

A national health policy framework:[1]
- identifies objectives and addresses major policy issues;
- defines respective roles of the public and private sectors in financing and provision;
- identifies policy instruments and organizational arrangements required in both the public and private sectors to meet system objectives;
- sets the agenda for capacity building and organizational development;
- provides guidance for prioritizing expenditure, thus linking analysis of problems to decisions about resource allocation.

[1] Cassels A. *A guide to sector-wide approaches for health development*. Geneva, World Health Organization/DANIDA/DFID/European Commission, 1997 (unpublished document WHO/ARA/97.12).

fessional standards" *(9)*. Ensuring probity in decisions on capital projects and other large purchasing decisions (equipment, pharmaceutical orders), where corruption may be particularly lucrative, is another frequent challenge to good stewardship.

Some recent developments create opportunities for better vision and more innovative stewardship. Greater autonomy in decisions relating to purchasing and service provision, for example, shifts some responsibility away from central or local government. But it creates new tasks for government in overseeing that both purchasing and provision are carried out in accordance with overall policy. Accumulated experience of practices such as contracting is now available *(10)* and rapid technological advances enable the fast, inexpensive handling of huge amounts of information, thus making it easier in principle for stewards to visualize the whole health system.

The notion of stewardship over all health actors and actions deserves renewed emphasis. Much conceptual and practical discussion is needed to improve the definition and measurement of how well stewardship is actually implemented in different settings. But several basic tasks can already be identified:

- formulating health policy – defining the vision and direction;
- exerting influence – approaches to regulation;
- collecting and using intelligence.

These tasks are discussed below.

HEALTH POLICY – VISION FOR THE FUTURE

An explicit health policy achieves several things: it defines a vision for the future which in turn helps establish benchmarks for the short and medium term. It outlines priorities and the expected roles of different groups. It builds consensus and informs people, and in doing so fulfils an important role of governance. The tasks of formulating and implementing health policy clearly fall to the health ministry.

Some countries appear to have issued no national health policy statement in the last decade; in others, policy exists in the form of documents which gather dust and are never translated into action. Too often, health policy and strategic planning have envisaged unre-

---

Box 6.2 Ghana's medium-term health policy framework

In Ghana, after an extensive process of consultation, the following strategies were identified as providing the means to better performance in health.

- Re-prioritization of health services to ensure that primary health care services (i.e. services with maximum benefits in terms of morbidity and mortality reduction) receive more emphasis in resource allocation.
- The strengthening and decentralization of management within the context of a national health service.
- Forging linkages between private and public providers of health care to ensure consensus and that all resources are focused on a common strategy.
- Expansion and rehabilitation of health infrastructure to increase coverage and improve quality.
- Strengthening human resource planning, management and training as a means of providing and retaining adequate numbers of good quality and well-motivated health teams to provide the services.
- Provision and management of adequate logistics such as drugs and other consumables, equipment, and vehicles at all levels of the health system.
- Strengthening the monitoring and regulatory systems within the health service to ensure more effective implementation of programmes.
- Empowering households and communities to take more responsibility for their health.
- Improving the financing of health care by ensuring the efficient and effective use of all available resources from government, nongovernmental organizations, and private, mission and donor sources. Ways of mobilizing additional resources with a view to making the services more accessible and affordable will also be explored.
- Promoting intersectoral action for health development, particularly in the areas of food and nutrition, employment, education, water and sanitation.

Source: *Medium-term health strategy: towards vision 2020 Republic of Ghana.* Accra, Ministry of Health, 1995.

alistic expansion of the publicly funded health care system, sometimes well in excess of national economic growth. Eventually, the policy and planning document is seen as infeasible and is ignored. Box 6.1 sketches how comprehensive health planning has given way to a more flexible 'framework' approach. Ghana's 1995 medium-term health strategy identified ten ways in which the health system would contribute towards better health (see Box 6.2).

Public consultation occurs in some countries at the beginning of the policy formulation process. A "rolling" framework is sometimes used, and periodically updated and amended. In countries where external assistance forms an important part of the health system's resources, an important expansion of this approach to policy-making and implementation is represented by sector-wide approaches (SWAPs). The essence of SWAPs is that, under government leadership, a partnership of funding agencies agrees to work together in support of a clear set of policy directions, often sharing many of the implementation procedures, such as supervision, monitoring, reporting, accounting, and purchasing. Box 6.3 summarizes the development of SWAPs. Health planning thus shows signs of moving beyond investment programming and towards consensus statements on broad lines of policy and system development.

A policy framework should recognize all three health system goals and identify strategies to improve the attainment of each. Few countries have explicit policies on the overall goodness and fairness of the health system. Yet the need to combine these two values in governance can be traced far back in history *(1)*. Box 6.4 describes the ancient *Hisba* system of stewardship in Islamic countries, highlighting both its ethical and economic purposes. Public statements about the desired balance among health outcomes, system responsiveness and fairness in financing are yet to be made anywhere. Policy should (and in partial

---

Box 6.3 SWAPs: are they good for stewardship?

A sector-wide approach (SWAP) is a method of working that brings together governments, donors, and other stakeholders within any sector. It is characterized by a set of operating principles rather than a specific package of policies or activities. The approach involves movement over time under government leadership towards: broadening policy dialogue; developing a single sector policy (that addresses private and public sector issues) and a common, realistic expenditure programme; common monitoring arrangements; and more coordinated procedures for funding and procurement. Being engaged in a SWAP implies commitment to this direction of change, rather than

the comprehensive attainment of all these different elements from the start. It implies changes to the ways in which both governments and donor agencies operate, and in their required staff skills and systems.

This approach has begun to take root primarily in some of the most highly aid-dependent countries. It has been driven by both government and donor concerns about the results of historical approaches to development assistance, which have often involved a combination of 'social sector-blind' macroeconomic adjustment policies and 'sector-fragmenting' projects. Many of the countries are in Africa, for example, Burkina Faso, Ethiopia, Ghana, Mali, Mozambique, Senegal, Uganda, the United Republic of Tanzania, and

Zambia. The other cluster of countries discussing or actively engaging in a SWAP is in Asia: Bangladesh, Cambodia, and Viet Nam are examples.

The evolution of a SWAP takes time. In Ghana, before the Ministry of Health single sector programme was endorsed by donors, the country had already gone through 10 years of institutional development, 4 years of major policy/strategy work, 3 years of strengthening core management functions, 2 years of negotiations, planning and design, and 1 year of slippage and delays.[1]

Cambodia and Viet Nam are at the earliest stage of discussing sector policy with donors. In other countries, progress has been mostly towards developing and agreeing to

operate within a single sector policy and medium-term expenditure framework. Joint review missions have become a feature in some countries. Least progress has been made towards common financing and procurement arrangements.

SWAPs have the potential to support good stewardship. Walt and colleagues argue that SWAPs are perceived as capable of strengthening governments' ability to oversee the entire health system, develop policies and engage with stakeholders beyond the public sector.[2] But, most importantly, SWAPs depend on vision and leadership by national government.

[1] Smithson P. Cited in Foster M. *Lessons of experience from sector-wide approaches in health.* Geneva, World Health Organization, Strategies for Cooperation and Partnership, 1999 (unpublished paper).
[2] Walt G et al. Managing external resources in the health sector: are there lessons for SWAPs? *Health Policy and Planning,* 1999, 14(3):273–284.

ways sometimes does) address the way in which the system's key functions are to be improved.

With respect to the provision of services, all providers should be recognized and their future contribution – greater in some cases, less in others – should be outlined. On financing, strategies to reduce dependence on out-of-pocket payments and to increase prepayment should be identified. Roles of the principal financing organizations – private and public, domestic and external – and of households should be recognized and their future directions determined. The machinery of stewardship, designed to regulate and monitor how these functions change in accordance with policy, should also be made explicit. This is likely to involve opportunities for consumer representatives to balance provider interests.

Danger exists when particular lines of policy, or whole reform strategies, become associated with a specific political party or minister of health. Regardless of whether the policy is good or bad, it becomes highly vulnerable. When that minister or party leaves office the policy dies, usually before it has either succeeded or failed, because the next minister or administration is seldom willing to work under the predecessor's banner. Rapid turnover of senior policy officials, and a politically charged environment, are both hazards to good stewardship *(11)*. Establishing good stewardship can reduce exposure to "personality capture" of particular policy directions, by creating an informed constituency of stakeholder support, and ensuring that the interests, skills and knowledge needed to maintain a particular policy direction are widely distributed.

All remaining stewardship tasks concern the implementation of policy, as distinct from its formulation and promotion.

SETTING THE RULES, ENSURING COMPLIANCE

Regulation is a widely recognized responsibility of health ministries and, in some countries, of social security agencies. It covers both the framing of the rules to govern the behaviour of actors in the health system, and ensuring compliance with them. In keeping with

---

Box 6.4 Stewardship: the Hisba system in Islamic countries

The institution of Hisba was developed to carry out the function of stewardship in Islamic countries more than 1400 years ago. The *Hisba* system is a moral as well as a socioeconomic institution, whose raison d'être is to ordain good and forbid evil. The functions of the *muhtasib* (the head of *Hisba* system) can be classified into three categories: those relating to (the rights of) God; those relating to (the rights of) people; and those relating to both.

The second and third categories are related to community affairs and municipal administration. The

main foundation of *Hisba* was to promote new social norms and develop the required system to ensure the adherence of various sectors of society to these norms.

The first *muhtasib* in Islam was a woman called Al Shifa, appointed in Medina, the capital of the Islamic state, by the second calif, Omar ibn Al Khattab, almost 1450 years ago, and given authority to control the markets. Another woman called Samra bint Nuhayk was given a similar authority in Mecca, the second city, by the same calif.

The *muhtasib* could appoint technically qualified staff to investigate

the conduct of different crafts, trades and public services, including health services. The *muhtasib* received complaints from the public but could also order an investigation on his or her own initiative.

Medical services were also regulated by the Hisba system. Physicians and other health specialists had to pass professional examinations and possess the necessary equipment before being licensed. The *muhtasib* had to ensure compliance of practising physicians to moral and ethical norms, including equitable provision of services and protection of the public interest. In

the field of pharmaceutical services, technical publications were prepared, including monographs describing standards and specifications for various drugs as well as methods of quality assurance. The system also included inspections and enforcement mechanisms.

Like many other institutions, the Hisba system underwent drastic modification with the advent of western colonization: its functions were transformed into a number of secular departments and its moral content reduced.

Contributed by the World Health Organization Regional Office for the Eastern Mediterranean.
Source: Al-Shaykh al-Imam Ibn Taymiya. *Public duties in Islam: the institution of the Hisba.* Markfield, UK, The Islamic Foundation, 1985.

the policy-making and intelligence tasks, regulation has to encompass all health actions and actors, and not just those of the health ministry or the public sector. While the public health care system is often replete with regulations, few countries (with either high or low income) have developed adequate strategies to regulate the private financing and provision of health services. The rethinking of a consistent set of regulatory approaches to private providers and sources of finance, in line with national goals and priorities, is a top priority task in most countries.

Regulation can either promote or restrict. Since the private sector comprises many different players, national policy needs to distinguish carefully where to promote and where to restrict. A single position on the private sector is unlikely to be appropriate. In promotive terms, explicit incentives may be provided for private practice such as the sale of public assets, preferential loans, or donations of land. Tax incentives may be offered to promote private provision, with no or very little government regulation of providers' market behaviour. China re-legalized private practice in the 1980s and promoted joint public/private ventures in hospital ownership. Thailand's finance ministry offers tax incentives to private hospital investors.

At the other extreme, significant barriers to market entry have sometimes been created, such as a legal ban on private practice. This is still the case in Cuba and was previously in Ethiopia, Greece (for hospitals), Mozambique, the United Republic of Tanzania and several other countries. Between these extremes are policies that allow relatively free market entry, provide modest incentives, or have limited prerequisites for those wishing to enter the private market, including some standards for market behaviour and some level of oversight and enforcement.

Incentives for greater private sector opportunities in health are often sought by government agencies other than the health ministry, and by private investors themselves. Finance, trade, and development ministries often advocate greater private investment in health in line with overall economic liberalization strategies.

Promotive policies seem to work, contributing to growth in private finance and provision *(12, 13)*. But they have also had serious side-effects: rising inequities, uneven quality of care, and inefficiency. The health ministry needs to know in advance what conditions it will require for such investments to contribute to the efficiency, quality, or equity goals of the health system, and how to defend the view that health is *not* just like all other sectors.

The harm caused by market abuses is difficult to remedy after the fact. The United States is probably the best-documented case of regulators trying to catch up with private health insurers *(14)*. State governments have extensive laws, regulations and enforcement authority over private insurers in the USA to ensure fair competition, assure quality and generally protect consumers from fraudulent marketing. This regulatory framework took many years to develop and is still far from perfect: it does not guarantee insurance for everyone. Recent regulatory changes have improved access to, but not the affordability of, private insurance by small employers and individuals. Private employers have devised various ways of avoiding the rules, so as to come under the looser federal regulations. But the system prevents many of the worst abuses – financially unsound or unscrupulous insurers – and helps to ameliorate many market failures. Chile and South Africa have similar experiences in regulating private health insurance practice. South Africa has recently changed earlier regulations governing medical schemes to reduce risk selection and increase risk pooling (see Box 6.5).

Chile has been unable to establish explicit contractual obligations for private insurers or prohibit risk selection by these private companies, due to the political influence of insurers and their clients. If there is a long delay between market entry and the enforcement of rules regarding market behaviour, experience suggests that the task of instituting those rules will become politically very difficult *(15, 16)*.

A more moderate form of incentives for private sector involvement are represented by contracts between public purchasers and private providers. In Lebanon, for example, 90% of hospital beds are in the private sector and nongovernmental organizations provide ambulatory care to about 10–15% of the population, particularly to the poor. Out of necessity, the Ministry of Health contracts with almost all private hospitals for a predetermined number of beds to serve public patients *(17)*. But the government does not use this regulatory tool to its advantage. Reimbursement policies allow unnecessary hospitalizations and overuse of services, which result in cost escalation; and private hospitals operate in a largely unregulated environment, which leads to uncontrolled investment. This in turn can lead to pressure for sustained public financial support, which will appear to justify further investment. Stewardship needs to ensure consistency in the incentive messages sent out by different levels of public policy.

Regulation requires resources. Regulatory oversight and contractual strategies entail high transaction costs for both government and providers or insurers, which may reduce the potential cost savings of these strategies. High levels of awareness of these costs accompanied the moves to separate the roles of purchasers and providers in the United Kingdom and New Zealand *(18)*. Often, lack of commitment and funds hamper government capacity to carry out regulatory responsibilities, old as well as new. This suggests that capacity building in contracting skills and regulatory oversight is critically needed both via recruitment of skilled staff and through training and technical aid to existing staff.

Box 6.5 South Africa: regulating the private insurance market to increase risk pooling

The government which came to power in 1994 after South Africa's first democratic elections found itself with a health sector which mirrored the inequalities existing in the wider society. A long-established and well-developed private health care industry accounted for 61% of health care financial resources, while providing for the needs of only the affluent 20% of the population. The vast majority of the population had to rely upon poorly distributed, underfunded and fragmented public services. Cost escalation in the private sector typically exceeded inflation during most of the late 1980s and 1990s. The private sector responded to this by limiting benefits, increasing co-payments and accelerating the exclusion of high-risk members from cover, thereby heightening the problem of inequality.

The new government's response to these challenges was to enact new legislation for medical schemes to offer a minimum benefits package and increased risk pooling. The fundamental principles and objectives at the core of the Act are as follows.

- *Community rating.* For a given product or option, the only grounds on which premiums may be varied are family size and income. Risk or age rating are prohibited.
- *Guaranteed access.* No-one who can afford the community rated premium may be excluded on grounds of age or health status.
- *Increased risk pooling.* Caps on the permissible contributions and accumulations through individual medical savings accounts will ensure that a greater proportion of contributions flows into the common risk pool.
- *Promoting lifetime coverage.* Community rating and guaranteed access will be combined with premium penalties for those who choose only to take out cover later in life, to provide powerful incentives for affordable lifetime membership.
- *Prescribed minimum benefits.* Every medical scheme must guarantee to cover in full the cost of treating a specified list of conditions and procedures in public facilities, thus greatly decreasing the impact of "dumping" patients onto the state.

A committee of inquiry was appointed by the health minister during 1995. It set up a small technical team to prepare new regulations for medical schemes. The team produced its first discussion document in 1996, and consulted widely with key stakeholders on its proposals. Discussion and debate continued until mid-1997, when a formal policy paper resulted.[1] After a period of intense, open debate during the legislative process, the new Medical Schemes Act and its accompanying Regulations came into force on 1 January 2000, three and a half years after the committee was formed. One important group will benefit immediately: HIV-positive members of medical schemes now have access to subsidized care, including drugs for opportunistic infections, whereas previously they were excluded or their entitlement was limited to very low benefit levels.

Contributed by T. Patrick Masobe, Department of Health, South Africa.
[1] *Reforming private health financing in South Africa: the quest for greater equity and efficiency.* Pretoria, Department of Health, 1997.

Shortcomings in staff skills or resources are often cited as the cause of outdated regulatory frameworks, or those which are not adequately enforced (4). Lack of legislative authority, too, is sometimes at fault. For example, in the late 1970s, Sri Lanka deregulated private practice by government doctors and liberalized the economy in general, which increased availability of capital (19). However, the health ministry failed to register effectively the growing number of private providers. It had no regulatory strategy, no staff responsible for private sector relations, and it lacked adequate legislative authority to take on many tasks. The only law on the books required registration of nursing homes, but not private clinics or doctors. A law has been pending since 1997 but has not yet been implemented. However, a new Ministry of Health unit for development and regulation of the private sector was set up in 1998.

In Egypt, most physicians work simultaneously for the government and in private practice. As a result, much of their work escapes oversight and regulation. Similar practice is widespread in Latin America. In India, mechanisms for monitoring, let alone regulating, the private sector have not kept pace with its expansion, despite concerns about quality of care. Health professionals are aware of practice-related laws but know that enforcement is weak or non-existent and that professional associations, which are nominally responsible for self-regulation, are also ineffective.

When public providers illegally use public facilities to provide special care to private patients, the public sector ends up subsidizing unofficial private practice. It is nearly impossible to completely prohibit private practice by health workers on the public payroll, but several steps can be taken to ensure that private practitioners compete on a fair basis and do not flourish by "moonlighting" at public expense (20, 21). Ensuring that patients, the public, and the media, as well as providers, know the rules is an important factor in regulating the public–private mix.

Effective public services themselves can be a regulatory tool. Developing effective public provision and financing systems becomes even more important if government policy seeks to restrict the development of a private health market, or when it lacks the resources to prevent undesirable market failures. The public sector must then respond to the changing needs of consumers, to the introduction of new medical technologies, and to reasonable expectations of health professionals. A strong public sector may even be a very good strategy for regulating private provision and for consumer protection, if it helps to keep the private sector more competitive in price and quality of service.

Too often, however, it is the public sector which is seen as uncompetitive in terms of quality and responsiveness, in spite of its free or subsidized services. If the public system deteriorates or does not continually improve, an unhealthy amount of resources and attention will be siphoned off trying to catch offenders in the "black market", and growing under-the-table payments will undermine equity goals.

Rules rarely enforced are invitations for abuse. Stricter oversight and regulation of private sector providers and insurers is now on the policy agenda of many countries. But progress is slow if not impossible. This suggests that countries must not only consider the impact of the private sector on the public sector and develop the regulatory framework to limit deleterious effects, but must make a continuing commitment to enforce the rules by investing in the knowledge and skills of regulatory staff. A study in Sri Lanka concluded, "the slow response in the 1980s makes the regulatory task in the 1990s more difficult: uncoordinated and unmonitored private sector growth has created a market context which is bigger, more complex, and with more established provider and user interests" (19).

Professional self-regulation, as distinct from personal self-interest, supports good practice. In establishing a professional organization, health workers assume several of the basic tasks of stewardship – identifying and certifying members, sharing experience, and sometimes offering in-service training. Small amounts of financial support to such organizations can ensure that basic information needed on non-government providers, particularly in ambulatory care settings, is available to the ministry of health. In several East African countries where religious groups are important providers of health services, central, nongovernmental coordinating bodies already perform this role. National medical associations are common; associations of traditional practitioners also exist.

Recent reforms in the Netherlands demonstrate the difficult balancing act between stronger regulation to protect consumers and increase equity, and looser rules to allow more competition (see Box 6.6).

Developing countries have also implemented policies which help ensure that private actors work on behalf of the larger public good. In addition to the South African example in Box 6.5, Bangladesh's National Drug Policy, adopted in 1982, prohibits importation and sale of all non-essential drugs. As a result, about 1666 products that were judged ineffective or harmful were banned, while about 300 were approved for marketing. The government also oversees production quality of all manufacturers and provides training to drug retailers on rational drug use. "Through a combination of public sector oversight and private initiative, essential drugs have been placed within reach of large numbers of the population, [and there are] reasonable and stable drug prices for products ... produced locally" *(22).*

Regulation requires dialogue. In countries with stronger oversight of the private sector, governments for the most part place their regulatory structure at arms-length from the regulated private players. If they do not, the private sector can subvert the system through "regulatory capture", i.e. coopting regulators to make the regulations more favourable to them. But "arms-length" does not mean no communication. Dialogue between public policy-makers or regulators and private sector players is a critical factor in making such regulations work. Governments must not only see well for good stewardship, they must also listen. Groups that have both public and private representation provide valuable input into policy development and rule-writing by assessing how private sector players can contribute to public policy goals without compromising their ability to succeed in the market. The drawback of such processes is that they may slow the pace of reform. And even with strong oversight and regulation, private sector players can weaken the regulatory apparatus through political pressure.

In conclusion, the following important lessons for the development of regulatory frameworks for private health markets are clear.

Box 6.6 Opening up the health insurance system in the Netherlands

The Netherlands' new health insurance system, authorized in 1990, for the first time required all private insurers to provide a comprehensive uniform benefits package. But it promoted competition by giving individuals a subsidy to help them buy compulsory health insurance from competing insurers. Insurers receive risk-adjusted per capita payments by the government and a separate flat rate premium from each insured person. The more efficient the insurer, the lower the premium paid by the insured. Insurers were also allowed to negotiate lower fees than officially approved provider fees, which was previously prohibited. As a result, private health insurers entered the market for the first time since 1941, and both insurers and providers became involved in quality improvement efforts, which became the focus for competition among insurers rather than competition only on price.[1] But the new system made the goal of reducing health-related inequalities more difficult, as better-off individuals can prepay for more inclusive benefit packages.[2]

[1] Van de Ven W, Schut F. Should catastrophic risks be included in a regulated competitive insurance market? *Social Science and Medicine,* 1994, 39(1): 1459–1472.
[2] Saltman RB, Figueras J, Sakellarides C, eds. *Critical challenges for health care reform in Europe.* Buckingham, UK, Open University Press, 1998.

- Frameworks should be instituted *prior* to any significant planned expansion through economic incentives and forcefully implemented as soon as the private market starts to respond to incentives.
- Regulatory policies must be continually reviewed to ensure consistency with changing political scenes.
- Improving quality, increasing access to care, and promoting efficiency each require different regulatory tools.
- Regulators must strike a balance between avoiding regulatory capture by private interests and maintaining productive dialogue with them to ensure that regulatory frameworks are realistic.
- Where governments choose to restrict the activities of the private sector, they must ensure that the public sector responds effectively to the needs of consumers.

Governments must make a continuing commitment to enforce regulations and rules by investing in the knowledge and skills of regulatory staff to keep pace with market developments.

EXERCISING INTELLIGENCE, SHARING KNOWLEDGE

Stewardship is about vision, intelligence and influence. Without a good understanding of what is happening in the entire health system, it is impossible for the ministry of health to develop strategies to influence the behaviour of the different interest groups in ways that support, or at least do not conflict with, the overall aims of health policy.

A good intelligence system in the sense of both information and understanding needs to be selective in the information it generates for decision-making at the top. But it must be drawn from grass-roots knowledge. Who are the principal service deliverers, and what challenges do they pose to health policy goals? Where are the main imbalances or bottlenecks in input production, and what policy options appear most suitable? Where are the major financing sources and what strategies will achieve greater and more equitable prepayment? What are the main uses of financing and what policies will ensure more efficient resource allocation?

Most health systems collect huge amounts of information that can clog the works. Such information may include accounts, personnel records, inventories, vehicle log books, activity reports (daily, by programme, department, ward, prescription and patient) at each health facility, and patient records. In many ministries of health, thousands of clerical hours each month are wasted in compiling information that is never used. As a general management rule, the amount of information passed up the system should be greatly reduced for each level.

For stewardship purposes, only periodic summaries, showing geographical or temporal variation, may be required. Information on the distribution and activity of public sector health inputs and on budgetary allocations may reveal important and unjustified variations. But of greater importance for stewardship are the missing pieces of information and analysis. Few low and middle income countries today have reliable information on the levels and sources of non-government finance or provision in the health system. As the national health accounts indicators in Annex Table 8 show, these are typically dominant in such countries. Little is known in most countries about peoples' expectations of the health system or about the structure of complex non-government provider markets. Without these data, assessments of responsiveness and fairness in financing, or of intermediate measures such as service quality and accessibility, are impossible. Without the full picture, good stewardship cannot be practised.

Intelligence requires resources. Stewardship requires a different type of information and understanding from that required in the daily management of service delivery. Should the ministry of health collect it? There is no reason to assume that the resource and skill cost of stewardship intelligence is greater than that of traditional health management systems. Of course, new skills in the area of regulation, coordination and communication are needed. But the ministry of health may already have several advantages.

First, the dispersed national network of public sector health workers and managers provides skilled people for undertaking inventory or survey work. District level health workers can rapidly compile an initial register of non-government providers. Second, the ministry of health has the moral authority to license and accredit providers, so it can engage its staff in the assessment process. Third, health workers have frequent contact with the population and are well placed to ask people about public goals and personal expectations. So the ministry of health can be a formidable potential resource for better stewardship, beginning with its engagement for better intelligence on the entire system.

However, not all of the intelligence gathering, or sharing, will be best done by the ministry. Research institutes, university departments, nongovernmental organizations *(23, 24)* and local or international consulting firms may be able to undertake inventory and survey work more speedily and accurately. To manage them, the ministry will need to draw on skills in contract setting and oversight.

Stewardship also requires information for influencing behaviour and events. Information dissemination provides support, for instance, to both policy-making and regulation. It also allows the ministry to build a constituency of public support for health policy, and thus a defence against incompetent or corrupt practice by interest groups in the health system. It helps to achieve a public debate on policy directions that is based on reliable evidence. A strategy for disseminating technical information can also form part of a capacity-building

---

Box 6.7 Responsiveness to patients' rights

Since the end of the 1970s there has been a slowly growing recognition of the rights of patients, such as respect for the dignity of the individual and for autonomy.

Rapid advances in medical and health sciences and in technology have hastened increases in patients' expectations: better-informed patients have begun to assert their rights in their dealings with professionals. To a growing extent, patients' rights are incorporated into statutory regulations: in laws on specific subjects, or in citizens' rights covering sectors broader than health care. Regulation may give patients direct legal rights in their relationships with health care providers, or may help to improve their position through

administrative health laws and hospital certification, for example. Self-regulation – voluntary arrangements in the form of professional codes or model contracts worked out in cooperation between consumers and health care providers' organizations – also have a role to play. Legislation opens new domains for self-regulation: framework laws on privacy and confidentiality, for example, may oblige institutions to elaborate their own guidelines for the protection of patients' data.

Three types of approaches can be distinguished in national legislation on patients' rights. Some countries have enacted a single comprehensive Law (e.g. San Marino in 1989, Finland and Uruguay in 1992, the Netherlands in 1994, Israel and

Lithuania in 1996, Argentina and Iceland in 1997, Denmark in 1998, and Norway in 1999). Other countries have integrated patients' rights into legislation regulating the health care system or into several health laws (e.g. Canada (New Brunswick) and Greece in 1992, France in 1992–94, Austria in 1993, Hong Kong in 1995, Belarus and Canada (Ontario) in 1996, Georgia and Guinea in 1997, and the USA in 1999). Charters on the rights of patients, which have varying status as national policy or are often embodied in the regulations of health care establishments, have been found more appropriate to the legal traditions of some countries, such as France (1974–95), Ireland (1991), the United Kingdom (1991–95) and Portugal (1997).

Informed consent, access to medical records, and the confidentiality of data are the classic rights of patients. New rules for the protection of personal data in medical data banks or automated hospital information systems are also being developed. In recent years the right to privacy has given rise to new individual concerns such as the right to be notified when personal data are first recorded in a data bank, the right to have inexact or incorrect data corrected or destroyed, and the right to be informed about the disclosure of information to third parties.

programme within the health system, and particularly within the ministry of health.

Information dissemination should focus on getting the most difficult tasks of stewardship into the open, both to inform and to consult. Priority setting in health, discussed in Chapter 3, has only recently been conducted as a public debate in a small number of countries. The debate is often noisy and confused because it lacks rules. The ministry's role is to clarify the rules: priority setting should take into account the burden of illness, the cost-effectiveness of available interventions, and the scale of existing action to address the problem. And it can listen to expressed preferences regarding the value basis of priority setting, as occurred in Sweden and Oregon, USA *(25)*. The rights and obligations of different players can be clarified through dissemination strategy in ways which reinforce the concerns of policy. For example, in situations with prevalent informal charging for care, providers may at least be required to display publicly the full costs of procedures, and patients invited to register complaints where additional charging occurs.

Many countries have already taken steps to safeguard the rights of patients, as shown in Box 6.7. Even without legislation, the notion of patients' rights and providers' obligations can be promoted and given substance by active stewardship. Where particular practices and procedures are widely practised and known to be harmful, the ministry as a steward has a clear responsibility to combat these with public information. Pharmaceutical sales by unregistered sellers, the dangers of excessive antibiotic prescription and of non-compliance with recommended dosages should all be objects of public stewardship, with active support from information campaigns targeted at different actors – patients, the providers in question, and local health authorities. Box 6.8 illustrates how for one key input – pharmaceuticals – actions at different levels are needed.

Box 6.8 Towards good stewardship – the case of pharmaceuticals

Most curative and many preventive health actions depend on medicines. However, medicines also involve powerful economic interests. In poor countries over 50% of household expenditure on health is spent on medicines: within government health budgets pharmaceuticals are usually the second largest item after wages. In industrialized countries drug costs are increasing by 8–12% per year, much faster than consumer prices. Many stakeholders are concerned with pharmaceuticals: manufacturers (both research-based and generic), consumer groups, professional associations, service providers of all types, donor agencies, and different departments of government.

The health system must make essential drugs available and affordable to all who need them, en-sure that drugs are of good quality, and that they are used in a therapeutically sound and cost-effective way. The following are the core roles of central government to achieve these objectives:

- ensuring the quality of medicines through effective regulation including systems for market approval, quality assurance, licensing of professionals and inspection of facilities;
- ensuring the affordability and adequate financing of essential drugs for the poor and disadvantaged;
- procuring essential drugs for public sector providers, or establishing central tendering with prime vendor or delivery contracts for regional and lower levels;
- developing and supporting a national programme to promote rational and cost-effective drug

use by health workers and the public;
- coordinating the activities of all stakeholders through the development, implementation and monitoring of a national policy.

Good stewardship at the international level includes supporting governments in fulfilling these core roles. External support may also be useful in the following areas:

- nongovernmental organizations, professional and consumer networks, religious bodies, universities, and private providers need information support and management training;
- national pharmaceuticals manufacturers need training, support and supervision in good manufacturing practice;
- regulations, training programmes and financial incentives are

needed to encourage rational drugs use in the private sector.

The international community must ensure that the overwhelming health problems of the world's poorest countries feature on the agenda of drug manufacturers; mechanisms such as the Global Alliance on Vaccine Initiatives and the Medicines for Malaria Venture are intended to do this.

In the technically and politically complex field of pharmaceuticals, external agencies may need guidance on the best types of support to give developing countries. For example, guidelines for good drug donation practice[1] are available to maximize the value of donated pharmaceuticals.

[1] *Guidelines for drug donations, 2nd ed.* Geneva, World Health Organization, 1999 (document WHO/EDM/PAR/99.4).

Broader information allowing comparisons of per capita health resources, and of health goal attainment by geographical area, are a way of spreading the stewards' concern about avoidable variations by creating public awareness. Without such awareness based on reliable information, government lacks an effective bulwark against incompetence and corruption in the form of personal or professional capture.

A recent study analysing initiatives in India, by the state governments of Delhi, Punjab and Rajasthan, to attract private investors into joint hospital ventures illustrates how the tasks of stewardship matter *(26)*. All three schemes failed: no joint venture resulted. Different factors came into play in each situation, but the report identifies failure in each of the above tasks of stewardship in the overall explanation. It specifically identifies:

- inadequate policy on the role of the private sector by each state;
- insufficient consultation with relevant stakeholders, and absence of mechanisms for coordination among the parties concerned;
- absent, weak or inappropriate regulation machinery related to private providers;
- ineffective performance monitoring and information sharing arrangements, making public–private partnerships vulnerable to inefficiency and high cost.

Requisite skills for carrying out these tasks were found to be lacking in the health departments of all three states.

STRATEGIES, ROLES AND RESOURCES: WHO SHOULD DO WHAT?

The previous sections discussed three basic tasks of stewardship and the principal role of the ministry of health in ensuring their implementation. This section considers *how* those tasks can be implemented, and what are the potential contributions of other groups and agencies to overall stewardship.

"Virtual" health systems, as described in Chapter 3, comprise many autonomous and semi-autonomous actors in different sectors of the economy, as well as those directly under the full authority of the ministry. The skills and strategies which have traditionally controlled public bureaucracies are inadequate for stewardship of contemporary health systems. Entrepreneurial, analytical and negotiating skills are needed to steward such systems. "Virtual" systems are held together by a shared policy vision and information, and by a variety of regulatory and incentive systems designed to reward goal achievement and punish capture, incompetence and fraud. An informed population of consumers helps in holding such a health system together.

Better stewardship requires an emphasis on *coordination, consultation and evidence-based communication* processes. For the ministry of health to understand the principal challenges to better performance it must have a full picture of what is happening. Initial engagement of other departments (education, finance, transport) may most effectively be done through government as a whole, rather than in bilateral approaches by the ministry of health, but the latter will need to provide evidence and continue the dialogue. Ministries of health can learn much from changing practice in other parts of government, where public roles have already greatly altered. And relevant international experience provides a major source of potential learning.

Ministries need to listen to a wider range of voices and to put the public case on health priorities and strategies forcefully and imaginatively. To ensure that the tasks of stewardship are carried out and delegated, the identity of all health actors should be known to the ministry of health, and regular lines of communication established. Special studies have sometimes been necessary *(26)* to assess the scale and content of private practice in health.

The ministry of health also needs communication capacity and strategies for ensuring that the media are aware of the health system's goals and progress or obstacles. Some ministries of health have offices responsible for private sector, media, and cross-sector liaison with other health players, and for consumer and public relations. In Thailand's experience, for example, skilful use of national media ensures that the Ministry of Public Health can amplify its own influence by judicious use of support (see Box 6.9).

Consultation is often a widely neglected part of the policy process, both in policy formulation and in implementation. A lack of consultation led to a public campaign of opposition by the British Medical Association to the reforms in Britain's national health service, introduced by the Thatcher administration in 1989 *(27)*.

Kenya introduced its cost-sharing policy with substantial increases in user fees in December 1989. The press featured a number of hardship stories as a result of cost-sharing. The following August, a presidential announcement was made abandoning the policy. Fee policy was subsequently re-introduced in a phased way, beginning at specialist hospitals, with a much greater emphasis on staff training and familiarizing the public *(28)*. Health system reforms in the United Republic of Tanzania and Zambia benefited from the Kenyan experience. They made great efforts to ensure that the reform programme was debated publicly, and that health workers were also involved in decisions about the reform process *(29)*. Finland's system of democratically elected municipal health boards is cited as a good example of how to ensure citizens' participation and empowerment in health *(30)*.

In many settings a sensible strategy to improve information for stewardship would be to begin with a review of key information needs for performance monitoring; develop strate-

---

Box 6.9 Thailand: the role of the media in health system stewardship

Thailand is becoming a more open and responsive society. The 1997 Constitution foresees full democratic participation by the individual, community and civic society. The Public Organization Act (1999) grants government units autonomy, in close collaboration with civic society. Several public hospitals are being given autonomous status. Remaining public hospitals are setting up boards consisting of local lay members.

The Public Information Act (1998) further promotes transparency and social accountability through guaranteed citizen rights to government information. Amidst these reforms the media have played an important role in reflecting the public needs, and

have helped in shaping several key health policies. A Council of Journalists sets standards for ethical conduct and fosters balanced public information in the media. Regular public opinion polls help serve as an effective interface between the public and policy-makers.

The Ministry of Public Health has a long history of engaging support from many stakeholders, including the press and broadcasting media. Recent efforts have mobilized medical bodies and nongovernmental organizations to put sustained and public pressure on the government to promulgate two important laws, the Tobacco Products Control Act (1992) and the Non-smoker Health Protection Act (1992). This legal framework aims towards eventually achieving a smoke-free Thai society.

Traffic accidents are Thailand's leading cause of death. Intensive messages by radio and television during the highest traffic peaks have significantly reduced deaths and injuries in recent years. Other health activities such as physical fitness, healthy diet, and traditional medicines have been covered by radio channels providing evidence-based and balanced information. The media and nongovernmental organizations have set up HIV/AIDS counselling, and the Ministry of Public Health has set up a help line to provide counselling on stress and suicide prevention, as well as a telephone hot line aiming at consumer protection.

The media reflect public dissatisfaction with both public and private hospital care. At the same time the

Health Systems Research Institute (HSRI) coordinates a national forum on hospital quality improvement and accreditation and is pressing for an independent hospital accreditation body. HSRI also has a programme to guide journalists wanting to specialize in the health field.

Thus, Thailand's media play an important role in health system stewardship, as information providers and change agents, linking the general public, consumer groups, civic society, the research community, professional organizations and the government in improving health of the people in a participatory way.

Contributed by Viroj Tangcharoensathian, Health Systems Research Institute, Bangkok, Thailand.

gies for improving data collecting; review the core policy vision and messages; review existing organizational and incentive arrangements; and establish coordination and communication processes. A massive investment in management information systems will not, of itself, bring about better stewardship. Advocacy strategies, too, are needed to influence other branches of government and non-government health system players. The scope of regulation has to be broader, bringing in and giving voice to consumers, private providers, professional associations, and external assistance agencies.

An improved information base for policy creates a major strength for communication. On occasions this may require a higher profile by the ministry of health – in its dealings with the ministry of finance, or with donors, for instance. But the health ministry may get its messages across more forcefully when it uses other channels, such as the press, television and radio, academic institutions, and professional or consumer groups, to put its case. The ministry of health has to recognize all those primarily motivated by health gain – whether they are in the public or private sector – as its partners in the health system. Regular communication is one of the fibres which holds the system together.

The wide range of partners involved in a health system gives rise to an important question: who should do what?

Much of the preceding has been concerned with the role of the ministry of health. But the local context and particular issue determine who the stakeholders are – who stands to win or lose by a line of policy. Seeking the support of stakeholders is an important task for the ministry of health. The political feasibility of policy depends on: the power of the players; their position; the intensity of their commitment; and their numbers *(31)*. As the agency responsible for formulating policy and steering its implementation, the ministry of health needs to bear this in mind.

Within the public sector, social security organizations and the education system are prominent among bodies whose activities affect health. The ministry of health can influence these either by dealing directly with them, or by working through higher political channels to ensure that health policies are supported, not contradicted by the practice of other parts of the public sector.

Where private sector activities are motivated by health gain, as for example in research and development in pharmaceuticals, medical technology, or motor vehicle safety, health ministries should at least ensure that their information and communication strategies include these partners. Where such inputs are internationally traded, regional and global organizations concerned with health should support the stewardship role of individual ministries of health by bringing governments, industry and consumer representatives together, promoting guidelines for good practice, and providing international information, monitoring and comparison.

Professional organizations can often play a much bigger role in self-regulation. With judicious support, ministries of health can assist professional bodies assume some of the burden of stewardship, such as licensing, credentials checking, and in-service training.

Consumer interests in health are weakly protected in countries at all levels of development. In countries such as Canada, New Zealand and Sweden, however, where public knowledge about health is taken seriously by government, numerically powerful and committed consumer groups have sprung up. Although they may oppose the ministry of health on some issues, on others the position of organized consumers will reinforce that of the ministry in dealings with input suppliers or professional groups. Modern communication strategies allow fast, easy access to health information in presentations suitable for nonspecialists: ministries should be energetic in making these resources available to the public.

External agencies, both public and nongovernmental, have special responsibilities in assisting stewardship. This report is directed to them and their expert advisers as well as to national policy-makers. External agencies have a dual mandate: they are accountable to their domestic chiefs and constituency as well as to governments in the developing countries in which they work. A focus on self-contained projects was a compromise which for many years made this dual mandate workable. Donors found projects an easy way to demonstrate their work to the home audience, and well-chosen projects also met a development priority need for the host country. The shift which began in the 1980s to more systemic support, through programmes and subsequently sector approaches, makes it much easier for external agencies to take a supportive role in government-led stewardship. Some donors now have a voice in the development of policy and strategy, and are abandoning their right to pick individual development projects in exchange for a fuller partnership with aid-receiving governments (32).

With their technical knowledge and resources, external agencies can ensure that the tasks of stewardship are recognized, and that the supporting investments in new skills needed to establish this function can be given priority. For stewardship is the irreducible core of public responsibility: government has to do this job and do it properly. Without stewardship, market failure and the exclusion of poorer consumers from access are ever-present dangers.

Donor agencies have a special responsibility not to make the stewardship role more difficult by acting in a semi-autonomous way. Donors – often numerous and anxious to ensure that their individual concerns are expressed in policy – can too easily find themselves at cross-purposes with each other and with government, compounding the difficulty of setting clear lines of policy (33). In this respect, the concept of sector-wide approaches offers a promising model. It puts government at the helm and establishes a dialogue on priorities, strategy and common implementation plans.

WHAT ARE THE CHALLENGES?

Many countries are falling far short of their potential, and most are making inadequate efforts to achieve responsiveness and fairness in financing. There are serious shortcomings in the performance of one or more functions in virtually all countries.

These failings result in very large numbers of preventable deaths and disabilities in each country; in unnecessary suffering; in injustice, inequality and denial of basic rights of individuals. The impact is undoubtedly most severe on the poor, who are driven deeper into poverty by lack of financial protection against ill-health.

Within all systems there are countless highly skilled, dedicated people working at all levels to improve the health of their communities. There is little argument that health systems in general have already contributed enormously to better health for most of the global population during the 20th century. As the new century begins, they have the power and the potential to achieve further extraordinary improvements.

Unfortunately, health systems can also misuse their power and squander their potential. Poorly structured, badly led, inefficiently organized and inadequately funded health systems may do more harm than good.

The ultimate responsibility for the overall performance of a country's health system lies with government, which in turn should involve all sectors of society in its stewardship. The careful and responsible management of the well-being of the population – stewardship – is the very essence of good government. The health of the people is always a national priority: government responsibility for it is continuous and permanent.

Stricter oversight and regulation of private sector providers and insurers must be placed high on national policy agendas. Good policy needs to differentiate between providers (public or private) who are contributing to health goals, and those who are doing damage or having no effect, and encourage or sanction appropriately. Policies to change the balance between providers' autonomy and accountability need to be monitored closely in terms of their effect on health, responsiveness and the distribution of the financing burden.

Consumers need to be better informed about what is good and bad for their health, why not all of their expectations can be met, but that they still have rights which all providers should respect. But consumer interests in health are weakly protected in countries at all levels of development. The notion of "patients' rights" should be promoted and machinery established to investigate violations quickly and fairly.

The most obvious route to increased prepayment is by raising the level of public finance for health, but this is difficult if not impossible for poor nations. But governments could encourage different forms of prepayment – job-based, community- based, or provider-based – as part of a preparatory process of consolidating small pools into larger ones. Governments need to promote community rating, a common benefit package and portability of benefits among schemes, and to use public funds to pay for the inclusion of poor people in such schemes. Insurance schemes designed to expand membership among the poor are an attractive way to channel external assistance in health, alongside government revenue. Alert stewardship is needed to prevent the capture of such schemes by lower-risk, better-off groups.

Mechanisms are needed in most low and middle income countries to separate revenue collection from payment at the time of service utilization, thus allowing the great majority of finance for health to come through prepayment. More pooling of finance allows cross-subsidies from rich to poor and from healthy to sick. Risk pooling strategies in each country need to be designed to increase such cross-subsidies. Payments to service providers of all types need to be redesigned to encourage providers to focus on achieving health system goals through the provision of cost-effective interventions to people with common conditions amenable to prevention or care.

On an international level, the largely private pharmaceutical and vaccine research and development industry must be encouraged to address global health priorities, and not concentrate on "lifestyle" products for more affluent populations.

Serious simultaneous imbalances exist in many countries in terms of human and physical resources, technology and pharmaceuticals. Many countries have too few qualified health personnel, others have too many. Health system staff in many low income nations are inadequately trained, poorly paid, and work in crumbling, obsolete facilities with chronic shortages of equipment. One result is a "brain drain" of talented but demoralized professionals who either go abroad or move into private practice.

Overall, governments have too little of the necessary information to draw up effective strategies. National health accounts offer an unbiased and comprehensive framework from which overall situation analyses can be made, and trends monitored. They should be much more widely created and used.

HOW TO IMPROVE PERFORMANCE

Stewardship is needed to achieve better health system performance. The following conclusions on stewardship apply in many industrialized countries as well as in low and middle income nations.

Stewardship of the health system is a government responsibility. To discharge it requires an inclusive, thought out policy vision which recognizes all principal players and assigns them roles. It uses a realistic resource scenario and focuses on achieving system goals. Intelligence requires a selective information system on key system functions and goal achievement, broken down into important population categories, such as income level, age, sex and ethnicity. Stewardship also calls for the ability to identify the principal policy challenges at any time, and to assess the options for dealing with them. Influence requires regulatory and advocacy strategies consistent with health system goals, and the capacity to implement them cost-effectively.

Service provision. Private provision of health services tends to be larger where countries' income levels are lower. But poorer countries seldom have clear lines of policy towards the private sector. They thus have important steps to take in recognizing the diverse forms of private provision and developing communications with the different groups of private providers.

In order to move towards higher quality care, a better information base on existing provision is commonly required. Local and national risk factors need to be understood. Information on numbers and types of providers is a basic – and often incompletely fulfilled – requirement. An understanding of provider market structure and utilization patterns is also needed, so that policy-makers know why this array of provision exists, as well as where it is growing. Information on the interventions offered and on major constraints on service implementation are also relevant to overall quality improvement.

An explicit, public process of priority setting should be undertaken to identify the contents of a benefit package which should be available to all, including those in private schemes, and which should reflect local disease priorities and cost-effectiveness, among other criteria. Rationing should take the form of excluding certain interventions from the benefit package, not leaving out any people. Supporting mechanisms – clinical protocols, registration, training, licensing and accreditation processes – need to be brought up to date and used. A regulatory strategy which distinguishes between the components of the private sector, and includes the promotion of self-regulation, needs to be developed. Aligning organizational structures and incentives with the overall objectives of policy is a task for stewardship, rather than one left only to service providers.

Monitoring is needed to assess behavioural change associated with decentralizing authority over resources and services, and the effects of different types of contractual relationships with public and private providers. Striking a balance between tight control and the independence needed to motivate providers is a delicate task, for which local – not textbook – solutions must be found. Experimentation and adaptation will be necessary in most settings. A supporting network for exchanging information will be necessary to create a "virtual health system" from a large set of semi-autonomous providers.

In middle income countries, where health service delivery is often segmented into parallel systems, quality-based competition among providers may be encouraged. A combination of public subsidy and regulated private providers, through extended insurance coverage

(Argentina, Colombia), and contracting directly to ministry providers (Brazil) has been implemented with some success. And in the high income economies, better regulation of private providers and greater attention to responsiveness (United Kingdom) and control of wastage due to over-prescribing, overuse of diagnostic technology and excessive interventions (France, Japan, the United States) are often needed.

Resource generation. Stewardship has to monitor several strategic balances and steer them in the right direction when they are out of equilibrium. A system of national health accounts (NHAs) provides the essential information base for monitoring the ratio of capital to recurrent expenditure, or of any one input to the total, and for observing trends. NHAs capture foreign as well as domestic, public as well as private inputs and usefully assemble data on physical quantities (numbers of nurses, CT scanners, district hospitals) as well as their costs. NHAs in some form now exist for most countries, but they are still often rudimentary and are not yet widely used as tools of stewardship.

NHA data allow the ministry of health to think critically about input purchases by all fundholders in the health system. The concept of strategic purchasing, introduced in Chapter 5, does not only apply to the purchase of health care services: it applies equally to the purchase of health system inputs. Where inputs such as trained personnel, diagnostic equipment, and vehicles are purchased directly with public funds the ministry of health has a direct responsibility to ensure that value for money is obtained – not only in terms of good prices, but also in ensuring that effective use is made of the items purchased.

Where health system inputs are purchased by other agencies (such as private insurers, providers, households or other public agencies) the ministry's stewardship role consists of using its regulatory and persuasive influence to ensure that these purchases improve, rather than worsen, the efficiency of the input mix. This does not, however, entail comprehensive central planning and programming. The role of stewardship in systems with a great deal of decentralized spending authority is to set the rules, rather than to adjudicate every decision. In Brazil, rules for allocating funds to states, prices for services, and reviews of major investment decisions have been put into practice *(34).* The central ministry may have to decide on major capital decisions, such as tertiary hospitals or medical schools. But regional and district health authorities should be entrusted with the larger number of lower-level purchasing decisions, using guidelines, criteria and procedures promoted by central government.

Ensuring a healthy balance between capital and recurrent spending in the health system requires analysis of both public and private spending trends and a consideration of both domestic and foreign funds. The budgetary information usually available to the ministry of health tells only part of the story. A clear policy framework, incentives, regulation and public information need to be brought to bear on important capital decisions in the entire system to counter ad hoc decisions and political influence.

In the field of human resources, similar combinations of strategy have had some success in tackling the geographical imbalances common within countries. In general, the content of training needs to be reassessed in relation to workers' actual job content, and overall supply often needs to be adjusted to meet employment opportunities. In countries such as China where the social return to medical training is negative, training institutions are being considered for privatization or closure. Certainly, public subsidies for training institutions often need to be reconsidered in the light of strategic purchasing. Re-balancing the intake levels of different training facilities is often possible without closure, and might free resources which could be used to retrain clearly surplus health workers (for example, specialist doctors in Egypt) in scarcer skills.

Stewardship of pharmaceuticals and vaccine inputs consists, at international level, of influencing the largely private research and development industry to address global health priorities. At national level the key tasks are to ensure cost-effective purchasing and quality control, rational prescribing, and that consumers are well informed. Health financing strategy also needs to ensure that poor people, in particular, get the drugs they need without financial barriers at the time they are sick.

Major equipment purchases are an easy way for the health system to waste resources, when they are underused, yield little health gain, and use up staff time and recurrent budget. They are also difficult to control. All countries need access to technology assessment information, though they do not necessarily need to produce this themselves. The stewardship role lies in ensuring that criteria for technology purchase in the public sector (which all countries need) are adhered to, and that the private sector does not receive incentives or public subsidy, including the subsidy inherent in being able to sell the services of that equipment to government, for its technology purchases unless these further the aim of national policy.

Providers frequently mobilize public support or subscriptions for technology purchase, and stewardship has to ensure that consumers understand why technology purchases have to be rationed like other services. The public case may be helped by identifying the opportunity cost of additional technology in terms of other needed services.

Health system financing. In all settings, very high levels of fairly distributed prepayment, and strategic purchasing of health interventions are desirable. Implementation strategies, however, are much more specific to each country's situation. Poor countries face the greatest challenge: most payment for health care is made at the time people are sick and using the health system. This is particularly true for the poorest people, who are unlikely to have any prepaid health insurance and who are frequently unable to benefit from subsidized services. Out-of-pocket payment for care, particularly by the poor, should not be relied on as a long-term source of health system finance.

Perhaps the most obvious route to increased prepayment is by raising the level of public finance for health, but two immediate obstacles appear. The poorest countries as a group manage to raise less, in public revenue, as a percentage of national income than middle and upper income countries. Indeed, this lack of institutional capacity is a facet of their poverty. And ministries of finance in poor countries, often aware that the existing health system is performing poorly, are sceptical of its claims on public revenues. Where there is no feasible organizational arrangement to boost prepayment levels, both donors and governments should explore ways of building enabling mechanisms for the development or consolidation of large risk pools. Insurance schemes designed to expand membership among the poor offer a path for government – with external funding partners – to a rapid improvement in the health of the most vulnerable.

In middle income countries substantial mandatory, income and risk-based schemes often coexist. The policy route to a fair prepaid system lies through strengthening such schemes, again ensuring increased public funding for the inclusion of poor people. Expansion of the beneficiary base through subsidies and merger of pre-existing schemes was how national coverage grew from small-scale schemes in Germany, Japan and the Republic of Korea.

Although most industrialized countries already have very high levels of prepayment, some of these strategies are also relevant to them. For its income level, the United States has an unusually high proportion of its population without health insurance protection: a combination of the above strategies will be necessary if the level and fairness of financial protection is to be substantially improved in the decade ahead.

To ensure that prepaid finance obtains the best possible value for money, strategic purchasing needs to replace much of the traditional machinery linking budget holders to service providers. Budget holders will no longer be passive financial intermediaries. Strategic purchasing means ensuring a coherent set of incentives for providers, whether public or private, to encourage them to offer priority interventions efficiently. Selective contracting and the use of several payment mechanisms are needed to set incentives for better responsiveness and improved health outcomes.

This report has broken new ground in presenting for the first time an overall index of national health systems' attainment, and an index of performance relative to potential. These are based on the fundamental goals of *good health, responsiveness to people's expectations* (where both level and distribution matter for each of these goals), and *fairness of contribution to financing the health system*. Achieving these goals depends on the effectiveness of four main functions: *service provision, resource generation, financing,* and *stewardship*.

The preliminary ranking of countries in terms of their health system performance is revealing. It suggests that, at very low levels of health expenditure, performance is both systematically worse and much more varied than at high spending levels, even when performance is judged relative to a country's human resources and how much is spent on health. Clearly the countries with limited resources and severe health problems present the greatest needs: to understand why health systems do not achieve as much as it seems they might, and to help them attain their potential. The findings reported here also show that while much achievement – particularly for the level of health and some aspects of responsiveness – depends greatly on how much a system spends, it is possible to achieve considerable health equality, respect for persons, and financial fairness even at low resource levels. Some systems achieve much more than others in these important respects.

Much more work lies ahead for all concerned to improve the concepts and generate the data on national health system performance. A widespread refocusing of policy is strongly suggested.

Service delivery, resource mix, health financing and, above all, stewardship all matter greatly. The better performance of these four common functions makes substantial gains in goal achievement possible in countries at all levels of development. The poor will be the principal beneficiaries.

REFERENCES

1. **Saltman RB, Ferroussier-Davis O.** On the concept of stewardship in health policy. *Bulletin of the World Health Organization*, 2000, **78**(6) (in press).

2. **Osborn D, Gaebler T.** *Reinventing government*. Reading, MA, Addison Wesley, 1993.

3. **Saltman RB, Figueras J, Sakellarides C, eds.** *Critical challenges for health care reform in Europe*. Buckingham, UK, Open University Press, 1998 (State of Health Series).

4. **Bossert T et al.** Transformation of ministries of health in the era of health reform: the case of Colombia. *Health Policy and Planning*, 1998, **13**(1): 59–77.

5. **Ogunbekun I et al.** Private health care in Nigeria: walking the tightrope. *Health Policy and Planning*, 1999, **14**(2): 174–181.

6. **Bennett S et al.** *Health insurance schemes for people outside formal sector employment*. Geneva, World Health Organization, 1998 (unpublished document WHO/ARA/CC/98.1).

7. **Killingsworth J et al.** Unofficial fees in Bangladesh: price, equity and institutional issues. *Health Policy and Planning,* 1999, **14**(2): 152–163.

8. **Halik J.** Respecting patients' rights in hospitals in Poland. In: *Health sector reform in Central and Eastern Europe: current trends and priority research: a FICOSSER research meeting, Velingrad, Bulgaria, 2–3 October 1998.* Warsaw, National Centre for Health System Management, 1999.

9. **Schuster M et al.** How good is the quality of good health care in the United States? *The Milbank Quarterly,* 1998, **76**(4): 517–563.

10. **Bennett S, McPake B, Mills A, eds.** *Private health providers in developing countries: serving the public interest?* London, Zed Books, 1996.

11. **Salinas H, Lenz R.** *Las no reformas de salud en Latinoamérica: razones que explican su fracaso* [*Non-reforms of health in Latin America: reasons explaining their failure*]. Santiago de Chile, 1999 (in Spanish).

12. **Nittayaramphong S, Tangcharoensathien V.** Thailand: private health care out of control? Health Policy and Planning, 1994, **9**(1):31–40.

13. **Turshen M.** *Privatizing health services in Africa.* New Brunswick, New Jersey, Rutgers University Press, 1999.

14. **Chollet DJ, Lewis M.** Private insurance: principles and practice. In: Schieber G, ed. *Innovations in health care financing.* Washington, DC, The World Bank, 1997 (World Bank Discussion Paper No. 365).

15. **Musgrove P.** *Public and private roles in health: theory and financing patterns.* Washington, DC, The World Bank, 1996 (World Bank Discussion Paper No. 339).

16. **Hsiao WC.** Abnormal economics in the health sector. *Health Policy,* 1995, **32**:125–139.

17. **Van Lerberghe W et al.** Reform follows failure: unregulated private care in Lebanon. *Health Policy and Planning,* 1997, **12**(4): 296–311.

18. **Borren P, Maynard A.** The market reform of the New Zealand health care system: searching for the Holy Grail in the Antipodes. *Health Policy,* 1994, **27**(3): 233–252.

19. **Russel S, Attanayake N.** *Sri Lanka: reforming the health sector. Does government have the capacity?* Birmingham, UK, University of Birmingham, 1997.

20. **Bennet S, Ngalande-Banda E.** *Public and private roles in health. A review and analysis of experience in sub-Saharan Africa.* Geneva, World Health Organization, 1994 (Current Concerns, ARA Paper No. 6, document WHO/ARA/CC/97.6).

21. **Broomberg J.** *Health care markets for export? Lessons for developing countries from European and American experience.* London School of Hygiene and Tropical Medicine, Department of Public Health and Policy, 1994.

22. **WHO Action Programme on Essential Drugs.** *Public–private roles in the pharmaceutical sector.* Geneva, World Health Organization, 1995 (unpublished discussion paper).

23. **Zurita B et al.** *Structural pluralism as a tool for equity, quality and efficiency in healthcare in Mexico: the role of FUNSALUD.* 2000 (unpublished paper).

24. **Smithson P.** Quarts into pint jugs? The financial viability of health sector investment in low income countries. *Health Policy and Planning,* 1995, **10**(Suppl.): 6–16.

25. **Ham C.** Priority setting in health care: learning from international experience. *Health Policy,* 1997, **42**(1): 49–66.

26. **Bhat R.** *Public–private partnerships in the health sector: the Indian experience.* 2000 (unpublished paper).

27. **Robinson R, Le Grand J, eds.** *Evaluating the NHS reforms.* London, King's Fund Institute, 1994.

28. **Quick JD, Musau SN.** *Impact of cost sharing in Kenya: 1989–1993. Effects of the Ministry of Health Facility Improvement Fund on revenue generation, recurrent expenditures, quality of care, and utilization patterns.* Nairobi, Management Sciences for Health, 1994.

29. **Kalumba K.** *Towards an equity-oriented policy of decentralization in health systems under conditions of turbulence: the case of Zambia.* Geneva, World Health Organization, 1997 (document WHO/ARA/97.2).

30. **Calnan M, Halik J, Sabbat J.** Citizen participation and patient choice in health reform. In: Saltman RB, Figueras J, Sakellarides C, eds. *Critical challenges for health care reform in Europe.* Buckingham, UK, Open University Press, 1998 (State of Health Series).

31. **Reich M.** In: *Diagnostic approaches to assessing strategies, weaknesses and change of health systems.* Washington, DC, Economic Development Institute, The World Bank, 1998 (Flagship Module 2).

32. **Hay R.** *International aid: economics and charity.* Oxford, Oxford Policy Institute, 2000 (Oxford Policy Brief No. 1).

33. **Walt G et al.** Health sector development: from aid coordination to resource management. *Health Policy and Planning,* 1999, **14**(3): 207–218.

34. *Brazil: social spending in selected states.* Washington, DC, The World Bank, 1999 (World Bank Report BR-17763: Chapter 3).

Statistical Annex

The tables in this annex present new concepts and measures which lay the empirical basis for assessing health system performance. The main body of the report provides detail on the different goals for health systems and the measures of performance. The material in these tables will be presented on an annual basis in each World health report. As with any innovative approach, methods and data sources can be refined and improved. It is hoped that careful scrutiny and use of results will lead to progressively better measurement of health system performance in the coming World health reports. All the main results are reported with uncertainty intervals in order to communicate to the user the plausible range of estimates for each country on each measure.

Statistical Annex

Explanatory Notes

The tables in this technical annex present new concepts and measures which lay the empirical basis for assessing health system performance. The main body of the report provides detail on the different goals for health systems and the measures of performance. Both the text of the report and the annex are based on the WHO framework for health system performance assessment.[1] The work leading to these annex tables was undertaken mostly by the WHO Global Programme on Evidence for Health Policy in collaboration with counterparts from the Regional Offices of WHO. This analytical effort was organized in eleven working groups. Membership of these working groups is listed in the Appendix. The material in these tables will be presented on an annual basis in each *World health report*. Because this is the first year of presentation for the material in Annex Tables 1 and 5-10, working papers have been prepared which provide details on the concepts, methods and results that are only briefly mentioned here. The footnotes to these technical notes include a complete listing of the detailed working papers.

As with any innovative approach, methods and data sources can be refined and improved. It is hoped that careful scrutiny and use of the results will lead to progressively better measurement of performance in the coming *World health reports*. All the main results are reported with uncertainty intervals in order to communicate to the user the plausible range of estimates for each country on each measure.

Although not provided in any table, extensive use has been made of estimates of income per capita in international dollars, average years of schooling for the population over age 15 years, percentage of the population in absolute poverty and the income Gini coefficient. In all cases, there are multiple and often conflicting sources of information from international agencies on these indicators; in addition, there are many countries for which there are no published estimates. To facilitate the analyses presented here, consistent and complete estimates of these key indicators have been developed through a variety of techniques including factor analysis, multiple imputation methods for missing data, remote sensing data from public use satellites and systematic reviews of household survey data. The details on methods and data sources for the final figures on income per capita, educational attainment, poverty and income distribution are outlined elsewhere.[2]

Annex Table 1

Annex Table 1 is designed as a guide for using Annex Tables 5-7, 9 and 10. Each measure of goal attainment and performance - disability-adjusted life expectancy, health equality in terms of child survival, responsiveness level, responsiveness distribution, fairness of financial contribution, performance on level of health, and overall health system performance -is reported as a league table ranked from the highest level of achievement or performance to the lowest level. Annex Table 1 lists countries alphabetically and provides the ranks on each of the measures reported in the other tables. The reader can use Annex Table 1 to identify quickly where a particular country falls in each table.

ANNEX TABLE 2

To assess the performance of health systems in terms of health achievement, it was crucial to develop the best possible assessment of the life table for each country. New life tables have been developed for all 191 Member States starting with a systematic review of all available evidence from surveys, censuses, sample registration systems, population laboratories and vital registration on levels and trends in child mortality and adult mortality. This review benefited greatly from the work undertaken on child mortality by UNICEF[3] and the UN Population Division 1998 demographic assessment.[4] To aid in demographic, cause of death and burden of disease analysis, the 191 Member States have been divided into 5 mortality strata on the basis of their level of child (5q0) and adult male mortality (45q15). The matrix defined by the six WHO Regions and the 5 mortality strata leads to 14 subregions, since not every mortality stratum is represented in every Region. These subregions are used in Tables 3 and 4 for presentation of results.

Because of increasing heterogeneity of patterns of adult and child mortality, WHO has developed a system of two-parameter logit life tables for each of the 14 subregions.[5] This system of model life tables has been used extensively in the development of life tables for each Member State and in projecting life tables to 1999 when the most recent data available are from earlier years. Details on the data, methods and results by country of this life table analysis are available in the corresponding technical paper.[6]

A major innovation that WHO is introducing this year to demographic and other analyses is the reporting of uncertainty intervals. To capture the uncertainty due to sampling, indirect estimation technique or projection to 1999, a total of 1000 life tables have been developed for each Member State. Uncertainty bounds are reported in Annex Table 1 by giving key life table values at the 10th percentile and the 90th percentile. This uncertainty analysis was facilitated by the development of new methods and software tools.[7] In countries with a substantial HIV epidemic, recent estimates of the level and uncertainty range of the magnitude of the HIV epidemic have been incorporated into the life table uncertainty analysis.[8]

ANNEX TABLES 3 AND 4

Causes of death for the 14 subregions and the world have been estimated based on data from national vital registration systems that capture 16.7 million deaths annually. In addition, information from sample registration systems, population laboratories and epidemiological analyses of specific conditions have been used to produce better estimates of the cause of death patterns.

Cause of death data have been carefully analysed to take into account incomplete coverage of vital registration in countries and the likely differences in cause of death patterns that would be expected in the uncovered and often poorer sub-populations. Techniques to undertake this analysis have been developed based on the global burden of disease study[9] and further refined using a much more extensive database and more robust modelling techniques.[10]

Special attention has been paid to problems of misattribution or miscoding of causes of death in cardiovascular diseases, cancer, injuries and general ill-defined categories. A correction algorithm for reclassifying ill-defined cardiovascular codes has been developed.[11] Cancer mortality by site has been evaluated using both vital registration data and population based cancer incidence registries. The latter have been analysed using a complete age, period cohort model of cancer survival in each region.[12]

Annex Table 4 provides estimates of the burden of disease using disability-adjusted life years (DALYs) as a measure of the health gap in the world in 1999. DALYs along with disability-adjusted life expectancy are summary measures of population health.[13] DALYs are a type of health gap that measures the difference between a population's health and a normative goal of living in full health. For a review of the development of DALYs and recent advances in the measurement of the burden of disease see Murray & Lopez.[14] DALYs have been estimated based on cause of death information for each Region and regional assessments of the epidemiology of major disabling conditions.

ANNEX TABLE 5

Annex Table 5 provides measurements of health attainment in terms of the average level of population health and the distribution of population health or health equality. Two measures are reported by WHO for the first time at the country level: disability-adjusted life expectancy and the index of equality of child survival.

Achievement of the average level of population health is reported in terms of disability-adjusted life expectancy (DALE). DALE is most easily understood as the expectation of life lived in equivalent full health. As a summary measure of the burden of disability from all causes in a population, DALE has two advantages over other summary measures. The first is that it is relatively easy to explain the concept of a lifespan without disability to a non-technical audience. The second is that it is easy to calculate DALE using the Sullivan method based on age-specific information on the prevalence of non-fatal health outcomes. In the global burden of disease study, DALE was estimated at the regional level, based on the estimates of all disabling sequelae included in the study. Disability weights were measured for each of these sequelae for five standard age groups, sex and eight regions.

National estimates of DALE are based on the life tables for each Member State summarized in Annex Table 2, population representative sample surveys assessing physical and cognitive disability and general health status, and detailed information on the epidemiology of major disabling conditions in each country. Use of household surveys is complicated by the variation in self-assessed health for a given level of observed health as a function of sex, age, socioeconomic status, exposure to health services, and culture.[15, 16] The methodological details for national estimates of DALE and the uncertainty in these estimates are provided elsewhere.[17]

Measurement of achievement in the distribution of health is based on the WHO framework for measuring health inequality.[18] The intention is ultimately to measure the distribution of health using the distribution of DALE across individuals. However, the analysis of the distribution of DALE in each country has not yet been completed. For selected countries, the distribution of life expectancy across small areas has been completed and reveals that there is often much greater variation in life expectancy and probably in DALE than expected.[19] In this *World health report,* the analysis of achievement in the distribution of health, presented in Annex Table 5, is the index of equality of child survival. It is based on the distribution of child survival across countries, and takes advantage of the widely available and extensive information on complete birth histories in the demographic and health surveys and small area vital registration data on child mortality.

Statistical methods based on maximum likelihood estimation of the extended beta-binomial distribution have been developed to distinguish between variation across mothers in the number of children who have died due to chance and that due to differences in the underlying risks of death.[20] This statistical method has been applied to demographic and health survey data and small area data from more than 60 countries to estimate the underlying distribution of the risk of child death.[21] For the purposes of calculating the index of equality of child survival, child mortality distributions have been transformed into distributions of expected survival time under age 5 years. The resulting distributions of survival time have been summarized for the creation of a composite index using the following formula:

$$\text{Equality of child survival} = \left(1 - \frac{\displaystyle\sum_{i=1}^{n}\sum_{j=1}^{n}\left|x_i - x_j\right|^3}{2n^2\,\overline{x}^{\,0.5}}\right)$$

where x is the survival time of a given child and $\overline{x}$ is the mean survival time across children.

The particular form of this summary measure of inequality has been selected on the basis of a survey of preferences for measuring health inequality of over one thousand respondents.[22] Because all measures of goal achievement are intended to be positive measures, the inequality index has been transformed into an index of equality by calculating one minus child survival inequality, as shown above. As the measure of inequality has a maximum value that can be greater than 1, in theory this transformed measure of equality of child survival could be negative. However, across the range of countries, no country has a degree of inequality that would lead to a measurement of equality less than zero. The value of 1 can be interpreted as complete equality and zero can be interpreted as a degree of inequality that is worse than has been seen in any country measured directly or estimated indirectly to date.

For countries without a demographic and health survey or small area data, the index of the distribution of health for child survival has been estimated using indirect techniques and information on important covariates of health inequality such as poverty, educational attainment and the level of child mortality.

ANNEX TABLE 6

The measurement of achievement in the level of responsiveness was based on a survey of nearly two thousand key informants in selected countries.[23] Key informants were asked to evaluate the performance of their health system regarding seven elements of responsiveness: dignity, autonomy and confidentiality (jointly termed respect of persons); and prompt attention, quality of basic amenities, access to social support networks during care and choice of care provider (encompassed by the term client orientation). The elements were scored from 0 to 10. Scores on each component were combined into a composite score for responsiveness based on results of the survey on preferences for health system performance assessment. For other countries, achievement in the level of responsiveness has been estimated using indirect techniques and information on important covariates of responsiveness.[24] To enhance the measurement of responsiveness, WHO is actively developing and field testing instruments to measure responsiveness from household respondents. This strategy of using household surveys will be supplemented with facility surveys to observe directly some components of responsiveness.[25]

The measurement of achievement in the distribution of responsiveness reflected in Annex Table 6 is based on a very simple approach. Respondents in the key informants survey were asked to identify groups who were disadvantaged with regard to responsiveness. The number of times a particular group was identified as disadvantaged was used to calculate a key informant intensity score. Four groups had high key informant intensity scores: poor people, women, old people, and indigenous groups or racially disadvantaged groups (in most instances minorities). The key informant intensity scores for these four groups were multiplied by the actual percentage of the population within these vulnerable groups in a country to calculate a simple measure of responsiveness inequality ranging from 0 to 1. The total score was calculated taking into account the fact that some individuals belong to more than one disadvantaged group. Annex Table 6 provides a measure of the equality of responsiveness, scaled such that 1 is complete equality and 0 is complete inequality. For other countries, achievement on the distribution of responsiveness has been estimated using indirect techniques and information on important covariates of the distribution of responsiveness including absolute poverty and access to health care.

ANNEX TABLE 7

The index presented in this table is meant to measure both fairness of financial contribution and financial risk protection;[1] the basic concepts and principles are outlined in detail elsewhere.[26] The measurement of achievement in fairness of financial contribution starts with the concept of a household's contribution to the financing of the health system. The health financing contribution of a household is defined as the ratio of total household spending on health to its permanent income above subsistence. Total household spending on health includes payments towards the financing of the health system through income taxes, value-added tax, excise tax, social security contributions, private voluntary insurance, and out-of-pocket payments. Permanent income above subsistence is estimated for a household as total expenditure plus tax payments not included in total expenditure minus expenditure on food.

The distribution of households' financial contribution is calculated using household survey data which includes information on income (individual level) and household expenditure (by goods and services including health). In addition, the calculations require government tax documents (including information on income tax, sales tax, and property tax), national health accounts, national accounts, and government budgets. Such in-depth analysis has been completed for selected countries where such information is available.[27] For other countries, the distribution of health financing contribution has been estimated using indirect methods and information on important covariates.[28]

To allow for comparisons of the fairness of financial contribution, the distribution of health financing contribution across households has been summarized using an index. This index is designed to weight highly households that have spent a very large share of their income beyond subsistence on health. The index therefore reflects inequality in household financial contribution but particularly reflects those households at risk of impoverishment from high levels of health expenditure. The index is of the form:

$$\text{Fairness of financial contribution} = \left[1 - 4 \frac{\sum_{i=1}^{n} \left| HFC_i - \overline{HFC} \right|^3}{0.125n} \right]$$

where HFC is the financial contribution of a given household and $\overline{HFC}$ is the average financial contribution across households.

The index is designed so that complete equality of household contributions is 1 and 0 is below the largest degree of inequality observed across countries.

ANNEX TABLE 8

National health accounts are designed to be a policy relevant, comprehensive, consistent, timely and standardized instrument that traces the levels and trends of consumption of medical goods and services (the expenditure approach), the value-added created by service and manufacturing industries producing these commodities (the production approach) and the incomes generated by this process as well as the taxes, mandatory contributions, premiums and direct payments that fund the system (the financial approach). The current developmental stage of WHO national health accounts leans more towards a measurement of the financing flows.[29]

Health care finance is divided into public and private flows. For public expenditure, the source most frequently used was Table B on expenditure by function published by the IMF in *Government finance statistics yearbook*. This rests on a body of exacting rules (not always strictly applied by the respondent countries) and deals in most cases only with central government expenditure. IMF and national sources have been used as far as possible to complement the central government data. United Nations *National accounts* (Tables 2.1 and 2.3) and consistent domestic sources have also been used. OECD *Health data* has supplied much of the information for the 29 OECD Member countries. Private expenditure on health has been estimated from United Nations and OECD *National accounts* (Tables 2.5 and 2.1, respectively) and from the ratio of medical care to total consumption as derived from household surveys, that ratio being applied to total private consumption. This concerns mainly out-of-pocket spending. Private insurance premiums, mandated employer health programmes, expenditure by non-profit institutions serving mainly households and, less frequently, private investment have been obtained from national sources. National health accounts prepared by a number of countries have been used to the extent that they were accessible. The plausibility of the estimates has been tested against financial and other analyses conducted in some countries or involving a group of countries.

A first complete table was reviewed by a large number of experts on individual countries and by policy analysts and statisticians of WHO Member States. Their observations led to a reassessment of certain sub-aggregates.

ANNEX TABLE 9

Overall health system attainment is presented in Annex Table 9. This composite measure of achievement in the level of health, the distribution of health, the level of responsiveness, the distribution of responsiveness and fairness of financial contribution has been constructed based on weights derived from the survey of over one thousand public health practitioners from over 100 countries.[22] The composite is constructed on a scale from 0 to 100, the maximum value. As explained in Box 2.4, the weights on the five components are 25% level of health, 25% distribution of health, 12.5% level of responsiveness, 12.5% distribution of responsiveness and 25% fairness of financial contribution. The mean value and uncertainty intervals have been estimated for overall health system achievement using the uncertainty intervals for each of the five components.[30] In addition, the table provides uncertainty intervals for the ranks as well as the value of overall health system achievement. Rank uncertainty is not only a function of the uncertainty of the measurement for each country but also the uncertainty of the measurement of adjacent countries in the league table.

ANNEX TABLE 10

The index of performance on the level of health reports how efficiently health systems translate expenditure into health as measured by disability-adjusted life expectancy (DALE). Performance on the level of health is defined as the ratio between achieved levels of health and the levels of health that could be achieved by the most efficient health system. More specifically, the numerator of the ratio is the difference between observed DALE in a country and the DALE that would be observed in the absence of a functioning modern health system given the other non-health system determinants that influence health, which are represented by education. The denominator of the ratio is the difference between the maximum possible DALE that could have been achieved for the observed levels of health expenditure per capita in each country and the DALE in the absence of a functioning health system. Econometric methods have been used to estimate the maximum DALE for a given level of health expenditure and other non-health system factors using frontier production analysis. The relationship between life expectancy and human capital at the turn of the century was used to estimate the minimum DALE that would have been expected in each country (at current levels of educational attainment) in the absence of an effective health system The details of the data, methods and results are provided elsewhere.[31] Annex Table 10 provides uncertainty intervals for both the absolute value of performance and the rank of each country.

Overall performance of health systems was measured using a similar process relating overall health system achievement to health system expenditure. Maximum attainable composite goal achievement was estimated using a frontier production model relating overall health system achievement to health expenditure and other non-health system determinants represented by educational attainment. Results of this analysis were largely invariant to model specification. More detail is provided in the corresponding technical paper.[32]

[1] Murray CJL, Frenk J. A WHO framework for health system performance assessment. *Bulletin of the World Health Organization*, 2000, **78**(6) (in press).

[2] Evans DE, Bendib L, Tandon A, Lauer J, Ebener S, Hutubessy R, Asada Y, Murray CJL. *Estimates of income per capita, literacy, educational attainment, absolute poverty, and income Gini coefficients for The World Health Report 2000*. Geneva, World Health Organization, 2000 (GPE Discussion Paper No. 7).

[3] Hill K, Rohini PO, Mahy M, Jones G. *Trends in child mortality in the developing world: 1960 to 1996*. New York, UNICEF, 1999.

[4] *World population prospects: the 1998 revision*. New York, United Nations, 1999.

[5] Murray CJL, Lopez AD, Ahmad O, Salomon J. *WHO system of model life tables*. Geneva, World Health Organization, 2000 (GPE Discussion Paper No. 8).

[6] Lopez AD, Salomon J, Ahmad O, Murray CJL. *Life tables for 191 countries: data, methods and results*. Geneva, World Health Organization, 2000 (GPE Discussion Paper No. 9).

[7] Salomon J, Murray CJL. *Methods for life expectancy and disability-adjusted life expectancy uncertainty analysis*. Geneva, World Health Organization, 2000 (GPE Discussion Paper No. 10).

[8] Salomon J, Gakidou EE, Murray CJL. *Methods for modelling the HIV/AIDS epidemic in sub-Saharan Africa*. Geneva, World Health Organization, 2000 (GPE Discussion Paper No. 3).

[9] Murray CJL, Lopez AD, eds. *The global burden of disease: a comprehensive assessment of mortality and disability from diseases, injuries and risk factors in 1990 and projected to 2020*. Cambridge, MA, Harvard School of Public Health on behalf of the World Health Organization and the World Bank, 1996 (Global Burden of Disease and Injury Series, Vol. 1).

[10] Salomon J, Murray CJL. *Compositional models for mortality by age, sex and cause*. Geneva, World Health Organization, 2000 (GPE Discussion Paper No. 11).

[11] Lozano R, Murray CJL, Lopez AD, Satoh T. *Miscoding and misclassification of ischaemic heart disease mortality*. Geneva, World Health Organization, 2000 (GPE Discussion Paper No. 12).

[12] Boschi-Pinto C, Murray CJL, Lopez AD, Lozano R. *Cancer survival by site for 14 regions of the world*. Geneva, World Health Organization, 2000 (GPE Discussion Paper No. 13).

[13] Murray CJL, Salomon J, Mathers C. *A critical review of summary measures of population health*. Geneva, World Health Organization, 2000 (GPE Discussion Paper No. 2).

[14] Murray CJL, Lopez AD. Progress and directions in refining the global burden of disease approach: response to Williams. *Health Economics*, 2000, **9**: 69-82.

[15] Moesgaard-Iburg K, Murray CJL, Salomon J. *Expectations for health distorts: self-reported and physician-assessed health status compared to observed health status*. Geneva, World Health Organization, 2000 (GPE Discussion Paper No. 14).

[16] Sadana R, Mathers C, Lopez A, Murray CJL. *Comparative analysis of more than 50 household surveys on health status*. Geneva, World Health Organization, 2000 (GPE Discussion Paper No. 15).

[17] Mathers C, Sadana R, Salomon J, Murray CJL, Lopez AD. *Estimates of DALE for 191 countries: methods and results*. Geneva, World Health Organization, 2000 (GPE Discussion Paper No. 16).

[18] Gakidou EE, Murray CJL, Frenk J. Defining and Measuring health inequality: an approach based on the distribution of health expectancy. *Bulletin of the World Health Organization*, 2000, **78**(1): 42-54.

[19] Lopez AD, Murray CJL, Ferguson B, Tomaskovic L. *Life expectancy for small areas in selected countries*. Geneva, World Health Organization, 2000 (GPE Discussion Paper No. 17).

[20] Gakidou EE, King G. *Using an extended beta-binomial model to estimate the distribution of child mortality risk*. Geneva, World Health Organization, 2000 (GPE Discussion Paper No. 18).

[21] Gakidou EE, Murray CJL. *Estimates of the distribution of child survival in 191 countries*. Geneva, World Health Organization, 2000 (GPE Discussion Paper No. 19).

[22] Gakidou EE, Frenk J, Murray CJL. *Measuring preferences on health system performance assessment*. Geneva, World Health Organization, 2000 (GPE Discussion Paper No. 20).

[23] de Silva A, Valentine N. *Measuring responsiveness: results of a key informants survey in 35 countries*. Geneva, World Health Organization, 2000 (GPE Discussion Paper No. 21).

[24] Valentine N, de Silva A, Murray CJL. *Estimates of responsiveness level and distribution for 191 countries: methods and results*. Geneva, World Health Organization, 2000 (GPE Discussion Paper No. 22).

[25] Darby C, Valentine N, Murray CJL. *WHO strategy on measuring responsiveness*. Geneva, World Health Organization, 2000 (GPE Discussion Paper No. 23).

[26] Murray CJL, Knaul F, Musgrove P, Xu K, Kawabata K. *Defining and measuring fairness of financial contribution*. Geneva, World Health Organization, 2000 (GPE Discussion Paper No. 24).

[27] Xu K, Lydon P, Ortiz de Iturbide J, Musgrove P, Knaul F, Kawabata K, Florez CE, John J, Wibulpolprasert S, Waters H, Tansel A. *Analysis of the fairness of financial contribution in 21 countries*. Geneva, World Health Organization, 2000 (GPE Discussion Paper No. 25).

[28] Xu K, Murray CJL, Lydon P, Ortiz de Iturbide J. *Estimates of the fairness of financial contribution for 191 countries*. Geneva, World Health Organization, 2000 (GPE Discussion Paper No. 26).

[29] Poullier JP, Hernández P. *Estimates of national health accounts. Aggregates for 191 countries in 1997*. Geneva, World Health Organization, 2000 (GPE Discussion Paper No. 27).

[30] Murray CJL, Frenk J, Tandon A, Lauer J. *Overall health system achievement for 191 countries*. Geneva, World Health Organization, 2000 (GPE Discussion Paper No. 28).

[31] Evans D, Tandon A, Murray CJL, Lauer J. *The comparative efficiency of national health systems in producing health: an analysis of 191 countries*. Geneva, World Health Organization, 2000 (GPE Discussion Paper No. 29).

[32] Tandon A, Murray CJL, Lauer J, Evans D. *Measuring overall health system performance for 191 countries*. Geneva, World Health Organization, 2000 (GPE Discussion Paper No. 30).

Annex Table 1 Health system attainment and performance in all Member States, ranked by eight measures, estimates for 1997

Member State	ATTAINMENT OF GOALS						Health expenditure per capita in international dollars	PERFORMANCE	
	Health		Responsiveness		Fairness in financial contribution	Overall goal attainment		On level of health	Overall health system performance
	Level (DALE)	Distribution	Level	Distribution					
Afghanistan	168	182	181 – 182	172 – 173	103 – 104	183	184	150	173
Albania	102	129	136	117	173 – 174	86	149	64	55
Algeria	84	110	90 – 91	50 – 52	74 – 75	99	114	45	81
Andorra	10	25	28	39 – 42	33 – 34	17	23	7	4
Angola	165	178	177	188	103 – 104	181	164	165	181
Antigua and Barbuda	48	58	47 – 48	39 – 42	116 – 120	71	43	123	86
Argentina	39	60	40	3 – 38	89 – 95	49	34	71	75
Armenia	41	63	92	111 – 112	181	81	102	56	104
Australia	2	17	12 – 13	3 – 38	26 – 29	12	17	39	32
Austria	17	8	12 – 13	3 – 38	12 – 15	10	6	15	9
Azerbaijan	65	99	130 – 131	125	116 – 120	103	162	60	109
Bahamas	109	67	18	3 – 38	138 – 139	64	22	137	94
Bahrain	61	72	43 – 44	3 – 38	61	58	48	30	42
Bangladesh	140	125	178	181	51 – 52	131	144	103	88
Barbados	53	36	39	3 – 38	107	38	36	87	46
Belarus	83	46	76 – 79	45 – 47	84 – 86	53	74	116	72
Belgium	16	26	16 – 17	3 – 38	3 – 5	13	15	28	21
Belize	94	95	105 – 107	90	146	104	88	34	69
Benin	157	132	175 – 176	160	140 – 141	143	171	136	97
Bhutan	138	158	163	137 – 138	89 – 95	144	135	73	124
Bolivia	133	118	151 – 153	178	68	117	101	142	126
Bosnia and Herzegovina	56	79	108 – 110	124	82 – 83	79	105	70	90
Botswana	187	146	76 – 79	111 – 112	89 – 95	168	85	188	169
Brazil	111	108	130 – 131	84 – 85	189	125	54	78	125
Brunei Darussalam	59	42	24	3 – 38	89 – 95	37	32	76	40
Bulgaria	60	53	161	2	170	74	96	92	102
Burkina Faso	178	137	174	164	173 – 174	159	173	162	132
Burundi	179	154	171	168	114	161	186	171	143
Cambodia	148	150	137 – 138	137 – 138	183	166	140	157	174
Cameroon	156	160	156	183	182	163	131	172	164
Canada	12	18	7 – 8	3 – 38	17 – 19	7	10	35	30
Cape Verde	118	123	154	134 – 135	89 – 95	126	150	55	113
Central African Republic	175	189	183	191	166	190	178	164	189
Chad	161	175	181 – 182	185	58 – 60	177	175	161	178
Chile	32	1	45	103	168	33	44	23	33
China	81	101	88 – 89	105 – 106	188	132	139	61	144
Colombia	74	44	82	93 – 94	1	41	49	51	22
Comoros	146	143	157 – 160	153 – 155	79 – 81	137	165	141	118
Congo	150	142	137 – 138	151	162	155	122	167	166
Cook Islands	67	92	65	89	45 – 47	88	61	95	107
Costa Rica	40	45	68	86 – 87	64 – 65	45	50	25	36
Côte d'Ivoire	155	181	157 – 160	153 – 155	116 – 120	157	153	133	137
Croatia	38	33	76 – 79	83	108 – 111	36	56	57	43
Cuba	33	41	115 – 117	98 – 100	23 – 25	40	118	36	39
Cyprus	25	31	11	44	131 – 133	28	39	22	24
Czech Republic	35	19	47 – 48	45 – 47	71 – 72	30	40	81	48
Democratic People's Republic of Korea	137	145	139	130 – 131	179	149	172	153	167
Democratic Republic of the Congo	174	174	142	169 – 170	169	179	188	185	188
Denmark	28	21	4	3 – 38	3 – 5	20	8	65	34
Djibouti	166	169	170	140	3 – 5	170	163	163	157
Dominica	26	35	84 – 86	77 – 78	99 – 100	42	70	59	35
Dominican Republic	79	97	95	72	154	66	92	42	51
Ecuador	93	133	76 – 79	182	88	107	97	96	111
Egypt	115	141	102	59	125 – 127	110	115	43	63
El Salvador	87	115	128	128 – 129	176	122	83	37	115

Member State	Health		Responsiveness		Fairness in financial contribution	Overall goal attainment	Health expenditure per capita in international dollars	On level of health	Overall health system performance
	Level (DALE)	Distribution	Level	Distribution					
Equatorial Guinea	152	151	143	118	134	152	129	174	171
Eritrea	169	167	186	169 – 170	108 – 111	176	187	148	158
Estonia	69	43	66	69	145	48	60	115	77
Ethiopia	182	176	179	179 – 180	138 – 139	186	189	169	180
Fiji	106	71	57 – 58	73 – 74	54 – 55	78	87	124	96
Finland	20	27	19	3 – 38	8 – 11	22	18	44	31
France	3	12	16 – 17	3 – 38	26 – 29	6	4	4	1
Gabon	144	136	118 – 119	101 – 102	84 – 86	141	95	143	139
Gambia	143	155	165 – 167	157	149	153	158	109	146
Georgia	44	61	165 – 167	141	105 – 106	76	125	84	114
Germany	22	20	5	3 – 38	6 – 7	14	3	41	25
Ghana	149	149	132 – 135	146	74 – 75	139	166	158	135
Greece	7	6	36	3 – 38	41	23	30	11	14
Grenada	49	82	63 – 64	84 – 85	147	68	67	49	85
Guatemala	129	106	115 – 117	159	157	113	130	99	78
Guinea	167	166	168 – 169	130 – 131	76 – 78	172	159	160	161
Guinea-Bissau	170	177	184	174	122 – 123	180	156	156	176
Guyana	98	126	114	105 – 106	45 – 47	116	109	104	128
Haiti	153	152	157 – 160	172 – 173	163	145	155	139	138
Honduras	92	119	129	163	178	129	100	48	131
Hungary	62	40	62	58	105 – 106	43	59	105	66
Iceland	19	24	15	3 – 38	12 – 15	16	14	27	15
India	134	153	108 – 110	127	42 – 44	121	133	118	112
Indonesia	103	156	63 – 64	70	73	106	154	90	92
Iran, Islamic Republic of	96	113	100	93 – 94	112 – 113	114	94	58	93
Iraq	126	130	103 – 104	114	56 – 57	124	117	75	103
Ireland	27	13	25	3 – 38	6 – 7	25	25	32	19
Israel	23	7	20 – 21	3 – 38	38 – 40	24	19	40	28
Italy	6	14	22 – 23	3 – 38	45 – 47	11	11	3	2
Jamaica	36	87	105 – 107	73 – 74	115	69	89	8	53
Japan	1	3	6	3 – 38	8 – 11	1	13	9	10
Jordan	101	83	84 – 86	53 – 57	49 – 50	84	98	100	83
Kazakhstan	122	52	90 – 91	60 – 61	167	62	112	135	64
Kenya	162	135	144	142	79 – 81	142	152	178	140
Kiribati	125	121	120 – 121	122	16	123	103	144	142
Kuwait	68	54	29	3 – 38	30 – 32	46	41	68	45
Kyrgyzstan	123	122	124	96	171	135	146	134	151
Lao People's Democratic Republic	147	147	145 – 147	143 – 144	159	154	157	155	165
Latvia	82	56	69 – 72	53 – 57	164 – 165	67	77	121	105
Lebanon	95	88	55	79 – 81	101 – 102	93	46	97	91
Lesotho	171	164	145 – 147	148 – 149	89 – 95	173	123	186	183
Liberia	181	191	175 – 176	176	84 – 86	187	181	176	186
Libyan Arab Jamahiriya	107	102	57 – 58	76	12 – 15	97	84	94	87
Lithuania	63	48	80 – 81	45 – 47	131 – 133	52	71	93	73
Luxembourg	18	22	3	3 – 38	2	5	5	31	16
Madagascar	172	168	168 – 169	179 – 180	116 – 120	167	190	173	159
Malawi	189	187	162	152	89 – 95	182	161	187	185
Malaysia	89	49	31	62	122 – 123	55	93	86	49
Maldives	130	134	98 – 99	101 – 102	51 – 52	128	76	147	147
Mali	183	180	187 – 188	187	150 – 151	178	179	170	163
Malta	21	38	43 – 44	3 – 38	42 – 44	31	37	2	5
Marshall Islands	121	120	98 – 99	134 – 135	20 – 22	119	80	140	141
Mauritania	158	163	165 – 167	123	153	169	141	151	162
Mauritius	78	77	56	3 – 38	124	90	69	113	84
Mexico	55	65	53 – 54	108 – 109	144	51	55	63	61

Annex Table 1 Health system attainment and performance in all Member States, ranked by eight measures, estimates for 1997

Member State	ATTAINMENT OF GOALS						Health expenditure per capita in international dollars	PERFORMANCE	
	Health		Responsiveness		Fairness in financial contribution	Overall goal attainment		On level of health	Overall health system performance
	Level (DALE)	Distribution	Level	Distribution					
Micronesia, Federated States of	104	112	112	128 – 129	23 – 25	111	81	110	123
Monaco	9	30	14	3 – 38	42 – 44	18	12	12	13
Mongolia	131	148	46	91	97	136	145	138	145
Morocco	110	111	151 – 153	67 – 68	125 – 127	94	99	17	29
Mozambique	180	190	189 – 190	175	38 – 40	185	160	168	184
Myanmar	139	162	151 – 153	158	190	175	136	129	190
Namibia	177	173	113	156	125 – 127	165	66	189	168
Nauru	136	51	42	39 – 42	17 – 19	75	42	166	98
Nepal	142	161	185	166 – 167	186	160	170	98	150
Netherlands	13	15	9	3 – 38	20 – 22	8	9	19	17
New Zealand	31	16	22 – 23	3 – 38	23 – 25	26	20	80	41
Nicaragua	117	96	140	139	164 – 165	101	104	74	71
Niger	190	184	189 – 190	184	160 – 161	188	185	177	170
Nigeria	163	188	149	177	180	184	176	175	187
Niue	85	100	126	145	35 – 36	102	127	108	121
Norway	15	4	7 – 8	3 – 38	8 – 11	3	16	18	11
Oman	72	59	83	49	56 – 57	59	62	1	8
Pakistan	124	183	120 – 121	115	62 – 63	133	142	85	122
Palau	112	66	52	39 – 42	30 – 32	63	47	125	82
Panama	47	93	59	88	76 – 78	70	53	67	95
Papua New Guinea	145	157	150	119	71 – 72	150	137	146	148
Paraguay	71	57	97	133	177	73	91	52	57
Peru	105	103	172	161	184	115	78	119	129
Philippines	113	50	49	48	128 – 130	54	124	126	60
Poland	45	5	50	65	150 – 151	34	58	89	50
Portugal	29	34	38	53 – 57	58 – 60	32	28	13	12
Qatar	66	55	26 – 27	3 – 38	70	47	27	53	44
Republic of Korea	51	37	35	43	53	35	31	107	58
Republic of Moldova	88	64	123	107	148	91	108	106	101
Romania	80	78	73 – 74	67 – 68	79 – 81	72	107	111	99
Russian Federation	91	69	69 – 72	86 – 87	185	100	75	127	130
Rwanda	185	185	145 – 147	143 – 144	58 – 60	171	177	181	172
Saint Kitts and Nevis	86	91	53 – 54	3 – 38	136 – 137	98	51	122	100
Saint Lucia	54	86	84 – 86	82	66 – 67	87	86	54	68
Saint Vincent and the Grenadines	43	89	103 – 104	98 – 100	99 – 100	92	90	38	74
Samoa	97	81	80 – 81	98 – 100	33 – 34	82	121	131	119
San Marino	11	9	32	3 – 38	30 – 32	21	21	5	3
Sao Tome and Principe	132	139	148	126	66 – 67	138	167	117	133
Saudi Arabia	58	70	67	50 – 52	37	61	63	10	26
Senegal	151	105	118 – 119	104	87	118	143	132	59
Seychelles	108	73	75	75	64 – 65	83	52	83	56
Sierra Leone	191	186	173	186	191	191	183	183	191
Singapore	30	29	20 – 21	3 – 38	101 – 102	27	38	14	6
Slovakia	42	39	60	63 – 64	96	39	45	88	62
Slovenia	34	23	37	53 – 57	82 – 83	29	29	62	38
Solomon Islands	127	117	132 – 135	120	17 – 19	108	134	20	80
Somalia	173	179	191	190	136 – 137	189	191	154	179
South Africa	160	128	73 – 74	147	142 – 143	151	57	182	175
Spain	5	11	34	3 – 38	26 – 29	19	24	6	7
Sri Lanka	76	80	101	77 – 78	76 – 78	80	138	66	76
Sudan	154	159	164	148 – 149	160 – 161	148	169	149	134
Suriname	77	94	87	79 – 81	172	105	72	77	110
Swaziland	164	140	108 – 110	110	156	164	116	184	177
Sweden	4	28	10	3 – 38	12 – 15	4	7	21	23
Switzerland	8	10	2	3 – 38	38 – 40	2	2	26	20

Member State	ATTAINMENT OF GOALS						Health expenditure per capita in international dollars	PERFORMANCE	
	Health		Responsiveness		Fairness in financial contribution	Overall goal attainment		On level of health	Overall health system performance
	Level (DALE)	Distribution	Level	Distribution					
Syrian Arab Republic	114	107	69 – 72	79 – 81	142 – 143	112	119	91	108
Tajikistan	120	124	125	136	112 – 113	127	126	145	154
Thailand	99	74	33	50 – 52	128 – 130	57	64	102	47
The former Yugoslav Republic of Macedonia	64	85	111	95	116 – 120	89	106	69	89
Togo	159	170	155	162	152	156	180	159	152
Tonga	75	84	61	97	108 – 111	85	73	114	116
Trinidad and Tobago	57	75	141	108 – 109	69	56	65	79	67
Tunisia	90	114	94	60 – 61	108 – 111	77	79	46	52
Turkey	73	109	93	66	49 – 50	96	82	33	70
Turkmenistan	128	131	88 – 89	113	121	130	128	152	153
Tuvalu	119	116	132 – 135	153 – 155	26 – 29	120	151	128	136
Uganda	186	138	187 – 188	165	128 – 130	162	168	179	149
Ukraine	70	47	96	63 – 64	140 – 141	60	111	101	79
United Arab Emirates	50	62	30	1	20 – 22	44	35	16	27
United Kingdom	14	2	26 – 27	3 – 38	8 – 11	9	26	24	18
United Republic of Tanzania	176	172	157 – 160	150	48	158	174	180	156
United States of America	24	32	1	3 – 38	54 – 55	15	1	72	37
Uruguay	37	68	41	53 – 57	35 – 36	50	33	50	65
Uzbekistan	100	144	105 – 107	71	131 – 133	109	120	112	117
Vanuatu	135	127	127	132	62 – 63	134	132	120	127
Venezuela, Bolivarian Republic of	52	76	69 – 72	92	98	65	68	29	54
Viet Nam	116	104	51	121	187	140	147	130	160
Yemen	141	165	180	189	135	146	182	82	120
Yugoslavia	46	90	115 – 117	116	158	95	113	47	106
Zambia	188	171	132 – 135	171	155	174	148	190	182
Zimbabwe	184	98	122	166 – 167	175	147	110	191	155

Source: Annex Tables 5–10.

Annex Table 2 Basic indicators for all Member States

Member State	POPULATION ESTIMATES							
	Total population (000)	Annual growth rate (%)	Dependency ratio (per 100)		Percentage of population aged 60+ years		Total fertility rate	
	1999	1990–1999	1990	1999	1990	1999	1990	1999
1 Afghanistan	21 923	4.5	89	86	5.0	4.9	6.9	6.7
2 Albania	3 113	-0.6	62	56	7.8	9.0	2.9	2.4
3 Algeria	30 774	2.4	84	69	5.5	5.7	4.6	3.7
4 Andorra	75	4.3	48	47	19.0	21.7	1.5	1.3
5 Angola	12 479	3.4	99	102	4.8	4.6	7.2	6.6
6 Antigua and Barbuda	67	0.6	63	58	9.1	9.7	2.0	1.7
7 Argentina	36 577	1.3	65	60	12.9	13.3	2.9	2.6
8 Armenia	3 525	-0.1	56	51	10.0	12.9	2.4	1.7
9 Australia	18 705	1.1	49	49	15.5	16.1	1.9	1.8
10 Austria	8 177	0.7	48	47	20.1	19.9	1.5	1.4
11 Azerbaijan	7 697	0.8	61	57	8.0	10.6	2.7	2.0
12 Bahamas	301	1.9	58	56	6.6	7.7	2.6	2.6
13 Bahrain	606	2.4	51	49	3.8	4.7	3.8	2.7
14 Bangladesh	126 947	1.7	90	64	4.9	5.1	4.3	3.0
15 Barbados	269	0.5	57	48	15.3	13.8	1.7	1.5
16 Belarus	10 274	0.0	51	49	16.5	19.1	1.8	1.4
17 Belgium	10 152	0.2	50	51	20.7	21.6	1.6	1.6
18 Belize	235	2.6	93	80	6.2	6.0	4.4	3.5
19 Benin	5 937	2.7	106	96	4.8	4.3	6.6	5.7
20 Bhutan	2 064	2.2	85	88	6.0	6.2	5.8	5.4
21 Bolivia	8 142	2.4	81	78	5.8	6.1	4.9	4.2
22 Bosnia and Herzegovina	3 839	-1.3	43	41	10.4	14.7	1.7	1.4
23 Botswana	1 597	2.5	93	81	3.6	4.0	5.1	4.2
24 Brazil	167 988	1.4	64	53	6.7	7.6	2.7	2.2
25 Brunei Darussalam	322	2.5	59	56	4.1	5.0	3.2	2.7
26 Bulgaria	8 279	-0.6	50	48	19.1	21.2	1.7	1.2
27 Burkina Faso	11 616	2.8	101	100	4.4	4.2	7.3	6.4
28 Burundi	6 565	2.1	95	97	4.8	4.0	6.8	6.1
29 Cambodia	10 945	2.6	73	80	4.8	4.8	5.0	4.5
30 Cameroon	14 693	2.8	94	90	5.6	5.5	5.9	5.2
31 Canada	30 857	1.2	47	47	15.5	16.7	1.7	1.6
32 Cape Verde	418	2.3	93	80	7.0	6.6	4.3	3.5
33 Central African Republic	3 550	2.1	90	87	6.2	5.9	5.5	4.8
34 Chad	7 458	2.9	96	96	5.6	5.3	6.6	5.9
35 Chile	15 019	1.5	57	56	9.0	10.0	2.6	2.4
36 China	1 273 640	1.0	50	47	8.6	10.0	2.2	1.8
37 Colombia	41 564	1.9	68	61	6.3	6.8	3.1	2.7
38 Comoros	676	2.8	98	83	4.1	4.3	6.0	4.7
39 Congo	2 864	2.9	96	98	5.3	4.9	6.3	5.9
40 Cook Islands	19	0.6	70	66	5.6	6.6	4.0	3.4
41 Costa Rica	3 933	2.9	69	61	6.4	7.3	3.2	2.8
42 Côte d'Ivoire	14 526	2.5	101	88	4.4	4.6	6.3	4.9
43 Croatia	4 477	-0.1	47	47	17.1	20.5	1.7	1.6
44 Cuba	11 160	0.5	46	45	11.7	13.4	1.7	1.6
45 Cyprus	778	1.5	58	54	14.8	15.6	2.4	2.0
46 Czech Republic	10 262	0.0	51	44	17.7	18.0	1.8	1.2
47 Democratic People's Republic of Korea	23 702	1.6	45	49	6.7	7.9	2.2	2.0
48 Democratic Republic of the Congo	50 335	3.4	100	104	4.6	4.4	6.7	6.3
49 Denmark	5 282	0.3	48	49	20.4	20.0	1.6	1.7
50 Djibouti	629	2.2	85	81	4.8	5.4	6.0	5.2
51 Dominica	71	-0.1	63	58	9.1	9.7	2.2	1.9
52 Dominican Republic	8 364	1.8	68	61	5.6	6.6	3.3	2.7
53 Ecuador	12 411	2.1	76	64	6.1	6.8	3.8	3.0
54 Egypt	67 226	2.0	78	67	6.0	6.3	4.2	3.2
55 El Salvador	6 154	2.1	82	69	6.5	7.1	3.7	3.1

	PROBABILITY OF DYING (per 1000)								LIFE EXPECTANCY AT BIRTH (years)			
	Under age 5 years				Between ages 15 and 59 years							
	Males		Females		Males		Females		Males		Females	
	1999	Uncertainty interval	1999	Uncertainty interval	1999	Uncertainty interval	1999	Uncertainty interval	1999	Uncertainty interval	1999	Uncertainty interval
1	279	243 – 317	249	214 – 286	348	315 – 379	326	298 – 350	45.3	42.7 – 47.8	47.2	44.5 – 49.9
2	61	51 – 73	49	40 – 60	175	159 – 191	84	74 – 94	65.1	63.7 – 66.4	72.7	71.3 – 73.9
3	50	40 – 63	48	38 – 58	139	122 – 157	118	103 – 134	68.2	66.7 – 69.7	68.8	67.3 – 70.2
4	5	3 – 8	5	3 – 8	129	108 – 154	54	43 – 68	75.4	73.9 – 76.6	82.2	81.0 – 83.3
5	209	190 – 238	192	173 – 216	427	395 – 457	375	347 – 405	46.3	44.0 – 48.4	49.1	46.9 – 51.1
6	22	19 – 24	20	18 – 23	173	161 – 185	100	96 – 104	71.4	70.3 – 72.5	76.8	76.0 – 77.8
7	23	20 – 27	20	17 – 22	178	173 – 183	92	88 – 96	70.6	70.2 – 71.1	77.8	77.3 – 78.3
8	19	13 – 26	16	11 – 23	166	147 – 187	81	67 – 97	72.3	71.0 – 73.4	77.1	75.7 – 78.4
9	7	6 – 7	5	5 – 6	94	91 – 98	53	49 – 58	76.8	76.5 – 77.1	82.2	81.6 – 82.8
10	6	5 – 7	6	5 – 7	131	120 – 143	66	62 – 69	74.4	73.7 – 75.0	80.4	80.0 – 80.7
11	32	26 – 40	25	20 – 31	217	198 – 238	101	89 – 115	67.8	66.4 – 69.0	75.3	74.1 – 76.4
12	24	20 – 28	21	18 – 25	239	223 – 256	129	118 – 141	67.0	66.0 – 67.9	73.6	72.7 – 74.5
13	23	19 – 25	20	18 – 23	137	125 – 147	99	92 – 107	70.6	69.9 – 71.5	73.6	72.9 – 74.3
14	113	101 – 129	116	103 – 133	300	283 – 317	259	242 – 278	57.5	56.0 – 58.7	58.1	56.3 – 59.5
15	11	11 – 12	10	7 – 14	169	142 – 200	91	77 – 104	72.7	70.4 – 75.2	77.8	76.3 – 79.5
16	16	12 – 21	11	8 – 14	375	341 – 412	126	110 – 142	62.4	60.7 – 63.9	74.6	73.5 – 75.5
17	9	8 – 9	6	5 – 7	121	117 – 126	62	53 – 71	74.5	74.1 – 74.9	81.3	80.9 – 81.7
18	30	26 – 35	25	21 – 30	200	186 – 214	119	108 – 132	69.6	68.6 – 70.6	75.0	73.8 – 75.9
19	157	141 – 174	148	134 – 165	381	350 – 409	338	310 – 365	51.3	49.5 – 53.4	53.3	51.3 – 55.3
20	113	101 – 128	114	102 – 130	258	243 – 269	214	202 – 228	59.6	58.5 – 60.8	60.8	59.3 – 62.1
21	91	81 – 101	81	75 – 88	281	264 – 297	245	231 – 258	60.7	59.6 – 62.0	62.2	61.3 – 63.2
22	22	19 – 25	17	15 – 20	158	146 – 170	99	91 – 109	71.2	70.3 – 72.0	75.0	74.1 – 75.8
23	99	92 – 106	97	92 – 102	786	767 – 804	740	718 – 761	39.5	38.5 – 40.5	39.3	38.2 – 40.4
24	47	38 – 57	42	33 – 51	295	272 – 318	157	142 – 174	63.7	62.1 – 65.1	71.7	70.3 – 73.0
25	12	9 – 14	9	7 – 11	153	139 – 167	94	84 – 105	74.5	73.7 – 75.2	79.8	79.1 – 80.4
26	21	19 – 23	16	15 – 18	242	233 – 253	98	94 – 102	67.4	66.9 – 68.0	74.7	74.4 – 75.1
27	182	159 – 206	171	151 – 197	532	493 – 573	486	448 – 528	44.1	41.8 – 46.4	45.7	43.2 – 48.1
28	170	148 – 197	166	144 – 193	582	509 – 653	546	473 – 620	43.2	39.8 – 46.6	43.8	40.0 – 47.5
29	138	127 – 149	129	113 – 148	394	377 – 414	323	306 – 343	52.2	50.9 – 53.3	55.4	53.6 – 56.9
30	123	109 – 136	120	106 – 132	477	439 – 520	419	384 – 462	49.9	47.8 – 52.1	52.0	49.7 – 54.2
31	6	5 – 7	5	4 – 6	104	98 – 109	59	55 – 64	76.2	75.8 – 76.5	81.9	81.5 – 82.3
32	55	50 – 60	50	46 – 54	228	205 – 248	126	110 – 142	64.2	62.9 – 65.8	71.8	70.2 – 73.6
33	153	138 – 166	143	129 – 155	608	572 – 645	555	520 – 593	43.3	41.4 – 45.2	44.9	42.8 – 46.9
34	184	159 – 213	165	143 – 192	439	406 – 472	386	356 – 416	47.3	44.8 – 49.6	50.1	47.6 – 52.4
35	11	9 – 13	8	7 – 10	132	119 – 146	66	61 – 70	73.4	71.9 – 74.9	79.9	79.2 – 80.7
36	35	29 – 43	40	33 – 48	170	158 – 182	125	115 – 135	68.1	67.3 – 68.9	71.3	70.4 – 72.2
37	31	28 – 34	26	24 – 28	221	207 – 235	128	120 – 136	68.1	67.2 – 69.0	74.1	73.3 – 74.9
38	113	100 – 124	92	83 – 103	323	293 – 352	295	269 – 321	56.0	54.3 – 57.9	58.1	56.5 – 59.8
39	112	99 – 127	102	89 – 119	415	378 – 453	378	342 – 413	53.6	51.5 – 55.8	55.2	53.0 – 57.4
40	29	27 – 32	24	23 – 26	154	142 – 166	101	94 – 107	69.2	68.3 – 70.2	73.3	72.4 – 74.2
41	13	9 – 17	14	11 – 19	121	106 – 137	79	68 – 90	74.2	73.1 – 75.1	78.9	77.8 – 79.8
42	145	132 – 161	124	114 – 139	524	495 – 553	497	467 – 525	47.2	45.5 – 49.0	48.3	46.7 – 50.2
43	9	7 – 11	7	5 – 8	194	180 – 209	76	67 – 84	69.3	68.7 – 69.9	77.3	76.8 – 77.8
44	10	9 – 11	8	6 – 10	143	132 – 155	99	86 – 114	73.5	72.4 – 74.7	77.4	76.2 – 78.5
45	9	6 – 12	8	6 – 11	102	89 – 117	57	48 – 67	74.8	73.8 – 75.7	78.8	77.9 – 79.5
46	6	5 – 8	5	4 – 6	173	160 – 188	73	65 – 82	71.3	70.7 – 71.9	78.2	77.6 – 78.7
47	100	91 – 109	99	91 – 109	305	291 – 319	229	214 – 244	58.0	57.0 – 58.9	60.6	59.5 – 61.8
48	170	155 – 185	153	141 – 167	515	483 – 543	482	449 – 509	45.1	43.5 – 46.7	46.5	45.0 – 48.3
49	7	5 – 9	6	5 – 6	138	125 – 152	89	82 – 97	72.9	72.2 – 73.7	78.1	77.6 – 78.7
50	169	154 – 202	162	147 – 190	556	513 – 596	524	483 – 563	45.0	42.5 – 47.0	45.0	42.6 – 47.2
51	9	8 – 10	7	6 – 8	123	115 – 131	55	54 – 57	74.0	73.0 – 75.1	80.2	79.4 – 81.2
52	52	48 – 58	46	42 – 51	177	164 – 189	147	141 – 150	71.4	70.2 – 72.6	72.8	72.5 – 73.3
53	40	36 – 44	33	30 – 36	200	186 – 214	144	134 – 153	67.4	66.4 – 68.3	70.3	69.5 – 71.1
54	74	66 – 84	72	63 – 81	187	176 – 202	148	133 – 164	64.2	63.1 – 65.1	65.8	64.4 – 67.2
55	42	38 – 46	35	31 – 40	238	224 – 252	144	133 – 154	66.9	65.9 – 67.8	73.0	72.0 – 73.9

Annex Table 2 Basic indicators for all Member States

Member State	POPULATION ESTIMATES								
	Total population (000)	Annual growth rate (%)	Dependency ratio (per 100)		Percentage of population aged 60+ years		Total fertility rate	
	1999	1990–1999	1990	1999	1990	1999	1990	1999
56 Equatorial Guinea	442	2.6	87	90	6.4	6.1	5.9	5.5
57 Eritrea	3 719	2.8	88	89	4.4	4.6	6.2	5.6
58 Estonia	1 412	-1.2	51	46	17.2	19.4	1.9	1.3
59 Ethiopia	61 095	2.7	94	96	4.7	4.5	6.8	6.2
60 Fiji	806	1.2	70	57	5.3	7.1	3.1	2.7
61 Finland	5 165	0.4	49	49	18.5	19.7	1.7	1.7
62 France	58 886	0.4	52	53	19.1	20.5	1.8	1.7
63 Gabon	1 197	2.8	76	84	9.2	8.7	5.1	5.3
64 Gambia	1 268	3.6	82	77	4.8	5.1	5.9	5.1
65 Georgia	5 006	-1.0	51	53	15.0	18.1	2.2	1.9
66 Germany	82 178	0.4	45	47	20.4	22.7	1.4	1.3
67 Ghana	19 678	3.0	93	87	4.6	4.9	6.0	5.0
68 Greece	10 626	0.4	49	49	20.0	23.6	1.5	1.3
69 Grenada	93	0.3	63	58	9.1	9.7	4.1	3.6
70 Guatemala	11 090	2.7	97	90	5.1	5.3	5.6	4.8
71 Guinea	7 360	2.8	97	89	4.3	4.4	6.3	5.4
72 Guinea-Bissau	1 187	2.2	85	88	6.6	6.4	6.0	5.6
73 Guyana	855	0.8	60	53	5.9	6.2	2.6	2.3
74 Haiti	8 087	1.8	93	81	5.8	5.5	5.4	4.3
75 Honduras	6 316	2.9	93	83	4.5	5.1	5.1	4.1
76 Hungary	10 076	-0.3	51	47	19.0	19.7	1.8	1.3
77 Iceland	279	1.0	55	54	14.6	14.9	2.2	2.1
78 India	998 056	1.8	69	63	6.9	7.5	3.8	3.0
79 Indonesia	209 255	1.5	65	55	6.3	7.3	3.1	2.5
80 Iran, Islamic Republic of	66 796	1.9	96	72	5.7	6.3	4.9	2.7
81 Iraq	22 450	2.4	89	81	4.5	4.8	5.9	5.1
82 Ireland	3 705	0.6	63	49	15.1	15.2	2.1	1.9
83 Israel	6 101	3.0	68	61	12.4	13.1	3.0	2.6
84 Italy	57 343	0.1	45	48	21.1	23.9	1.3	1.2
85 Jamaica	2 560	0.9	74	63	10.0	9.3	2.8	2.4
86 Japan	126 505	0.3	44	46	17.4	22.6	1.6	1.4
87 Jordan	6 482	3.8	100	82	4.8	4.5	5.8	4.7
88 Kazakhstan	16 269	-0.3	60	54	9.6	11.2	2.8	2.2
89 Kenya	29 549	2.6	109	87	4.5	4.4	6.1	4.2
90 Kiribati	82	1.4	76	72	4.6	5.1	4.9	4.2
91 Kuwait	1 897	-1.3	61	58	2.1	3.4	3.6	2.8
92 Kyrgyzstan	4 669	0.7	74	71	8.3	8.9	3.8	3.1
93 Lao People's Democratic Republic	5 297	2.7	87	90	5.0	5.2	6.5	5.6
94 Latvia	2 389	-1.3	50	48	17.7	20.0	1.9	1.3
95 Lebanon	3 236	2.7	67	64	8.1	8.3	3.3	2.6
96 Lesotho	2 108	2.3	83	79	6.2	6.4	5.1	4.7
97 Liberia	2 930	1.4	98	87	4.7	4.5	6.8	6.2
98 Libyan Arab Jamahiriya	5 471	2.4	91	71	4.1	5.1	4.9	3.7
99 Lithuania	3 682	-0.2	50	49	16.1	18.3	1.9	1.4
100 Luxembourg	426	1.3	44	48	18.9	19.4	1.6	1.7
101 Madagascar	15 497	3.2	82	90	5.1	4.4	6.2	5.3
102 Malawi	10 640	1.5	100	99	4.3	4.2	7.3	6.6
103 Malaysia	21 830	2.3	67	63	5.8	6.5	3.8	3.1
104 Maldives	278	2.9	99	89	5.4	5.4	6.4	5.2
105 Mali	10 960	2.4	101	101	4.8	5.5	7.1	6.4
106 Malta	386	1.0	51	47	14.7	16.3	2.0	1.9
107 Marshall Islands	62	3.4	76	72	4.6	5.1	6.1	5.4
108 Mauritania	2 598	2.8	93	88	4.9	4.9	6.0	5.4
109 Mauritius	1 150	0.9	54	47	8.3	8.9	2.2	1.9
110 Mexico	97 365	1.8	74	62	5.9	6.8	3.4	2.7

	PROBABILITY OF DYING (per 1000)								LIFE EXPECTANCY AT BIRTH (years)			
	Under age 5 years				Between ages 15 and 59 years							
	Males		Females		Males		Females		Males		Females	
	1999	Uncertainty interval	1999	Uncertainty interval	1999	Uncertainty interval	1999	Uncertainty interval	1999	Uncertainty interval	1999	Uncertainty interval
56	146	129 – 164	131	115 – 145	384	350 – 413	309	281 – 334	51.4	49.4 – 53.5	55.4	53.6 – 57.4
57	144	133 – 159	134	121 – 146	520	481 – 556	514	477 – 548	46.6	44.8 – 48.5	46.5	44.7 – 48.3
58	12	8 – 15	11	7 – 16	341	308 – 377	120	100 – 143	64.4	62.8 – 65.9	75.3	73.9 – 76.5
59	188	171 – 207	177	162 – 194	596	556 – 641	545	505 – 591	41.4	39.3 – 43.5	43.1	40.8 – 45.3
60	25	14 – 42	19	11 – 31	247	194 – 307	141	106 – 186	64.0	61.0 – 66.4	69.2	66.6 – 71.3
61	5	4 – 5	4	4 – 5	148	145 – 150	59	55 – 64	73.4	72.9 – 73.8	80.7	80.1 – 81.4
62	7	6 – 8	5	4 – 6	146	141 – 151	59	56 – 62	74.9	74.4 – 75.3	83.6	83.1 – 84.1
63	94	81 – 109	85	73 – 99	397	366 – 431	336	306 – 368	54.6	52.5 – 56.6	57.5	55.4 – 59.6
64	103	94 – 114	93	85 – 102	351	321 – 378	295	270 – 319	56.0	54.3 – 57.8	58.9	57.4 – 60.6
65	20	14 – 27	16	11 – 22	209	184 – 237	85	70 – 102	69.4	67.8 – 70.9	76.7	75.3 – 77.9
66	6	6 – 7	5	5 – 5	136	128 – 144	67	64 – 70	73.7	73.3 – 74.2	80.1	79.9 – 80.4
67	118	102 – 135	109	95 – 126	376	339 – 413	343	309 – 378	54.2	51.8 – 56.4	55.6	53.2 – 57.7
68	8	7 – 9	7	6 – 7	117	113 – 120	50	47 – 52	75.5	75.3 – 75.7	80.5	80.1 – 80.9
69	27	24 – 30	22	20 – 25	206	192 – 220	109	105 – 113	69.1	68.1 – 70.2	75.9	75.1 – 76.8
70	58	53 – 63	44	40 – 48	326	307 – 343	223	210 – 237	60.2	59.2 – 61.1	64.7	63.9 – 65.6
71	217	201 – 230	193	180 – 208	413	379 – 443	369	338 – 395	46.2	44.4 – 48.1	48.9	47.2 – 50.8
72	207	190 – 236	196	175 – 215	457	423 – 489	411	380 – 440	45.0	42.7 – 47.0	47.0	45.0 – 49.0
73	75	66 – 84	58	51 – 65	242	227 – 256	153	142 – 164	65.6	64.3 – 66.9	72.2	71.1 – 73.3
74	120	110 – 135	111	101 – 126	481	459 – 503	360	341 – 382	50.6	49.1 – 51.7	55.1	53.4 – 56.3
75	42	38 – 46	37	33 – 42	219	205 – 233	168	157 – 180	68.2	67.2 – 69.2	70.8	69.8 – 71.8
76	12	9 – 15	10	9 – 12	292	263 – 325	127	123 – 131	66.3	64.9 – 67.6	75.1	74.5 – 75.7
77	5	4 – 7	3	2 – 4	81	71 – 91	54	45 – 61	76.1	74.8 – 77.4	80.4	78.9 – 81.9
78	97	84 – 110	104	91 – 118	275	261 – 289	217	205 – 229	59.6	58.4 – 60.6	61.2	59.9 – 62.3
79	63	53 – 70	53	49 – 58	240	224 – 257	197	183 – 210	66.6	65.3 – 67.9	69.0	67.9 – 70.1
80	48	41 – 55	42	36 – 48	160	143 – 178	129	120 – 139	66.8	65.5 – 68.0	67.9	67.1 – 68.6
81	67	60 – 79	54	50 – 61	243	220 – 259	208	190 – 220	61.6	60.4 – 62.8	62.8	62.1 – 63.7
82	7	5 – 9	6	4 – 8	116	101 – 133	67	56 – 78	73.3	72.4 – 74.2	78.3	77.4 – 79.0
83	8	7 – 8	7	7 – 8	101	97 – 105	59	52 – 67	76.2	75.6 – 76.8	79.9	79.5 – 80.4
84	6	6 – 7	5	5 – 6	109	102 – 116	51	46 – 55	75.4	75.1 – 75.6	82.1	81.9 – 82.3
85	29	25 – 32	25	21 – 30	135	123 – 146	99	90 – 110	75.2	74.2 – 76.4	77.4	76.4 – 78.4
86	5	5 – 6	5	4 – 5	95	92 – 99	48	46 – 49	77.6	77.3 – 77.8	84.3	83.9 – 84.7
87	29	24 – 36	25	21 – 30	172	160 – 191	132	125 – 148	66.3	65.1 – 66.9	67.5	66.5 – 68.0
88	48	39 – 58	36	29 – 44	407	389 – 424	177	161 – 193	58.8	57.6 – 59.9	69.9	68.7 – 71.0
89	100	89 – 112	99	87 – 110	591	545 – 634	546	500 – 592	47.3	45.1 – 49.5	48.1	45.6 – 50.5
90	62	57 – 67	58	54 – 62	276	257 – 295	196	184 – 208	61.4	60.7 – 62.1	65.5	64.8 – 66.2
91	19	15 – 23	17	14 – 21	119	106 – 134	83	74 – 94	71.9	70.9 – 72.8	75.2	74.2 – 76.1
92	73	61 – 87	68	56 – 81	293	271 – 316	152	139 – 168	61.6	60.0 – 63.0	69.0	67.4 – 70.4
93	143	127 – 163	126	112 – 145	341	321 – 361	302	284 – 323	54.0	52.2 – 55.6	56.6	54.7 – 58.1
94	21	14 – 32	16	11 – 22	349	307 – 393	131	111 – 155	63.6	61.3 – 65.5	74.6	73.0 – 75.9
95	31	24 – 37	25	19 – 32	172	150 – 195	136	116 – 160	66.2	65.0 – 67.5	67.3	65.8 – 68.5
96	147	130 – 164	134	119 – 151	604	549 – 653	565	510 – 615	44.1	41.6 – 46.7	45.1	42.4 – 47.9
97	214	195 – 240	196	176 – 218	513	480 – 544	461	433 – 491	42.5	40.4 – 44.5	44.9	42.9 – 46.8
98	39	32 – 49	35	27 – 43	192	169 – 215	141	121 – 161	65.0	63.7 – 66.3	67.0	65.7 – 68.4
99	16	12 – 21	9	7 – 12	284	254 – 317	95	83 – 109	67.0	65.2 – 68.6	77.9	76.9 – 78.8
100	6	5 – 9	6	4 – 9	139	126 – 151	69	66 – 72	74.5	73.7 – 75.4	81.4	80.4 – 82.5
101	179	163 – 198	157	141 – 172	486	457 – 515	440	410 – 467	45.0	43.2 – 46.7	47.7	45.9 – 49.4
102	222	207 – 248	215	196 – 233	664	631 – 689	618	587 – 643	37.3	35.4 – 39.0	38.4	36.7 – 40.1
103	15	13 – 17	13	11 – 15	172	159 – 188	125	115 – 137	67.6	66.8 – 68.3	69.9	69.2 – 70.5
104	90	81 – 102	86	76 – 98	214	198 – 228	208	194 – 223	63.3	62.1 – 64.5	62.6	61.3 – 63.8
105	240	222 – 260	229	214 – 249	500	468 – 529	432	401 – 459	41.3	39.5 – 43.2	44.0	42.2 – 45.8
106	9	7 – 13	6	4 – 8	94	81 – 108	45	38 – 54	75.7	74.7 – 76.5	80.8	80.0 – 81.5
107	60	56 – 66	51	48 – 55	227	209 – 245	175	163 – 186	64.0	63.2 – 64.9	67.1	66.4 – 67.9
108	189	174 – 204	168	157 – 180	367	335 – 396	312	284 – 336	49.5	47.8 – 51.6	53.0	51.3 – 54.8
109	26	17 – 39	15	10 – 21	247	211 – 284	116	99 – 134	66.7	64.7 – 68.6	74.1	72.8 – 75.1
110	26	19 – 36	23	18 – 28	194	176 – 214	109	102 – 116	71.0	69.7 – 72.2	77.1	76.4 – 77.9

Annex Table 2 Basic indicators for all Member States

Member State	Total population (000) 1999	Annual growth rate (%) 1990–1999	Dependency ratio (per 100) 1990	Dependency ratio (per 100) 1999	Percentage of population aged 60+ years 1990	Percentage of population aged 60+ years 1999	Total fertility rate 1990	Total fertility rate 1999
111 Micronesia, Federated States of	116	2.1	76	72	4.6	5.1	5.1	4.6
112 Monaco	33	1.2	48	49	19.7	21.3	1.7	1.7
113 Mongolia	2 621	1.9	84	65	5.8	5.8	4.1	2.5
114 Morocco	27 867	1.7	74	60	6.1	6.7	3.8	2.9
115 Mozambique	19 286	3.5	91	93	5.2	5.1	6.5	6.1
116 Myanmar	45 059	1.2	66	50	6.4	7.4	3.2	2.3
117 Namibia	1 695	2.6	87	83	5.7	5.9	5.4	4.8
118 Nauru	11	1.9	76	72	4.6	5.1	4.6	4.0
119 Nepal	23 385	2.5	87	82	5.7	5.5	5.3	4.3
120 Netherlands	15 735	0.6	45	47	17.3	18.3	1.6	1.5
121 New Zealand	3 828	1.5	53	53	15.3	15.5	2.1	2.0
122 Nicaragua	4 938	2.9	96	86	4.4	4.6	5.0	4.3
123 Niger	10 400	3.3	101	103	4.0	4.0	7.6	6.7
124 Nigeria	108 945	2.5	93	87	4.5	4.9	6.0	5.0
125 Niue	2	-2.0	70	66	5.6	6.6	3.2	2.7
126 Norway	4 442	0.5	54	54	21.0	19.7	1.8	1.9
127 Oman	2 460	3.6	95	89	3.8	4.1	7.0	5.7
128 Pakistan	152 331	2.8	85	83	4.7	4.9	5.8	4.9
129 Palau	19	2.5	76	72	4.6	5.1	2.9	2.5
130 Panama	2 812	1.8	67	59	7.3	8.0	3.0	2.6
131 Papua New Guinea	4 702	2.3	75	72	4.7	5.0	5.1	4.5
132 Paraguay	5 358	2.7	84	77	5.4	5.3	4.7	4.1
133 Peru	25 230	1.8	73	63	6.1	7.1	3.7	2.9
134 Philippines	74 454	2.3	78	68	5.3	5.6	4.1	3.5
135 Poland	38 740	0.2	54	47	14.9	16.3	2.0	1.5
136 Portugal	9 873	0.0	51	47	19.0	20.8	1.6	1.4
137 Qatar	589	2.2	40	40	2.0	4.4	4.4	3.6
138 Republic of Korea	46 480	0.9	45	39	7.7	10.2	1.7	1.7
139 Republic of Moldova	4 380	0.0	57	51	12.8	14.1	2.4	1.7
140 Romania	22 402	-0.4	51	46	15.7	18.6	1.9	1.2
141 Russian Federation	147 196	-0.1	49	45	16.0	18.3	1.8	1.4
142 Rwanda	7 235	0.4	100	92	4.1	3.9	6.8	6.0
143 Saint Kitts and Nevis	39	-0.9	63	58	9.1	9.7	2.8	2.4
144 Saint Lucia	152	1.4	63	58	9.1	9.7	2.6	2.3
145 Saint Vincent and the Grenadines	113	0.8	63	58	9.1	9.7	2.3	1.9
146 Samoa	177	1.1	80	75	5.2	6.2	4.7	4.4
147 San Marino	26	1.4	48	47	19.0	21.7	1.8	1.5
148 Sao Tome and Principe	144	2.2	105	105	6.7	6.7	6.7	6.1
149 Saudi Arabia	20 899	3.0	80	77	4.0	4.6	6.6	5.6
150 Senegal	9 240	2.6	94	90	4.7	4.2	6.3	5.4
151 Seychelles	77	1.1	61	61	9.5	9.5	2.3	2.0
152 Sierra Leone	4 717	1.9	88	89	5.1	4.8	6.5	5.9
153 Singapore	3 522	1.7	37	41	8.4	10.3	1.7	1.7
154 Slovakia	5 382	0.3	55	46	14.8	15.3	2.0	1.4
155 Slovenia	1 989	0.4	45	43	17.1	18.8	1.5	1.3
156 Solomon Islands	430	3.3	94	86	4.3	4.7	5.7	4.7
157 Somalia	9 672	2.5	102	101	4.3	3.9	7.3	7.2
158 South Africa	39 900	1.8	69	63	5.3	5.7	3.7	3.2
159 Spain	39 634	0.1	50	46	19.2	21.6	1.4	1.1
160 Sri Lanka	18 639	1.0	61	50	8.0	9.5	2.4	2.1
161 Sudan	28 883	2.0	85	76	4.5	5.1	5.2	4.5
162 Suriname	415	0.4	68	58	6.8	8.0	2.7	2.2
163 Swaziland	980	3.0	95	85	4.3	4.4	5.4	4.6
164 Sweden	8 892	0.4	56	56	22.8	22.3	2.0	1.6
165 Switzerland	7 344	0.8	45	47	19.1	19.3	1.5	1.5

	PROBABILITY OF DYING (per 1000)								LIFE EXPECTANCY AT BIRTH (years)			
	Under age 5 years				Between ages 15 and 59 years							
	Males		Females		Males		Females		Males		Females	
	1999	Uncertainty interval	1999	Uncertainty interval	1999	Uncertainty interval	1999	Uncertainty interval	1999	Uncertainty interval	1999	Uncertainty interval
111	44	40 – 48	31	29 – 34	194	179 – 209	137	128 – 145	66.4	65.6 – 67.4	70.1	69.3 – 70.9
112	9	5 – 15	7	4 – 10	146	118 – 178	59	46 – 73	74.7	72.8 – 76.4	83.6	82.2 – 84.7
113	123	103 – 144	104	88 – 123	263	245 – 278	181	169 – 193	58.9	57.2 – 60.7	64.8	63.2 – 66.3
114	69	63 – 76	61	54 – 67	177	161 – 197	139	127 – 153	65.0	63.7 – 66.2	66.8	65.6 – 67.9
115	196	170 – 225	189	164 – 218	580	523 – 633	514	454 – 571	41.8	39.1 – 44.7	44.0	41.1 – 47.4
116	142	131 – 157	126	112 – 142	253	235 – 268	231	221 – 243	58.4	57.0 – 59.8	59.2	57.8 – 60.3
117	113	101 – 126	112	100 – 124	682	614 – 741	649	578 – 711	43.3	40.3 – 46.3	43.0	39.7 – 46.5
118	19	18 – 21	15	14 – 17	511	493 – 528	260	250 – 270	56.4	56.2 – 56.6	63.3	62.9 – 63.6
119	119	105 – 134	107	95 – 119	297	276 – 317	274	256 – 291	57.3	55.8 – 58.8	57.8	56.5 – 59.3
120	7	7 – 7	6	5 – 6	103	97 – 109	66	62 – 70	75.0	74.9 – 75.2	81.1	80.5 – 81.7
121	9	8 – 10	7	6 – 8	125	116 – 133	74	70 – 79	73.9	73.5 – 74.4	79.3	78.8 – 79.9
122	50	46 – 54	44	40 – 48	239	224 – 254	163	152 – 173	64.8	63.8 – 65.7	68.8	67.9 – 69.7
123	331	310 – 355	339	318 – 363	470	436 – 502	362	329 – 393	37.2	35.3 – 39.1	40.6	38.6 – 42.7
124	173	152 – 199	170	148 – 196	473	435 – 513	429	393 – 468	46.8	44.4 – 49.1	48.2	45.6 – 50.6
125	33	19 – 57	30	17 – 53	185	144 – 234	149	113 – 193	68.3	64.8 – 71.1	70.9	67.4 – 73.5
126	6	5 – 7	5	4 – 6	109	99 – 115	60	57 – 64	75.1	74.8 – 75.4	82.1	81.6 – 82.6
127	18	16 – 20	18	16 – 19	135	122 – 150	94	90 – 100	70.4	69.4 – 71.5	73.8	73.2 – 74.2
128	100	90 – 109	98	92 – 111	194	173 – 216	147	131 – 161	62.6	61.1 – 64.2	64.9	62.1 – 66.1
129	23	21 – 25	16	15 – 17	236	222 – 251	132	125 – 139	64.5	63.9 – 65.1	69.7	69.1 – 70.3
130	35	30 – 40	32	28 – 36	163	152 – 175	116	107 – 125	72.6	71.6 – 73.6	75.8	74.9 – 76.8
131	129	114 – 139	106	92 – 123	377	358 – 395	325	306 – 345	53.4	52.2 – 54.7	56.6	54.9 – 58.0
132	37	33 – 42	33	28 – 37	200	191 – 209	132	122 – 142	69.6	68.9 – 70.3	74.1	73.1 – 75.0
133	52	48 – 56	45	42 – 48	224	210 – 239	159	149 – 168	65.6	64.6 – 66.6	69.1	68.3 – 69.9
134	48	44 – 52	41	36 – 46	232	218 – 246	147	137 – 158	64.1	63.3 – 64.9	69.3	68.5 – 70.2
135	13	13 – 14	11	10 – 11	242	219 – 268	88	83 – 92	67.9	66.5 – 69.1	76.6	76.0 – 77.2
136	9	7 – 10	7	5 – 8	162	152 – 171	64	60 – 68	72.0	71.3 – 72.7	79.5	79.1 – 79.9
137	19	16 – 22	19	17 – 21	122	110 – 128	89	85 – 96	71.6	71.1 – 72.7	74.6	74.0 – 75.2
138	12	8 – 16	10	8 – 13	215	181 – 253	92	76 – 111	69.2	67.4 – 70.7	76.3	75.1 – 77.4
139	20	16 – 25	17	13 – 21	293	274 – 313	146	132 – 162	64.8	63.8 – 65.7	71.9	71.0 – 72.7
140	29	27 – 32	22	20 – 24	285	248 – 325	119	114 – 125	65.1	64.5 – 65.7	73.5	72.9 – 74.0
141	24	19 – 30	19	14 – 24	352	326 – 378	131	116 – 147	62.7	61.3 – 63.9	74.0	72.8 – 75.0
142	189	172 – 206	163	149 – 178	602	526 – 662	581	506 – 642	41.2	38.6 – 44.5	42.3	39.4 – 45.7
143	34	30 – 38	28	24 – 32	272	255 – 288	160	155 – 164	65.0	64.2 – 65.9	71.2	70.7 – 71.8
144	27	24 – 31	19	16 – 21	209	195 – 223	114	111 – 117	68.9	67.9 – 70.0	74.9	74.2 – 75.6
145	28	25 – 31	26	22 – 29	170	158 – 183	118	114 – 122	71.9	70.7 – 73.2	75.2	74.4 – 76.0
146	28	25 – 30	25	23 – 27	217	203 – 231	126	119 – 134	65.4	64.7 – 66.1	70.7	70.0 – 71.5
147	7	4 – 12	6	4 – 9	109	86 – 136	51	40 – 64	75.3	73.6 – 76.8	82.0	80.8 – 83.1
148	82	79 – 85	51	49 – 52	241	208 – 277	212	186 – 240	62.1	59.9 – 64.5	64.9	63.1 – 66.7
149	21	19 – 23	20	18 – 23	131	124 – 136	107	99 – 116	71.0	70.6 – 71.6	72.6	71.9 – 73.4
150	134	121 – 149	126	114 – 140	362	334 – 390	308	283 – 334	53.5	51.6 – 55.5	56.2	54.3 – 58.1
151	21	21 – 22	12	12 – 12	234	205 – 266	131	114 – 149	64.9	63.3 – 66.4	70.5	69.2 – 71.8
152	326	298 – 367	298	271 – 336	599	569 – 627	557	527 – 584	33.2	30.7 – 35.2	35.4	33.0 – 37.5
153	4	3 – 6	3	2 – 4	126	110 – 144	67	58 – 77	75.1	74.0 – 76.0	80.8	79.9 – 81.5
154	12	10 – 14	10	8 – 12	216	202 – 231	84	76 – 94	68.9	68.2 – 69.5	76.7	76.0 – 77.2
155	6	4 – 7	4	3 – 5	171	157 – 185	66	59 – 74	71.6	71.0 – 72.2	79.5	78.9 – 80.0
156	49	45 – 53	47	43 – 50	274	256 – 292	227	215 – 239	62.0	61.4 – 62.7	64.0	63.5 – 64.5
157	206	174 – 245	196	173 – 235	522	482 – 556	487	451 – 522	44.0	41.4 – 46.5	44.7	41.8 – 46.9
158	85	76 – 92	67	60 – 74	601	562 – 641	533	493 – 575	47.3	45.4 – 49.0	49.7	47.7 – 51.8
159	6	6 – 7	6	5 – 8	129	117 – 144	54	48 – 61	75.3	74.0 – 76.4	82.1	81.5 – 82.7
160	25	21 – 29	19	16 – 22	269	254 – 280	141	131 – 152	65.8	65.2 – 66.7	73.4	72.5 – 74.2
161	117	97 – 147	103	86 – 127	396	364 – 427	350	319 – 380	53.1	50.7 – 55.1	54.7	52.4 – 56.6
162	34	30 – 39	27	23 – 32	220	206 – 235	134	123 – 145	68.1	67.1 – 69.2	73.6	72.6 – 74.5
163	107	94 – 119	97	85 – 110	612	556 – 660	568	510 – 618	45.8	43.4 – 48.5	46.8	44.0 – 49.8
164	5	3 – 6	4	4 – 5	89	79 – 99	60	56 – 63	77.1	76.6 – 77.7	81.9	81.3 – 82.4
165	6	4 – 9	6	4 – 8	111	96 – 126	58	49 – 69	75.6	74.6 – 76.6	83.0	82.0 – 83.9

Annex Table 2 Basic indicators for all Member States

	Member State	POPULATION ESTIMATES							
		Total population (000)	Annual growth rate (%)	Dependency ratio (per 100)		Percentage of population aged 60+ years		Total fertility rate	
		1999	1990–1999	1990	1999	1990	1999	1990	1999
166	Syrian Arab Republic	15 725	2.7	102	81	4.4	4.7	5.7	3.9
167	Tajikistan	6 104	1.6	89	83	6.2	6.7	4.9	4.0
168	Thailand	60 856	1.0	57	46	6.7	8.5	2.3	1.7
169	The former Yugoslav Republic of Macedonia	2 011	0.6	51	49	11.5	14.4	2.2	2.1
170	Togo	4 512	2.8	95	96	5.1	4.8	6.6	5.9
171	Tonga	98	0.3	70	66	5.6	6.6	4.7	4.0
172	Trinidad and Tobago	1 289	0.7	66	48	8.7	9.4	2.4	1.6
173	Tunisia	9 460	1.7	72	58	6.6	8.4	3.6	2.5
174	Turkey	65 546	1.7	65	52	7.1	8.4	3.2	2.4
175	Turkmenistan	4 384	2.0	79	74	6.2	6.5	4.3	3.5
176	Tuvalu	11	2.8	70	66	5.6	6.6	3.4	2.9
177	Uganda	21 143	2.8	104	109	4.0	3.2	7.1	7.0
178	Ukraine	50 658	-0.3	51	48	18.5	20.7	1.8	1.4
179	United Arab Emirates	2 398	2.5	47	45	2.4	4.7	4.2	3.3
180	United Kingdom	58 744	0.2	54	54	20.9	20.9	1.8	1.7
181	United Republic of Tanzania	32 793	2.8	96	93	4.1	4.1	6.1	5.3
182	United States of America	276 218	0.9	52	52	16.6	16.4	2.0	2.0
183	Uruguay	3 313	0.7	60	60	16.4	17.1	2.5	2.4
184	Uzbekistan	23 942	1.7	82	74	6.5	6.9	4.1	3.3
185	Vanuatu	186	2.5	91	83	5.4	4.9	4.9	4.2
186	Venezuela, Bolivarian Republic of	23 706	2.2	72	64	5.7	6.5	3.5	2.9
187	Viet Nam	78 705	1.9	77	65	7.2	7.5	3.8	2.5
188	Yemen	17 488	4.7	106	102	4.1	3.8	7.6	7.4
189	Yugoslavia	10 637	0.5	49	50	15.2	18.4	2.1	1.8
190	Zambia	8 976	2.4	107	99	3.9	3.4	6.2	5.4
191	Zimbabwe	11 529	1.7	89	80	4.3	4.2	5.0	3.7

	PROBABILITY OF DYING (per 1000)								LIFE EXPECTANCY AT BIRTH (years)			
	Under age 5 years				Between ages 15 and 59 years				Males		Females	
	Males		Females		Males		Females					
	1999	Uncertainty interval	1999	Uncertainty interval	1999	Uncertainty interval	1999	Uncertainty interval	1999	Uncertainty interval	1999	Uncertainty interval
56	44	35 – 55	40	32 – 49	198	176 – 222	140	121 – 160	64.6	63.1 – 65.9	67.1	65.6 – 68.5
57	69	61 – 79	59	51 – 69	234	218 – 251	149	137 – 162	65.1	63.8 – 66.4	70.1	68.7 – 71.3
58	40	35 – 45	27	24 – 30	261	244 – 277	181	171 – 189	66.0	64.9 – 67.0	70.4	69.8 – 71.1
59	27	21 – 34	23	18 – 29	165	149 – 184	95	83 – 108	69.8	68.6 – 70.8	74.1	73.0 – 75.0
70	142	124 – 161	122	108 – 138	480	436 – 517	441	399 – 478	48.9	46.7 – 51.3	50.8	48.6 – 53.3
71	29	26 – 31	23	21 – 25	167	155 – 180	103	97 – 110	68.3	67.4 – 69.2	72.8	72.0 – 73.7
72	10	7 – 13	7	5 – 10	217	196 – 240	140	123 – 159	68.7	67.6 – 69.6	73.4	72.4 – 74.3
73	36	31 – 41	31	26 – 35	158	146 – 169	128	114 – 141	67.0	66.3 – 67.8	67.9	67.0 – 69.0
74	45	42 – 50	42	39 – 46	180	168 – 191	157	148 – 167	69.7	68.8 – 70.6	69.9	69.1 – 70.8
75	83	62 – 108	77	58 – 102	293	257 – 330	173	148 – 201	61.0	58.3 – 63.3	65.3	62.7 – 67.6
76	45	41 – 49	32	30 – 34	238	221 – 254	204	194 – 214	63.9	63.2 – 64.7	65.5	65.0 – 66.1
77	165	151 – 180	153	142 – 167	622	590 – 649	592	559 – 618	41.9	40.4 – 43.5	42.4	40.9 – 44.2
78	16	14 – 20	12	10 – 15	326	311 – 341	121	110 – 132	64.4	63.6 – 65.1	74.4	73.7 – 75.0
79	19	16 – 23	16	15 – 18	117	106 – 127	80	74 – 86	72.2	71.4 – 73.0	75.6	74.9 – 76.4
80	7	7 – 7	6	5 – 6	111	108 – 113	67	66 – 69	74.7	74.4 – 75.0	79.7	79.4 – 80.0
81	157	143 – 170	148	134 – 161	568	542 – 597	525	500 – 553	44.4	42.9 – 46.0	45.6	44.0 – 47.2
82	8	8 – 8	8	7 – 8	148	139 – 157	85	83 – 87	73.8	73.0 – 74.6	79.7	79.4 – 80.0
83	20	18 – 23	16	13 – 19	184	171 – 194	88	80 – 95	70.5	69.8 – 71.4	77.8	77.2 – 78.6
84	48	38 – 60	38	30 – 49	227	206 – 247	137	121 – 155	65.8	64.2 – 67.1	71.2	69.8 – 72.5
85	64	59 – 70	57	53 – 61	333	313 – 353	239	226 – 252	58.7	58.2 – 59.3	63.0	62.5 – 63.6
86	22	21 – 24	23	19 – 26	163	151 – 176	94	84 – 105	70.9	70.0 – 71.9	76.2	74.9 – 77.3
87	39	36 – 44	31	28 – 35	225	211 – 239	153	142 – 163	64.7	63.9 – 65.5	68.8	68.1 – 69.6
88	113	101 – 137	108	92 – 127	288	259 – 314	257	234 – 281	57.3	55.0 – 58.9	58.0	56.1 – 59.7
89	29	25 – 32	22	20 – 26	153	143 – 165	90	83 – 99	71.8	70.9 – 72.6	76.4	75.4 – 77.1
90	174	160 – 190	163	149 – 178	729	690 – 765	682	640 – 721	38.0	36.0 – 39.9	39.0	36.7 – 41.2
91	122	108 – 134	113	101 – 125	730	683 – 773	710	663 – 754	40.9	38.6 – 43.2	40.0	37.5 – 42.5

Annex Table 3 Deaths by cause, sex and mortality stratum in WHO Regions[a], estimates for 1999

Cause[b]	SEX Both sexes (000)	% total	Males (000)	% total	Females (000)	% total	AFRICA High child, high adult (000)	High child, very high adult (000)	THE AMERICAS Very low child, very low adult (000)	Low child, low adult (000)	High child, high adult (000)
Population (000)	5 961 628		3 002 288		2 959 340		286 350	330 085	318 235	424 932	69 898
TOTAL DEATHS	55 965	100	29 158	100	26 807	100	4 381	6 055	2 641	2 490	556
I. Communicable diseases, maternal and perinatal conditions and nutritional deficiencies	17 380	31.1	8 734	30.0	8 645	32.2	2 931	4 429	185	519	175
Infectious and parasitic diseases	9 986	17.8	5 178	17.8	4 809	17.9	1 933	3 290	60	195	81
Tuberculosis	1 669	3.0	1 003	3.4	666	2.5	128	229	2	36	21
STDs excluding HIV	178	0.3	83	0.3	95	0.4	38	36	0	3	0
Syphilis	153	0.3	83	0.3	69	0.3	33	31	0	3	0
Chlamydia	16	0.0	0	0.0	16	0.1	3	3	0	0	0
Gonorrhoea	9	0.0	0	0.0	9	0.0	2	2	0	0	0
HIV/AIDS	2 673	4.8	1 302	4.5	1 371	5.1	458	1 696	19	45	17
Diarrhoeal diseases	2 213	4.0	1 119	3.8	1 094	4.1	371	394	2	49	23
Childhood diseases	1 554	2.8	798	2.7	755	2.8	373	367	0	20	1
Pertussis	295	0.5	157	0.5	138	0.5	67	66	0	14	0
Poliomyelitis	2	0.0	1	0.0	1	0.0	0	0	0	0	0
Diphtheria	4	0.0	2	0.0	2	0.0	0	0	0	0	0
Measles	875	1.6	451	1.5	424	1.6	258	256	0	1	0
Tetanus	377	0.7	188	0.6	189	0.7	47	44	0	5	0
Meningitis	171	0.3	90	0.3	81	0.3	19	22	1	11	2
Hepatitis	124	0.2	74	0.3	50	0.2	17	20	5	5	2
Malaria	1 086	1.9	553	1.9	532	2.0	481	472	0	2	0
Tropical diseases	171	0.3	94	0.3	77	0.3	43	51	0	23	0
Trypanosomiasis	66	0.1	37	0.1	30	0.1	29	35	0	0	0
Chagas disease	21	0.0	11	0.0	10	0.0	0	0	0	21	0
Schistosomiasis	14	0.0	8	0.0	6	0.0	3	3	0	2	0
Leishmaniasis	57	0.1	32	0.1	25	0.1	6	8	0	0	0
Lymphatic filariasis	0	0.0	0	0.0	0	0.0	0	0	0	0	0
Onchocerciasis	0	0.0	0	0.0	0	0.0	0	0	0	0	0
Leprosy	3	0.0	2	0.0	1	0.0	0	0	0	1	0
Dengue	13	0.0	6	0.0	7	0.0	0	0	0	0	0
Japanese encephalitis	6	0.0	3	0.0	3	0.0	0	0	0	0	0
Trachoma	0	0.0	0	0.0	0	0.0	0	0	0	0	0
Intestinal nematode infections	16	0.0	8	0.0	7	0.0	2	3	0	2	2
Ascariasis	3	0.0	2	0.0	2	0.0	1	1	0	0	0
Trichuriasis	2	0.0	1	0.0	1	0.0	0	1	0	0	0
Hookworm disease	7	0.0	4	0.0	3	0.0	1	1	0	1	0
Respiratory infections	4 039	7.2	2 046	7.0	1 993	7.4	492	594	101	159	39
Acute lower respiratory infections	3 963	7.1	2 013	6.9	1 950	7.3	486	587	101	157	37
Acute upper respiratory infections	47	0.1	23	0.1	24	0.1	3	3	0	2	2
Otitis media	20	0.0	9	0.0	11	0.0	3	4	0	0	0
Maternal conditions	497	0.9	0	0.0	497	1.9	102	153	0	12	6
Perinatal conditions	2 356	4.2	1 273	4.4	1 084	4.0	319	296	15	103	35
Nutritional deficiencies	493	0.9	236	0.8	257	1.0	85	95	9	50	13
Protein-energy malnutrition	272	0.5	133	0.5	139	0.5	52	58	4	34	9
Iodine deficiency	9	0.0	6	0.0	4	0.0	1	1	0	0	0
Vitamin A deficiency	61	0.1	30	0.1	31	0.1	17	20	0	0	0
Anaemias	133	0.2	60	0.2	73	0.3	14	16	5	16	4

Cause[b]	EASTERN MEDITERRANEAN		EUROPE			SOUTH-EAST ASIA		WESTERN PACIFIC	
	Mortality stratum		Mortality stratum			Mortality stratum		Mortality stratum	
	Low child, Low adult	High child, high adult	Very low child, very low adult	Low child, low adult	Low child, high adult	Low child, low adult	High child, high adult	Very low child, very low adult	Low child, low adult
Population (000)	136 798	348 468	410 233	215 276	246 336	288 750	1 219 492	152 882	1 513 894
	(000)	(000)	(000)	(000)	(000)	(000)	(000)	(000)	(000)
TOTAL DEATHS	900	3 318	4 084	1 817	3 156	1 944	12 326	1 115	11 182
I. Communicable diseases, maternal and perinatal conditions and nutritional deficiencies	132	1 364	240	184	107	574	5 025	120	1 396
Infectious and parasitic diseases	60	697	53	72	52	266	2 651	19	558
Tuberculosis	13	99	6	19	35	152	571	4	355
STDs excluding HIV	0	19	0	0	0	1	80	0	2
Syphilis	0	18	0	0	0	0	65	0	2
Chlamydia	0	0	0	0	0	0	10	0	0
Gonorrhoea	0	0	0	0	0	0	5	0	0
HIV/AIDS	0	29	7	4	4	36	324	1	33
Diarrhoeal diseases	28	272	2	25	3	27	951	1	66
Childhood diseases	12	179	0	11	2	26	516	2	45
Pertussis	2	35	0	4	1	2	93	2	10
Poliomyelitis	0	0	0	0	0	0	1	0	0
Diphtheria	0	0	0	0	0	0	3	0	0
Measles	8	89	0	4	0	18	223	0	17
Tetanus	1	54	0	3	1	6	196	0	18
Meningitis	3	22	2	4	3	10	59	0	13
Hepatitis	0	4	4	1	0	4	31	5	26
Malaria	0	44	0	0	0	10	59	0	16
Tropical diseases	1	8	0	1	0	1	40	0	2
Trypanosomiasis	0	2	0	0	0	0	0	0	0
Chagas disease	0	0	0	0	0	0	0	0	0
Schistosomiasis	1	1	0	1	0	1	0	0	2
Leishmaniasis	0	3	0	0	0	0	40	0	0
Lymphatic filariasis	0	0	0	0	0	0	0	0	0
Onchocerciasis	0	0	0	0	0	0	0	0	0
Leprosy	0	0	0	0	0	0	2	0	0
Dengue	0	0	0	0	0	0	12	0	0
Japanese encephalitis	0	0	0	0	0	0	1	0	4
Trachoma	0	0	0	0	0	0	0	0	0
Intestinal nematode infections	0	1	0	0	0	1	5	0	1
Ascariasis	0	0	0	0	0	0	1	0	0
Trichuriasis	0	0	0	0	0	0	1	0	0
Hookworm disease	0	0	0	0	0	0	3	0	0
Respiratory infections	37	306	166	73	36	108	1 415	96	418
Acute lower respiratory infections	37	301	164	60	33	106	1 382	95	417
Acute upper respiratory infections	0	3	2	13	3	1	14	1	0
Otitis media	0	2	0	0	0	1	10	0	0
Maternal conditions	3	36	1	2	1	14	144	0	21
Perinatal conditions	26	287	11	34	17	180	671	2	361
Nutritional deficiencies	6	38	9	4	1	16	143	1	21
Protein-energy malnutrition	3	23	3	1	0	7	73	1	4
Iodine deficiency	0	1	0	0	0	0	6	0	0
Vitamin A deficiency	0	5	0	0	0	0	19	0	0
Anaemias	1	7	6	2	1	7	47	0	3

Annex Table 3 Deaths by cause, sex and mortality stratum in WHO Regions[a], estimates for 1999

Cause[b]	Both sexes (000)	Both sexes % total	Males (000)	Males % total	Females (000)	Females % total	AFRICA High child, high adult (000)	AFRICA High child, very high adult (000)	THE AMERICAS Very low child, very low adult (000)	THE AMERICAS Low child, low adult (000)	THE AMERICAS High child, high adult (000)
Population (000)	5 961 628		3 002 288		2 959 340		286 350	330 085	318 235	424 932	69 898
II. Noncommunicable conditions	33 484	59.8	17 039	58.4	16 445	61.3	1 074	1 226	2 283	1 648	324
Malignant neoplasms	7 065	12.6	3 915	13.4	3 150	11.7	234	289	632	335	65
Mouth and oropharynx	282	0.5	185	0.6	97	0.4	5	6	11	10	1
Esophagus	381	0.7	250	0.9	131	0.5	19	25	16	13	1
Stomach	801	1.4	489	1.7	312	1.2	21	27	19	42	12
Colon/rectum	509	0.9	263	0.9	246	0.9	6	6	76	24	2
Liver	589	1.1	410	1.4	179	0.7	44	56	6	6	3
Pancreas	194	0.3	102	0.4	91	0.3	6	8	32	6	2
Trachea/bronchus/lung	1 193	2.1	860	2.9	333	1.2	14	16	180	41	5
Melanoma and other skin cancers	74	0.1	38	0.1	36	0.1	2	3	3	3	0
Breast	467	0.8	0	0.0	467	1.7	12	15	56	27	5
Cervix	237	0.4	0	0.0	237	0.9	24	32	6	18	6
Corpus uteri	79	0.1	0	0.0	79	0.3	1	1	9	10	0
Ovary	105	0.2	0	0.0	105	0.4	4	4	15	3	2
Prostate	255	0.5	255	0.9	0	0.0	14	18	45	22	2
Bladder	138	0.2	100	0.3	39	0.1	8	10	16	6	0
Lymphoma	295	0.5	170	0.6	125	0.5	13	15	47	15	4
Leukaemia	268	0.5	142	0.5	127	0.5	7	8	27	15	4
Other neoplasms	102	0.2	53	0.2	49	0.2	2	2	9	10	2
Diabetes mellitus	777	1.4	335	1.2	441	1.6	18	20	74	98	44
Nutritional/endocrine disorders	306	0.5	155	0.5	151	0.6	22	24	27	54	11
Neuropsychiatric disorders	911	1.6	473	1.6	438	1.6	38	43	120	44	13
Unipolar major depression	1	0.0	1	0.0	1	0.0	0	0	0	0	0
Bipolar affective disorder	5	0.0	2	0.0	3	0.0	0	0	0	0	0
Psychoses	18	0.0	9	0.0	9	0.0	0	0	1	0	0
Epilepsy	95	0.2	61	0.2	35	0.1	11	13	2	6	2
Alcohol dependence	60	0.1	52	0.2	8	0.0	0	1	6	10	3
Alzheimer and other dementias	271	0.5	98	0.3	173	0.6	2	2	60	5	0
Parkinson disease	84	0.2	42	0.1	42	0.2	1	2	14	0	0
Multiple sclerosis	17	0.0	7	0.0	10	0.0	0	0	3	1	0
Drug dependence	5	0.0	5	0.0	1	0.0	0	0	0	0	0
Post traumatic stress disorder	0	0.0	0	0.0	0	0.0	0	0	0	0	0
Obsessive-compulsive disorders	0	0.0	0	0.0	0	0.0	0	0	0	0	0
Panic disorder	0	0.0	0	0.0	0	0.0	0	0	0	0	0
Sense organ disorders	2	0.0	1	0.0	2	0.0	0	1	0	0	0
Glaucoma	0	0.0	0	0.0	0	0.0	0	0	0	0	0
Cataracts	1	0.0	0	0.0	1	0.0	0	0	0	0	0
Cardiovascular diseases	16 970	30.3	8 059	27.6	8 911	33.2	447	488	1 086	760	96
Rheumatic heart disease	376	0.7	154	0.5	222	0.8	17	18	6	6	2
Ischaemic heart disease	7 089	12.7	3 556	12.2	3 533	13.2	153	159	551	294	41
Cerebrovascular disease	5 544	9.9	2 530	8.7	3 014	11.2	153	180	187	207	24
Inflammatory cardiac disease	454	0.8	238	0.8	216	0.8	17	17	30	12	2
Respiratory diseases	3 575	6.4	1 897	6.5	1 678	6.3	104	122	162	121	19
Chronic obstructive pulmonary disease	2 660	4.8	1 420	4.9	1 240	4.6	50	59	118	39	5
Asthma	186	0.3	92	0.3	94	0.4	9	10	6	6	2

Cause[b]	EASTERN MEDITERRANEAN		EUROPE			SOUTH-EAST ASIA		WESTERN PACIFIC	
	Mortality stratum		Mortality stratum			Mortality stratum		Mortality stratum	
	Low child, Low adult	High child, high adult	Very low child, very low adult	Low child, low adult	Low child, high adult	Low child, low adult	High child, high adult	Very low child, very low adult	Low child, low adult
Population (000)	136 798	348 468	410 233	215 276	246 336	288 750	1 219 492	152 882	1 513 894
	(000)	(000)	(000)	(000)	(000)	(000)	(000)	(000)	(000)
II. Noncommunicable conditions	709	1 609	3 642	1 479	2 655	1 089	6 281	920	8 542
Malignant neoplasms	74	200	1 066	248	480	283	886	336	1 937
Mouth and oropharynx	2	14	25	7	16	12	113	6	53
Esophagus	2	10	28	7	15	9	59	12	166
Stomach	4	14	71	26	75	39	73	56	322
Colon/rectum	3	7	140	22	57	10	28	43	84
Liver	4	13	24	7	2	33	39	34	319
Pancreas	3	5	51	9	3	6	13	20	27
Trachea/bronchus/lung	12	21	209	50	99	44	75	61	366
Melanoma and other skin cancers	1	1	7	4	1	14	2	3	31
Breast	1	12	91	15	36	23	91	13	70
Cervix	4	12	8	8	11	10	51	3	44
Corpus uteri	1	1	16	4	11	3	6	3	11
Ovary	1	4	25	4	1	5	20	5	11
Prostate	2	7	70	8	12	2	29	10	13
Bladder	3	6	36	7	1	4	16	6	19
Lymphoma	9	18	53	11	13	8	48	14	27
Leukaemia	5	14	36	10	14	10	53	9	55
Other neoplasms	1	3	27	3	4	5	10	9	14
Diabetes mellitus	16	38	87	28	21	37	143	17	136
Nutritional/endocrine disorders	9	20	24	7	4	14	3	9	77
Neuropsychiatric disorders	15	47	152	24	33	41	150	20	171
Unipolar major depression	0	0	0	0	0	0	0	0	1
Bipolar affective disorder	0	0	0	0	0	0	4	0	0
Psychoses	0	1	1	0	0	2	9	0	4
Epilepsy	1	6	6	4	4	5	19	1	16
Alcohol dependence	0	1	12	3	1	4	7	1	9
Alzheimer and other dementias	1	5	77	2	1	20	41	8	46
Parkinson disease	1	2	20	1	0	2	12	4	26
Multiple sclerosis	0	0	4	1	2	0	5	0	1
Drug dependence	0	0	4	0	0	0	0	0	0
Post traumatic stress disorder	0	0	0	0	0	0	0	0	0
Obsessive-compulsive disorders	0	0	0	0	0	0	0	0	0
Panic disorder	0	0	0	0	0	0	0	0	0
Sense organ disorders	0	0	0	0	0	0	0	0	0
Glaucoma	0	0	0	0	0	0	0	0	0
Cataracts	0	0	0	0	0	0	0	0	0
Cardiovascular diseases	462	907	1 802	981	1 841	428	3 752	392	3 527
Rheumatic heart disease	11	28	11	14	15	12	116	3	117
Ischaemic heart disease	196	405	823	372	968	160	2 078	121	767
Cerebrovascular disease	116	212	471	255	623	193	804	166	1 952
Inflammatory cardiac disease	20	41	26	22	25	13	144	7	80
Respiratory diseases	42	114	201	62	124	104	473	55	1 871
Chronic obstructive pulmonary disease	28	61	144	41	90	46	249	22	1 708
Asthma	4	10	12	5	9	20	34	7	50

Annex Table 3 Deaths by cause, sex and mortality stratum in WHO Regions[a], estimates for 1999

Cause[b]	SEX						AFRICA		THE AMERICAS		
	Both sexes		Males		Females		Mortality stratum		Mortality stratum		
							High child, high adult	High child, very high adult	Very low child, very low adult	Low child, low adult	High child, high adult
Population (000)	*5 961 628*		*3 002 288*		*2 959 340*		*286 350*	*330 085*	*318 235*	*424 932*	*69 898*
	(000)	% total	(000)	% total	(000)	% total	(000)	(000)	(000)	(000)	(000)
Digestive diseases	2 049	3.7	1 241	4.3	808	3.0	96	114	93	137	47
Peptic ulcer disease	266	0.5	161	0.6	105	0.4	6	8	6	11	3
Cirrhosis of the liver	909	1.6	614	2.1	294	1.1	32	39	30	62	28
Appendicitis	43	0.1	27	0.1	16	0.1	1	2	1	2	1
Diseases of the genitourinary system	900	1.6	497	1.7	403	1.5	57	63	52	48	15
Nephritis/nephrosis	697	1.2	372	1.3	325	1.2	39	41	29	35	12
Benign prostatic hypertrophy	45	0.1	45	0.2	0	0.0	3	4	1	1	0
Skin diseases	61	0.1	27	0.1	34	0.1	10	13	4	4	1
Musculoskeletal diseases	107	0.2	37	0.1	69	0.3	6	8	12	7	2
Rheumatoid arthritis	19	0.0	7	0.0	12	0.0	1	1	2	0	0
Osteoarthritis	1	0.0	0	0.0	1	0.0	0	0	0	0	0
Congenital abnormalities	652	1.2	348	1.2	304	1.1	39	40	14	29	8
Oral diseases	1	0.0	0	0.0	0	0.0	0	0	0	0	0
Dental caries	0	0.0	0	0.0	0	0.0	0	0	0	0	0
Periodontal disease	0	0.0	0	0.0	0	0.0	0	0	0	0	0
Edentulism	0	0.0	0	0.0	0	0.0	0	0	0	0	0
III. Injuries	5 101	9.1	3 385	11.6	1 716	6.4	376	400	172	322	58
Unintentional	3 412	6.1	2 284	7.8	1 128	4.2	224	232	113	183	35
Road traffic accidents	1 230	2.2	908	3.1	323	1.2	91	97	48	87	13
Poisoning	257	0.5	170	0.6	87	0.3	15	16	12	3	1
Falls	347	0.6	206	0.7	142	0.5	9	11	20	17	4
Fires	258	0.5	111	0.4	147	0.5	16	13	4	4	1
Drowning	447	0.8	294	1.0	153	0.6	42	37	4	18	3
Other unintentional injuries	865	1.5	589	2.0	276	1.0	51	58	24	51	12
Intentional	1 689	3.0	1 101	3.8	588	2.2	152	168	59	140	22
Self-inflicted	893	1.6	545	1.9	348	1.3	32	37	38	21	3
Homicide and violence	527	0.9	392	1.3	135	0.5	65	72	21	107	14
War	269	0.5	164	0.6	105	0.4	55	59	0	12	6

[a] See list of Member States by WHO Region and mortality stratum (pp. 204–205).

[b] Estimates for specific causes may not sum to broader cause groupings due to omission of residual categories.

Cause[b]	EASTERN MEDITERRANEAN Mortality stratum		EUROPE Mortality stratum			SOUTH-EAST ASIA Mortality stratum		WESTERN PACIFIC Mortality stratum	
	Low child, Low adult	High child, high adult	Very low child, very low adult	Low child, low adult	Low child, high adult	Low child, low adult	High child, high adult	Very low child, very low adult	Low child, low adult
Population (000)	136 798	348 468	410 233	215 276	246 336	288 750	1 219 492	152 882	1 513 894
	(000)	(000)	(000)	(000)	(000)	(000)	(000)	(000)	(000)
Digestive diseases	38	105	186	77	101	102	426	45	483
Peptic ulcer disease	1	10	18	6	13	20	71	5	88
Cirrhosis of the liver	10	42	69	41	51	45	248	15	196
Appendicitis	0	3	1	0	1	1	24	0	7
Diseases of the genitourinary system	41	71	59	36	26	45	191	26	171
Nephritis/nephrosis	36	61	39	30	11	36	167	23	137
Benign prostatic hypertrophy	0	3	2	1	3	1	18	0	8
Skin diseases	1	4	8	1	2	5	4	1	3
Musculoskeletal diseases	1	3	18	2	4	10	5	5	24
Rheumatoid arthritis	0	0	4	0	0	2	4	2	2
Osteoarthritis	0	0	0	0	0	0	0	0	0
Congenital abnormalities	9	97	12	11	15	22	238	4	115
Oral diseases	0	0	0	0	0	0	0	0	0
Dental caries	0	0	0	0	0	0	0	0	0
Periodontal disease	0	0	0	0	0	0	0	0	0
Edentulism	0	0	0	0	0	0	0	0	0
III. Injuries	59	346	201	154	395	281	1 020	76	1 241
Unintentional	51	241	141	102	240	199	794	48	809
Road traffic accidents	30	90	45	39	46	123	231	16	274
Poisoning	7	19	6	11	70	7	32	1	56
Falls	3	24	48	12	16	18	64	8	94
Fires	3	23	3	5	12	7	148	2	18
Drowning	4	28	4	10	25	16	94	6	154
Other unintentional injuries	4	56	34	24	71	29	224	15	213
Intentional	7	105	60	52	155	82	226	28	432
Self-inflicted	5	30	54	21	91	36	135	27	363
Homicide and violence	1	37	5	7	50	11	71	1	66
War	1	38	1	23	15	35	20	0	4

Annex Table 4 Burden of disease in disability-adjusted life years (DALYs) by cause, sex and mortality stratum in WHO Regions[a], estimates for 199[?]

Cause[b]	Both sexes (000)	Both sexes % total	Males (000)	Males % total	Females (000)	Females % total	AFRICA High child, high adult (000)	AFRICA High child, very high adult (000)	THE AMERICAS Very low child, very low adult (000)	THE AMERICAS Low child, low adult (000)	THE AMERICAS High child, high adult (000)
Population (000)	5 961 628		3 002 288		2 959 340		286 350	330 085	318 235	424 932	69 898
TOTAL DALYs	1 438 154	100	751 600	100	686 555	100	158 439	214 921	38 627	70 969	16 346
I. Communicable diseases, maternal and perinatal conditions and nutritional deficiencies	615 105	42.8	296 674	39.5	318 431	46.4	110 969	162 607	2 851	16 073	6 371
Infectious and parasitic diseases	353 779	24.6	175 376	23.3	178 403	26.0	73 124	120 024	1 307	7 360	2 918
Tuberculosis	33 287	2.3	19 030	2.5	14 257	2.1	3 158	5 563	16	627	471
STDs excluding HIV	19 747	1.4	6 686	0.9	13 060	1.9	3 780	4 068	155	917	136
Syphilis	6 081	0.4	3 558	0.5	2 523	0.4	1 587	1 602	2	104	7
Chlamydia	7 969	0.6	944	0.1	7 024	1.0	1 046	1 187	135	557	87
Gonorrhoea	5 686	0.4	2 181	0.3	3 504	0.5	1 147	1 278	17	255	41
HIV/AIDS	89 819	6.2	42 623	5.7	47 196	6.9	15 778	58 671	563	1 628	621
Diarrhoeal diseases	72 063	5.0	36 413	4.8	35 650	5.2	11 867	12 454	102	1 642	770
Childhood diseases	54 638	3.8	27 986	3.7	26 652	3.9	12 864	12 878	10	477	46
Pertussis	10 905	0.8	5 662	0.7	5 243	0.8	2 460	2 477	10	173	6
Poliomyelitis	1 725	0.1	946	0.1	779	0.1	55	224	0	126	26
Diphtheria	151	0.0	75	0.0	76	0.0	13	11	0	2	0
Measles	29 838	2.1	15 328	2.0	14 510	2.1	8 762	8 701	0	23	8
Tetanus	12 020	0.8	5 975	0.8	6 045	0.9	1 574	1 465	0	154	6
Meningitis	9 824	0.7	4 661	0.6	5 164	0.8	1 685	1 935	54	529	139
Hepatitis	2 790	0.2	1 689	0.2	1 101	0.2	544	628	70	83	59
Malaria	44 998	3.1	22 758	3.0	22 240	3.2	18 600	18 238	0	53	23
Tropical diseases	12 966	0.9	8 443	1.1	4 523	0.7	3 289	3 824	0	781	89
Trypanosomiasis	2 048	0.1	1 111	0.1	937	0.1	917	1 074	0	0	1
Chagas disease	676	0.0	400	0.1	277	0.0	0	0	0	624	53
Schistosomiasis	1 932	0.1	1 174	0.2	758	0.1	755	882	0	122	11
Leishmaniasis	1 983	0.1	1 200	0.2	782	0.1	113	143	0	27	23
Lymphatic filariasis	4 918	0.3	3 777	0.5	1 141	0.2	852	982	0	7	1
Onchocerciasis	1 085	0.1	623	0.1	461	0.1	508	575	0	2	0
Leprosy	476	0.0	253	0.0	223	0.0	37	42	0	52	8
Dengue	465	0.0	220	0.0	245	0.0	11	13	0	0	0
Japanese encephalitis	1 046	0.1	519	0.1	527	0.1	0	0	0	0	0
Trachoma	1 239	0.1	336	0.0	903	0.1	207	227	0	0	0
Intestinal nematode infections	2 653	0.2	1 351	0.2	1 303	0.2	400	460	1	169	124
Ascariasis	505	0.0	253	0.0	252	0.0	94	108	0	13	30
Trichuriasis	481	0.0	284	0.0	197	0.0	92	106	0	113	42
Hookworm disease	1 699	0.1	869	0.1	830	0.1	189	217	0	153	20
Respiratory infections	101 127	7.0	50 852	6.7	50 275	7.3	15 352	17 419	566	2 480	1 158
Acute lower respiratory infections	96 682	6.7	48 891	6.5	47 792	6.9	14 858	16 871	500	2 315	1 054
Acute upper respiratory infections	1 600	0.1	784	0.1	816	0.1	108	106	11	49	70
Otitis media	2 183	0.2	985	0.1	1 198	0.2	346	402	32	102	20
Maternal conditions	26 101	1.8	0	0.0	26 101	3.8	4 954	7 571	49	861	297
Perinatal conditions	89 508	6.2	48 911	6.5	40 597	5.9	12 351	11 746	576	3 707	1 283
Nutritional deficiencies	44 539	3.1	21 478	2.8	23 062	3.4	5 189	5 848	353	1 665	715
Protein-energy malnutrition	13 578	0.9	6 826	0.9	6 752	1.0	2 731	3 073	43	617	264
Iodine deficiency	1 032	0.1	597	0.1	435	0.1	107	112	9	37	8
Vitamin A deficiency	108	0.0	55	0.0	53	0.0	18	21	0	5	1
Anaemias	26 272	1.8	11 729	1.6	14 544	2.1	1 511	1 708	282	920	422

Cause[b]	EASTERN MEDITERRANEAN		EUROPE			SOUTH-EAST ASIA		WESTERN PACIFIC	
	Mortality stratum		Mortality stratum			Mortality stratum		Mortality stratum	
	Low child, Low adult	High child, high adult	Very low child, very low adult	Low child, low adult	Low child, high adult	Low child, low adult	High child, high adult	Very low child, very low adult	Low child, low adult
Population (000)	136 798	348 468	410 233	215 276	246 336	288 750	1 219 492	152 882	1 513 894
	(000)	(000)	(000)	(000)	(000)	(000)	(000)	(000)	(000)
TOTAL DALYs	20 895	101 688	48 999	36 484	50 868	56 604	355 876	15 235	252 204
I. Communicable diseases, maternal and perinatal conditions and nutritional deficiencies	5 858	52 472	2 861	6 515	3 620	21 762	168 893	942	53 311
Infectious and parasitic diseases	2 337	26 485	1 230	2 614	1 672	9 672	85 629	304	19 105
Tuberculosis	225	2 035	47	450	761	3 453	10 648	26	5 806
STDs excluding HIV	103	899	192	252	273	1 159	7 566	69	180
Syphilis	7	641	2	2	2	17	2 050	1	58
Chlamydia	68	182	167	198	216	686	3 292	60	85
Gonorrhoea	27	74	21	51	54	454	2 221	8	37
HIV/AIDS	10	2 162	519	108	98	1 102	7 764	28	767
Diarrhoeal diseases	977	9 146	111	875	145	1 057	28 960	43	3 912
Childhood diseases	399	6 161	12	390	75	989	18 460	23	1 852
Pertussis	83	1 332	11	143	43	88	3 546	16	517
Poliomyelitis	6	13	0	1	0	94	1 001	0	178
Diphtheria	1	10	0	1	0	4	106	0	2
Measles	273	3 020	1	147	0	611	7 697	6	588
Tetanus	35	1 786	1	99	31	192	6 110	0	566
Meningitis	156	1 316	74	227	137	818	1 749	11	994
Hepatitis	8	101	41	14	2	106	600	56	479
Malaria	47	2 727	2	0	0	323	2 748	0	2 235
Tropical diseases	52	333	0	16	0	256	4 018	0	308
Trypanosomiasis	0	56	0	0	0	0	0	0	0
Chagas disease	0	0	0	0	0	0	0	0	0
Schistosomiasis	34	64	0	15	0	18	0	0	30
Leishmaniasis	14	196	0	0	0	15	1 452	0	0
Lymphatic filariasis	3	8	0	0	0	222	2 566	0	278
Onchocerciasis	0	0	0	0	0	0	0	0	0
Leprosy	3	7	0	0	0	31	287	0	9
Dengue	0	1	0	0	0	3	437	0	0
Japanese encephalitis	0	1	0	0	0	47	171	0	828
Trachoma	68	169	0	0	0	23	39	0	505
Intestinal nematode infections	46	103	0	2	1	239	989	0	119
Ascariasis	19	24	0	0	0	5	181	0	31
Trichuriasis	0	3	0	0	0	1	119	0	5
Hookworm disease	26	67	0	0	0	157	705	0	166
Respiratory infections	980	9 936	724	1 987	798	3 014	35 130	401	11 183
Acute lower respiratory infections	921	9 625	645	1 435	637	2 904	33 746	372	10 798
Acute upper respiratory infections	10	114	24	502	122	28	405	12	40
Otitis media	40	166	36	28	25	73	624	14	276
Maternal conditions	704	2 016	54	215	182	624	7 109	15	1 451
Perinatal conditions	1 134	10 621	454	1 269	647	6 362	26 353	91	12 914
Nutritional deficiencies	704	3 415	400	430	322	2 194	14 672	131	8 502
Protein-energy malnutrition	39	1 196	36	93	47	366	4 837	16	218
Iodine deficiency	28	109	9	13	9	2	354	3	233
Vitamin A deficiency	5	15	0	0	0	6	25	0	12
Anaemias	607	1 835	337	308	257	1 749	8 462	111	7 764

Annex Table 4　Burden of disease in disability-adjusted life years (DALYs) by cause, sex and mortality stratum in WHO Regions[a], estimates for 199

Cause[b]	SEX						AFRICA		THE AMERICAS		
							Mortality stratum		Mortality stratum		
	Both sexes		Males		Females		High child, high adult	High child, very high adult	Very low child, very low adult	Low child, low adult	High child, high adult
Population (000)	5 961 628		3 002 288		2 959 340		286 350	330 085	318 235	424 932	69 898
	(000)	% total	(000)	% total	(000)	% total	(000)	(000)	(000)	(000)	(000)
II.　Noncommunicable conditions	621 742	43.2	322 583	42.9	299 159	43.6	30 080	33 601	31 085	43 789	8 035
Malignant neoplasms	84 500	5.9	46 145	6.1	38 355	5.6	3 277	3 903	5 689	4 107	818
Mouth and oropharynx	3 993	0.3	2 725	0.4	1 268	0.2	78	93	120	127	10
Esophagus	3 921	0.3	2 518	0.3	1 403	0.2	200	255	138	134	8
Stomach	8 683	0.6	5 395	0.7	3 288	0.5	267	332	160	437	127
Colon/rectum	5 182	0.4	2 707	0.4	2 474	0.4	77	88	663	257	21
Liver	7 819	0.5	5 720	0.8	2 099	0.3	670	851	61	63	35
Pancreas	1 788	0.1	1 014	0.1	774	0.1	68	82	245	67	23
Trachea/bronchus/lung	11 628	0.8	8 347	1.1	3 281	0.5	149	166	1 509	425	47
Melanoma and other skin cancers	749	0.1	393	0.1	355	0.1	33	41	35	35	3
Breast	6 529	0.5	3	0.0	6 525	0.9	174	221	636	386	64
Cervix	3 354	0.2	0	0.0	3 354	0.5	302	384	94	282	83
Corpus uteri	860	0.1	0	0.0	860	0.1	14	16	72	133	3
Ovary	1 439	0.1	0	0.0	1 439	0.2	53	62	145	41	26
Prostate	1 736	0.1	1 736	0.2	0	0.0	94	120	296	152	14
Bladder	1 207	0.1	925	0.1	282	0.0	69	85	135	49	4
Lymphoma	4 538	0.3	2 831	0.4	1 707	0.2	313	333	431	224	61
Leukaemia	5 522	0.4	2 985	0.4	2 538	0.4	177	180	265	330	88
Other neoplasms	1 366	0.1	733	0.1	633	0.1	42	44	82	164	36
Diabetes mellitus	15 070	1.0	6 972	0.9	8 098	1.2	411	446	1 628	1 596	625
Nutritional/endocrine disorders	14 667	1.0	7 998	1.1	6 669	1.0	1 725	1 755	757	3 386	588
Neuropsychiatric disorders	158 721	11.0	77 771	10.3	80 950	11.8	7 466	8 554	9 424	14 538	2 508
Unipolar major depression	59 030	4.1	20 956	2.8	38 074	5.5	2 662	3 027	2 623	4 240	646
Bipolar affective disorder	16 368	1.1	8 340	1.1	8 028	1.2	765	873	665	1 172	181
Psychoses	12 054	0.8	5 675	0.8	6 380	0.9	260	298	851	1 228	191
Epilepsy	7 634	0.5	4 502	0.6	3 132	0.5	841	1 024	153	577	209
Alcohol dependence	18 743	1.3	16 512	2.2	2 231	0.3	982	1 131	1 863	3 762	656
Alzheimer and other dementias	10 002	0.7	4 166	0.6	5 836	0.8	173	193	1 141	577	82
Parkinson disease	1 587	0.1	705	0.1	882	0.1	33	41	217	29	4
Multiple sclerosis	1 568	0.1	687	0.1	881	0.1	51	58	120	98	16
Drug dependence	5 657	0.4	4 486	0.6	1 171	0.2	209	239	563	1 048	165
Post traumatic stress disorder	2 197	0.2	837	0.1	1 360	0.2	109	126	108	162	27
Obsessive-compulsive disorders	11 703	0.8	5 074	0.7	6 630	1.0	541	621	573	839	133
Panic disorder	5 493	0.4	1 838	0.2	3 654	0.5	254	290	273	388	60
Sense organ disorders	12 005	0.8	5 390	0.7	6 614	1.0	1 142	1 239	41	588	80
Glaucoma	3 021	0.2	1 190	0.2	1 830	0.3	227	245	28	90	12
Cataracts	8 942	0.6	4 184	0.6	4 757	0.7	909	988	12	487	66
Cardiovascular diseases	157 185	10.9	81 848	10.9	75 337	11.0	5 731	6 198	7 273	7 891	1 001
Rheumatic heart disease	7 755	0.5	3 311	0.4	4 444	0.6	481	523	54	116	33
Ischaemic heart disease	58 981	4.1	32 792	4.3	26 189	3.8	1 632	1 737	3 298	2 915	381
Cerebrovascular disease	49 856	3.5	24 738	3.3	25 118	3.7	1 712	1 974	1 410	2 208	243
Inflammatory cardiac disease	8 894	0.6	4 915	0.7	3 979	0.6	423	401	382	291	47
Respiratory diseases	70 017	4.9	36 038	4.8	33 980	4.9	3 177	3 647	2 587	3 189	428
Chronic obstructive pulmonary disease	38 156	2.6	20 635	2.7	17 521	2.5	809	891	1 267	869	86
Asthma	12 881	0.9	6 898	0.9	5 983	0.9	972	1 129	492	678	144

Cause[b]	EASTERN MEDITERRANEAN Mortality stratum		EUROPE Mortality stratum			SOUTH-EAST ASIA Mortality stratum		WESTERN PACIFIC Mortality stratum	
	Low child, Low adult	High child, high adult	Very low child, very low adult	Low child, low adult	Low child, high adult	Low child, low adult	High child, high adult	Very low child, very low adult	Low child, low adult
Population (000)	136 798	348 468	410 233	215 276	246 336	288 750	1 219 492	152 882	1 513 894
	(000)	(000)	(000)	(000)	(000)	(000)	(000)	(000)	(000)
II. Noncommunicable conditions	12 568	38 471	41 818	25 387	36 827	22 973	133 563	12 626	150 920
Malignant neoplasms	920	3 053	9 181	3 084	5 597	4 275	13 575	2 882	24 139
Mouth and oropharynx	32	205	294	108	222	212	1 592	62	838
Esophagus	12	122	246	73	156	93	854	98	1 530
Stomach	47	186	534	286	826	515	1 008	462	3 496
Colon/rectum	41	95	1 133	254	617	142	385	397	1 013
Liver	37	171	187	65	15	530	432	289	4 413
Pancreas	29	59	384	96	26	76	213	151	269
Trachea/bronchus/lung	112	225	1 774	550	1 062	501	909	448	3 752
Melanoma and other skin cancers	4	11	77	41	10	146	12	27	275
Breast	7	181	954	198	492	411	1 510	173	1 122
Cervix	26	149	103	104	154	176	813	36	647
Corpus uteri	6	15	122	55	124	54	63	31	151
Ovary	19	69	233	59	14	95	369	61	192
Prostate	16	44	455	71	119	15	183	68	88
Bladder	24	43	312	76	16	45	118	45	186
Lymphoma	167	397	458	208	201	163	1 034	117	431
Leukaemia	118	375	345	203	213	262	1 431	102	1 434
Other neoplasms	24	67	181	49	69	88	226	69	226
Diabetes mellitus	293	905	1 176	876	769	716	3 212	303	2 115
Nutritional/endocrine disorders	492	1 324	568	506	246	670	194	200	2 256
Neuropsychiatric disorders	3 231	8 429	12 611	6 430	7 425	8 651	28 704	4 164	36 585
Unipolar major depression	1 312	3 227	3 376	1 964	2 297	3 104	12 165	1 255	17 132
Bipolar affective disorder	377	929	844	526	590	860	3 520	307	4 758
Psychoses	399	985	1 061	554	599	1 047	2 520	381	1 681
Epilepsy	44	289	337	343	373	534	1 509	68	1 333
Alcohol dependence	73	198	2 562	1 192	1 140	926	1 386	714	2 159
Alzheimer and other dementias	61	205	1 737	427	649	473	1 590	580	2 113
Parkinson disease	17	45	310	38	33	57	259	82	421
Multiple sclerosis	28	76	145	58	145	65	469	14	226
Drug dependence	258	628	788	359	385	406	118	258	234
Post traumatic stress disorder	53	132	131	78	84	112	461	48	566
Obsessive-compulsive disorders	271	667	718	423	471	607	2 444	261	3 132
Panic disorder	121	299	343	198	226	291	1 108	127	1 514
Sense organ disorders	257	625	61	33	48	839	4 521	24	2 506
Glaucoma	29	71	41	15	22	262	857	16	1 105
Cataracts	227	547	19	17	26	575	3 664	7	1 400
Cardiovascular diseases	4 367	10 399	10 254	8 726	15 010	4 815	42 692	2 584	30 243
Rheumatic heart disease	251	687	80	299	244	362	2 730	21	1 874
Ischaemic heart disease	1 484	3 588	4 757	2 986	7 113	1 732	20 133	721	6 505
Cerebrovascular disease	1 041	2 277	2 857	2 727	5 584	2 041	8 639	1 160	15 982
Inflammatory cardiac disease	381	932	283	557	470	299	3 314	81	1 034
Respiratory diseases	1 047	3 345	2 911	1 461	2 472	3 133	12 409	754	29 456
Chronic obstructive pulmonary disease	460	1 187	1 441	688	1 323	970	5 385	186	22 593
Asthma	324	852	587	370	438	1 008	2 290	242	3 356

Annex Table 4 Burden of disease in disability-adjusted life years (DALYs) by cause, sex and mortality stratum in WHO Regions[a], estimates for 199

Cause[b]	SEX						AFRICA		THE AMERICAS		
							Mortality stratum		Mortality stratum		
	Both sexes		Males		Females		High child, high adult	High child, very high adult	Very low child, very low adult	Low child, low adult	High child, high adult
Population (000)	5 961 628		3 002 288		2 959 340		286 350	330 085	318 235	424 932	69 898
	(000)	% total	(000)	% total	(000)	% total	(000)	(000)	(000)	(000)	(000)
Digestive diseases	36 829	2.6	23 809	3.2	13 020	1.9	1 966	2 316	1 023	2 388	740
Peptic ulcer disease	5 061	0.4	3 295	0.4	1 766	0.3	149	198	59	156	40
Cirrhosis of the liver	16 254	1.1	11 300	1.5	4 953	0.7	518	625	474	1 190	453
Appendicitis	1 222	0.1	776	0.1	446	0.1	40	48	16	33	10
Diseases of the genitourinary system	16 085	1.1	9 619	1.3	6 466	0.9	1 208	1 358	392	837	242
Nephritis/nephrosis	10 997	0.8	5 837	0.8	5 159	0.8	749	806	178	479	165
Benign prostatic hypertrophy	2 447	0.2	2 447	0.3	0	0.0	165	194	79	184	26
Skin diseases	855	0.1	495	0.1	359	0.1	177	217	20	45	13
Musculoskeletal diseases	20 918	1.4	7 783	1.0	13 134	1.9	709	806	1 526	2 903	427
Rheumatoid arthritis	4 051	0.3	1 114	0.1	2 937	0.4	70	87	359	573	85
Osteoarthritis	15 820	1.1	6 270	0.8	9 550	1.4	544	605	1 087	2 224	314
Congenital abnormalities	36 557	2.5	19 562	2.6	16 995	2.5	3 180	3 257	633	1 764	438
Oral diseases	4 928	0.3	2 487	0.3	2 440	0.4	172	200	180	846	148
Dental caries	4 622	0.3	2 334	0.3	2 288	0.3	157	182	166	824	146
Periodontal disease	301	0.0	150	0.0	150	0.0	16	18	14	19	3
Edentulism	0	0.0	0	0.0	0	0.0	0	0	0	0	0
III. Injuries	201 307	13.9	132 343	17.5	68 965	10.0	17 389	18 714	4 691	11 107	1 940
Unintentional	152 464	10.6	101 190	13.4	51 275	7.5	11 843	12 683	2 943	6 483	1 320
Road traffic accidents	39 573	2.7	29 416	3.9	10 157	1.5	3 011	3 207	1 612	2 901	429
Poisoning	6 457	0.4	4 132	0.5	2 325	0.3	449	498	270	86	30
Falls	30 950	2.1	20 068	2.7	10 882	1.6	993	1 150	419	1 414	312
Fires	10 483	0.7	4 042	0.5	6 441	0.9	725	540	105	148	32
Drowning	12 987	0.9	8 583	1.1	4 404	0.6	1 356	1 156	108	532	95
Other unintentional injuries	20 573	1.4	14 093	1.9	6 480	0.9	1 436	1 646	360	1 221	294
Intentional	48 843	3.4	31 153	4.1	17 690	2.6	5 545	6 031	1 749	4 624	620
Self-inflicted	25 095	1.7	14 876	2.0	10 220	1.5	1 821	1 961	966	1 006	130
Homicide and violence	15 308	1.1	10 818	1.4	4 490	0.7	1 969	2 170	627	3 000	338
War	8 439	0.6	5 460	0.7	2 980	0.4	1 755	1 900	155	617	151

[a] See list of Member States by WHO Region and mortality stratum (pp. 204–205).

[b] Estimates for specific causes may not sum to broader cause groupings due to omission of residual categories.

Cause[b]	EASTERN MEDITERRANEAN		EUROPE			SOUTH-EAST ASIA		WESTERN PACIFIC	
	Mortality stratum		Mortality stratum			Mortality stratum		Mortality stratum	
	Low child, Low adult	High child, high adult	Very low child, very low adult	Low child, low adult	Low child, high adult	Low child, low adult	High child, high adult	Very low child, very low adult	Low child, low adult
Population (000)	136 798	348 468	410 233	215 276	246 336	288 750	1 219 492	152 882	1 513 894
	(000)	(000)	(000)	(000)	(000)	(000)	(000)	(000)	(000)
Digestive diseases	525	2 355	1 806	1 310	1 843	2 140	9 991	436	7 988
Peptic ulcer disease	15	264	133	121	290	374	1 751	38	1 473
Cirrhosis of the liver	138	834	979	672	888	922	5 132	203	3 227
Appendicitis	2	111	16	18	33	36	760	4	95
Diseases of the genitourinary system	605	1 574	405	694	433	838	4 170	177	3 154
Nephritis/nephrosis	466	1 167	200	507	192	586	3 380	107	2 014
Benign prostatic hypertrophy	55	152	120	52	78	102	523	48	670
Skin diseases	5	72	28	11	35	76	107	5	42
Musculoskeletal diseases	223	580	2 078	1 466	1 898	967	2 159	823	4 353
Rheumatoid arthritis	48	123	502	295	364	108	299	196	943
Osteoarthritis	169	418	1 508	1 151	1 481	777	1 833	599	3 111
Congenital abnormalities	463	5 446	616	646	890	1 171	10 889	210	6 955
Oral diseases	188	489	218	165	180	248	1 077	79	737
Dental caries	183	475	199	154	167	233	970	72	694
Periodontal disease	5	13	17	10	12	16	108	6	43
Edentulism	0	0	0	0	0	0	0	0	0
III. Injuries	2 469	10 745	4 320	4 582	10 421	11 869	53 420	1 667	47 974
Unintentional	2 199	8 260	2 994	3 352	6 548	9 523	46 653	1 086	36 577
Road traffic accidents	881	2 298	1 423	1 355	1 589	4 377	7 460	414	8 615
Poisoning	172	529	140	277	1 396	188	977	21	1 424
Falls	254	1 318	785	624	906	1 515	13 742	201	7 316
Fires	81	688	57	150	271	275	6 806	28	579
Drowning	109	672	78	274	610	486	2 654	68	4 789
Other unintentional injuries	104	1 176	436	571	1 447	735	5 408	143	5 595
Intentional	270	2 484	1 326	1 230	3 873	2 346	6 768	581	11 397
Self-inflicted	206	868	1 089	599	2 200	1 207	4 123	513	8 407
Homicide and violence	27	688	182	217	1 240	413	1 771	62	2 601
War	37	928	55	414	432	726	874	6	389

Annex Table 5 Health attainment, level and distribution in all Member States, estimates for 1997 and 1999

									LEVEL[a]	
			Disability-adjusted life expectancy **(years)**							
		Total population		**Males**				**Females**		
Rank	**Member State**	**At birth**	**At birth**	**Uncertainty interval**	**At age 60**	**Uncertainty interval**	**At birth**	**Uncertainty interval**	**At age 60**	**Uncertainty interval**
1	Japan	74.5	71.9	71.6 - 72.3	17.5	17.3 - 18.1	77.2	76.9 - 78.0	21.6	21.3 - 22.4
2	Australia	73.2	70.8	70.5 - 71.3	16.8	16.6 - 17.3	75.5	75.2 - 76.2	20.2	19.9 - 20.9
3	France	73.1	69.3	69.0 - 69.7	16.8	16.5 - 17.4	76.9	76.5 - 77.8	21.7	21.4 - 22.7
4	Sweden	73.0	71.2	70.9 - 71.8	16.8	16.5 - 17.3	74.9	74.4 - 75.7	19.6	19.4 - 20.5
5	Spain	72.8	69.8	69.1 - 70.6	16.8	16.4 - 17.6	75.7	75.3 - 76.6	20.1	19.8 - 21.0
6	Italy	72.7	70.0	69.7 - 70.5	16.2	16.0 - 16.8	75.4	75.0 - 76.2	19.9	19.6 - 20.7
7	Greece	72.5	70.5	70.2 - 70.9	16.9	16.6 - 17.3	74.6	74.2 - 75.2	18.8	18.6 - 19.5
8	Switzerland	72.5	69.5	69.0 - 70.2	16.0	15.7 - 16.7	75.5	75.0 - 76.5	20.6	20.3 - 21.6
9	Monaco	72.4	68.5	67.5 - 69.6	16.4	15.9 - 17.2	76.3	75.6 - 77.3	21.5	21.1 - 22.5
10	Andorra	72.3	69.3	68.6 - 70.2	16.3	15.9 - 17.0	75.2	74.6 - 76.2	20.0	19.6 - 20.9
11	San Marino	72.3	69.5	68.6 - 70.5	15.7	15.3 - 16.5	75.0	74.4 - 76.0	19.6	19.2 - 20.5
12	Canada	72.0	70.0	69.7 - 70.5	16.0	15.8 - 16.6	74.0	73.6 - 74.9	18.9	18.6 - 19.8
13	Netherlands	72.0	69.6	69.3 - 70.1	15.4	15.3 - 16.0	74.4	74.0 - 75.3	19.7	19.4 - 20.6
14	United Kingdom	71.7	69.7	69.4 - 70.1	15.7	15.5 - 16.2	73.7	73.5 - 74.4	18.6	18.3 - 19.2
15	Norway	71.7	68.8	68.5 - 69.3	15.1	15.0 - 15.7	74.6	74.2 - 75.3	19.7	19.4 - 20.6
16	Belgium	71.6	68.7	68.4 - 69.2	15.8	15.6 - 16.4	74.6	74.2 - 75.3	19.6	19.3 - 20.4
17	Austria	71.6	68.8	68.4 - 69.4	15.2	15.0 - 15.8	74.4	74.1 - 75.1	18.7	18.4 - 19.4
18	Luxembourg	71.1	68.0	67.6 - 68.7	15.8	15.2 - 16.8	74.2	73.7 - 75.2	19.7	19.0 - 21.0
19	Iceland	70.8	69.2	68.6 - 70.1	14.9	14.2 - 15.9	72.3	71.7 - 73.4	17.0	16.4 - 18.3
20	Finland	70.5	67.2	66.9 - 67.7	14.5	14.2 - 15.0	73.7	73.4 - 74.4	18.5	18.3 - 19.3
21	Malta	70.5	68.4	67.9 - 69.2	14.8	14.5 - 15.6	72.5	72.0 - 73.4	17.3	17.0 - 18.2
22	Germany	70.4	67.4	67.1 - 67.9	14.3	14.1 - 14.9	73.5	73.2 - 74.1	18.5	18.2 - 19.1
23	Israel	70.4	69.2	68.9 - 69.7	15.6	15.3 - 16.3	71.6	71.2 - 72.4	16.9	16.7 - 17.8
24	United States of America	70.0	67.5	67.0 - 68.1	15.0	14.7 - 15.7	72.6	72.2 - 73.3	18.4	18.1 - 19.2
25	Cyprus	69.8	68.7	68.2 - 69.4	15.9	15.6 - 16.6	70.9	70.4 - 71.7	17.3	17.0 - 18.1
26	Dominica	69.8	67.2	66.2 - 68.2	15.0	14.3 - 15.6	72.3	71.0 - 73.4	17.9	17.2 - 18.7
27	Ireland	69.6	67.5	67.0 - 68.2	13.9	13.6 - 14.6	71.7	71.2 - 72.5	16.6	16.3 - 17.4
28	Denmark	69.4	67.2	66.8 - 67.9	14.2	13.9 - 14.8	71.5	71.2 - 72.2	17.2	16.9 - 18.0
29	Portugal	69.3	65.9	65.6 - 66.6	14.0	13.7 - 14.6	72.7	72.4 - 73.4	17.7	17.3 - 18.5
30	Singapore	69.3	67.4	66.9 - 68.2	14.4	14.1 - 15.2	71.2	70.7 - 72.2	16.8	16.5 - 17.8
31	New Zealand	69.2	67.1	66.8 - 67.6	14.4	14.1 - 15.0	71.2	70.8 - 72.0	17.0	16.8 - 17.9
32	Chile	68.6	66.0	65.2 - 67.0	14.3	13.6 - 15.3	71.3	70.9 - 72.2	17.8	17.3 - 18.8
33	Cuba	68.4	67.4	66.8 - 68.1	15.4	14.9 - 16.1	69.4	68.9 - 70.3	16.1	15.8 - 16.9
34	Slovenia	68.4	64.9	64.6 - 65.4	12.7	12.6 - 13.4	71.9	71.5 - 72.6	16.8	16.5 - 17.6
35	Czech Republic	68.0	65.2	64.9 - 65.7	12.7	12.6 - 13.2	70.8	70.5 - 71.5	16.4	16.2 - 17.1
36	Jamaica	67.3	66.8	65.5 - 68.0	18.9	18.1 - 19.7	67.9	66.5 - 69.3	18.2	17.3 - 19.1
37	Uruguay	67.0	64.1	63.1 - 65.0	15.3	14.8 - 15.8	69.9	68.8 - 71.0	18.3	17.6 - 19.0
38	Croatia	67.0	63.3	63.1 - 63.8	11.4	11.3 - 11.9	70.6	70.3 - 71.3	16.0	15.8 - 16.7
39	Argentina	66.7	63.8	63.5 - 64.3	14.7	14.4 - 15.3	69.6	69.2 - 70.3	18.1	17.8 - 19.0
40	Costa Rica	66.7	65.2	64.6 - 66.0	14.2	13.9 - 15.0	68.1	67.5 - 69.1	16.6	16.2 - 17.6
41	Armenia	66.7	65.0	64.4 - 65.9	14.5	14.2 - 15.5	68.3	67.6 - 69.3	15.5	15.1 - 16.5
42	Slovakia	66.6	63.5	63.2 - 64.0	12.7	12.6 - 13.1	69.7	69.4 - 70.3	16.0	15.9 - 16.7
43	Saint Vincent and the Grenadines	66.4	65.0	63.8 - 66.2	15.9	15.2 - 16.7	67.8	66.4 - 69.0	16.7	15.9 - 17.5
44	Georgia	66.3	63.1	62.2 - 64.0	13.8	13.5 - 14.6	69.4	68.7 - 70.3	16.6	16.2 - 17.4
45	Poland	66.2	62.3	61.6 - 63.0	12.5	12.1 - 13.1	70.1	69.7 - 70.7	16.6	16.4 - 17.3
46	Yugoslavia	66.1	64.2	63.1 - 65.3	15.1	14.4 - 15.7	68.1	66.9 - 69.2	17.5	16.8 - 18.1
47	Panama	66.0	64.9	63.6 - 66.1	17.3	16.4 - 18.1	67.2	65.9 - 68.5	17.4	16.5 - 18.3
48	Antigua and Barbuda	65.8	63.4	62.0 - 64.6	14.4	13.7 - 15.2	68.3	66.9 - 69.6	16.8	15.9 - 17.6
49	Grenada	65.5	62.4	61.1 - 63.6	14.1	13.5 - 14.8	68.5	67.2 - 69.7	16.9	16.2 - 17.7
50	United Arab Emirates	65.4	65.0	64.0 - 65.9	11.7	10.9 - 12.5	65.8	64.6 - 67.0	12.6	11.8 - 13.5
51	Republic of Korea	65.0	62.3	61.6 - 63.1	12.1	11.6 - 12.7	67.7	66.7 - 68.7	15.2	14.5 - 15.8
52	Venezuela, Bolivarian Republic of	65.0	62.9	62.4 - 63.6	13.4	13.1 - 14.2	67.1	66.5 - 68.1	15.7	15.2 - 16.7
53	Barbados	65.0	62.4	61.2 - 63.8	14.5	13.8 - 15.8	67.6	66.9 - 68.7	16.6	15.8 - 17.9

Expectation of disability at birth (years)		Percentage of lifespan lived with disability				DISTRIBUTION[b]		
						Equality of child survival[c]		
Males	Females	Males	Females	Rank	Member State	Index	Uncertainty interval
5.7	7.1	7.3	8.4	1	Chile	0.999	0.999 - 0.999
6.0	6.7	7.8	8.1	2	United Kingdom	0.999	0.999 - 0.999
5.6	6.7	7.5	8.0	3	Japan	0.999	0.999 - 0.999
5.9	7.0	7.7	8.5	4	Norway	0.999	0.999 - 0.999
5.5	6.4	7.3	7.7	5	Poland	0.999	0.999 - 0.999
5.4	6.7	7.1	8.2	6	Greece	0.979	0.962 - 0.996
5.0	5.9	6.7	7.4	7	Israel	0.979	0.961 - 0.996
6.1	7.5	8.1	9.1	8	Austria	0.978	0.959 - 0.996
6.2	7.3	8.3	8.7	9	San Marino	0.978	0.961 - 0.995
6.1	7.0	8.0	8.5	10	Switzerland	0.978	0.959 - 0.996
5.8	7.0	7.7	8.6	11	Spain	0.978	0.960 - 0.996
6.2	7.8	8.1	9.6	12	France	0.978	0.961 - 0.996
5.4	6.7	7.2	8.2	13	Ireland	0.978	0.960 - 0.995
5.0	6.0	6.7	7.5	14	Italy	0.978	0.960 - 0.996
6.3	7.6	8.4	9.2	15	Netherlands	0.978	0.960 - 0.995
5.8	6.7	7.8	8.2	16	New Zealand	0.978	0.961 - 0.996
5.6	6.0	7.5	7.4	17	Australia	0.977	0.959 - 0.996
6.5	7.2	8.7	8.8	18	Canada	0.977	0.959 - 0.995
6.8	8.1	9.0	10.0	19	Czech Republic	0.977	0.958 - 0.995
6.2	7.0	8.4	8.6	20	Germany	0.977	0.959 - 0.995
7.3	8.3	9.6	10.3	21	Denmark	0.977	0.958 - 0.996
6.3	6.6	8.6	8.3	22	Luxembourg	0.977	0.958 - 0.995
7.1	8.3	9.3	10.4	23	Slovenia	0.977	0.958 - 0.995
6.3	7.0	8.6	8.8	24	Iceland	0.976	0.954 - 0.996
6.1	7.9	8.2	10.0	25	Andorra	0.975	0.953 - 0.996
6.8	8.0	9.2	10.0	26	Belgium	0.975	0.956 - 0.994
5.8	6.6	8.0	8.4	27	Finland	0.975	0.952 - 0.996
5.7	6.6	7.9	8.4	28	Sweden	0.975	0.953 - 0.996
6.1	6.8	8.4	8.6	29	Singapore	0.971	0.946 - 0.995
7.7	9.6	10.2	11.8	30	Monaco	0.970	0.946 - 0.994
6.8	8.1	9.2	10.2	31	Cyprus	0.968	0.944 - 0.993
7.4	8.6	10.1	10.8	32	United States of America	0.966	0.950 - 0.983
6.2	8.0	8.4	10.3	33	Croatia	0.962	0.932 - 0.992
6.7	7.6	9.4	9.6	34	Portugal	0.959	0.928 - 0.993
6.3	7.5	8.8	9.5	35	Dominica	0.953	0.917 - 0.990
8.4	9.5	11.2	12.3	36	Barbados	0.947	0.906 - 0.988
6.4	7.9	9.1	10.2	37	Republic of Korea	0.947	0.906 - 0.989
6.0	6.6	8.7	8.6	38	Malta	0.946	0.903 - 0.989
6.8	8.2	9.6	10.6	39	Slovakia	0.945	0.902 - 0.988
9.0	10.8	12.1	13.7	40	Hungary	0.941	0.894 - 0.987
7.3	8.8	10.1	11.4	41	Cuba	0.938	0.890 - 0.987
5.4	7.0	7.8	9.1	42	Brunei Darussalam	0.936	0.886 - 0.986
6.8	7.4	9.5	9.8	43	Estonia	0.934	0.883 - 0.985
6.3	7.3	9.1	9.5	44	Colombia	0.912	0.873 - 0.952
5.6	6.5	8.2	8.5	45	Costa Rica	0.906	0.835 - 0.979
7.6	8.2	10.6	10.8	46	Belarus	0.905	0.834 - 0.979
7.8	8.6	10.7	11.4	47	Ukraine	0.905	0.833 - 0.979
8.0	8.5	11.2	11.1	48	Lithuania	0.903	0.830 - 0.978
6.7	7.4	9.7	9.7	49	Malaysia	0.901	0.825 - 0.978
7.3	9.8	10.0	13.0	50	Philippines	0.892	0.856 - 0.928
6.4	8.3	9.3	10.9	51	Nauru	0.884	0.797 - 0.972
8.1	9.0	11.4	11.8	52	Kazakhstan	0.880	0.877 - 0.989
10.3	10.2	14.2	13.1	53	Bulgaria	0.877	0.786 - 0.970

Annex Table 5 Health attainment, level and distribution in all Member States, estimates for 1997 and 1999

								LEVEL[a]			
			Disability-adjusted life expectancy (years)								
		Total population	Males				Females				
Rank	Member State	At birth	At birth	Uncertainty interval	At age 60	Uncertainty interval	At birth	Uncertainty interval	At age 60	Uncertainty interval
54	Saint Lucia	65.0	62.4	61.1 - 63.6	14.1	13.5 - 14.8	67.6	66.4 - 68.7	15.8	15.2 - 16.5
55	Mexico	65.0	62.4	61.6 - 63.3	14.7	14.4 - 15.6	67.6	67.1 - 68.5	16.8	16.4 - 17.9
56	Bosnia and Herzegovina	64.9	63.4	62.3 - 64.5	13.3	12.7 - 14.1	66.4	65.2 - 67.5	15.3	14.5 - 15.9
57	Trinidad and Tobago	64.6	62.8	62.2 - 63.5	12.0	11.8 - 12.6	66.4	65.9 - 67.1	13.9	13.7 - 14.6
58	Saudi Arabia	64.5	65.1	64.3 - 65.9	12.7	12.1 - 13.4	64.0	62.6 - 65.2	12.8	12.2 - 13.5
59	Brunei Darussalam	64.4	63.4	63.0 - 64.5	12.4	12.0 - 13.6	65.4	64.7 - 66.9	12.6	11.9 - 14.4
60	Bulgaria	64.4	61.2	60.8 - 61.6	12.2	12.0 - 12.7	67.7	67.4 - 68.3	15.1	14.8 - 15.7
61	Bahrain	64.4	63.9	63.0 - 64.8	11.6	11.0 - 12.3	64.9	63.8 - 66.0	12.6	11.8 - 13.3
62	Hungary	64.1	60.4	59.6 - 61.2	11.7	11.4 - 12.3	67.9	67.5 - 68.5	15.5	15.3 - 16.3
63	Lithuania	64.1	60.6	59.7 - 61.6	13.4	13.1 - 14.2	67.5	66.9 - 68.3	16.2	15.9 - 17.0
64	The former Yugoslav Republic of Macedonia	63.7	61.8	61.2 - 62.6	11.7	11.4 - 12.5	65.6	65.1 - 66.5	13.5	13.2 - 14.3
65	Azerbaijan	63.7	60.6	59.9 - 61.4	12.7	12.4 - 13.5	66.7	66.1 - 67.7	15.7	15.4 - 16.7
66	Qatar	63.5	64.2	63.4 - 65.1	10.8	10.1 - 11.4	62.8	61.2 - 64.3	10.2	8.9 - 11.3
67	Cook Islands	63.4	62.2	61.0 - 63.4	12.2	11.5 - 12.8	64.5	63.1 - 65.9	13.7	13.0 - 14.5
68	Kuwait	63.2	63.0	61.6 - 64.3	11.1	10.2 - 12.0	63.4	61.6 - 65.1	11.8	10.6 - 12.9
69	Estonia	63.1	58.1	57.3 - 59.0	11.2	10.9 - 11.9	68.1	67.4 - 69.0	15.8	15.5 - 16.6
70	Ukraine	63.0	58.5	58.1 - 59.0	11.5	11.4 - 12.0	67.5	67.1 - 68.0	15.5	15.3 - 16.1
71	Paraguay	63.0	60.7	59.2 - 62.0	14.2	13.3 - 15.1	65.3	63.9 - 66.7	16.0	15.1 - 17.0
72	Oman	63.0	61.8	60.8 - 62.8	10.6	9.9 - 11.3	64.1	62.8 - 65.3	12.1	11.2 - 12.8
73	Turkey	62.9	64.0	62.9 - 65.0	16.2	15.5 - 16.8	61.8	60.6 - 63.0	15.2	14.6 - 15.9
74	Colombia	62.9	60.3	59.2 - 61.5	13.5	12.7 - 14.2	65.5	64.2 - 66.7	15.4	14.6 - 16.2
75	Tonga	62.9	61.4	60.2 - 62.6	11.5	10.9 - 12.2	64.3	62.9 - 65.6	13.3	12.6 - 14.1
76	Sri Lanka	62.8	59.3	58.3 - 60.3	12.7	12.1 - 13.4	66.3	65.2 - 67.4	16.0	15.4 - 16.7
77	Suriname	62.7	60.2	58.9 - 61.4	14.4	13.8 - 15.2	65.2	64.0 - 66.5	15.5	14.6 - 16.3
78	Mauritius	62.7	59.0	57.9 - 60.2	10.2	9.8 - 11.2	66.3	65.7 - 67.3	13.5	13.2 - 14.4
79	Dominican Republic	62.5	62.1	60.7 - 63.6	17.1	16.1 - 18.2	62.9	61.8 - 63.7	16.1	15.2 - 16.8
80	Romania	62.3	58.8	58.4 - 59.2	12.0	11.8 - 12.6	65.8	65.4 - 66.5	14.6	14.3 - 15.3
81	China	62.3	61.2	60.7 - 62.0	11.6	11.3 - 12.3	63.3	62.8 - 64.2	13.5	13.2 - 14.4
82	Latvia	62.2	57.1	55.9 - 58.2	11.4	11.0 - 12.2	67.2	66.4 - 68.2	15.9	15.5 - 16.7
83	Belarus	61.7	56.2	55.4 - 57.1	10.1	9.8 - 10.8	67.2	66.7 - 68.0	15.1	14.8 - 15.9
84	Algeria	61.6	62.5	61.4 - 63.5	12.9	12.3 - 13.6	60.7	59.4 - 62.0	12.0	11.3 - 12.6
85	Niue	61.6	61.0	59.2 - 62.6	12.2	11.7 - 13.3	62.2	60.4 - 63.8	13.2	12.7 - 15.2
86	Saint Kitts and Nevis	61.6	58.7	57.4 - 59.9	12.8	12.2 - 13.3	64.4	63.2 - 65.6	14.3	13.7 - 15.0
87	El Salvador	61.5	58.6	57.4 - 59.7	13.9	13.1 - 14.6	64.5	63.2 - 65.7	15.8	14.9 - 16.6
88	Republic of Moldova	61.5	58.5	58.0 - 59.0	10.7	10.6 - 11.2	64.5	64.0 - 65.2	13.0	12.8 - 13.7
89	Malaysia	61.4	61.3	60.2 - 62.1	9.7	9.2 - 10.2	61.6	60.5 - 62.7	9.7	9.1 - 10.3
90	Tunisia	61.4	62.0	61.2 - 62.9	11.2	10.8 - 11.7	60.7	59.7 - 61.8	10.3	9.8 - 10.8
91	Russian Federation	61.3	56.1	55.4 - 56.9	10.5	10.3 - 11.2	66.4	65.8 - 67.2	14.9	14.6 - 15.7
92	Honduras	61.1	60.0	58.8 - 61.2	15.0	14.2 - 15.7	62.3	61.1 - 63.5	14.4	13.5 - 15.1
93	Ecuador	61.0	59.9	58.9 - 60.9	12.6	11.9 - 13.2	62.1	61.1 - 63.3	12.9	12.3 - 13.7
94	Belize	60.9	58.5	56.9 - 60.1	13.6	12.7 - 14.4	63.3	61.5 - 65.0	15.2	14.3 - 16.2
95	Lebanon	60.6	61.2	60.2 - 62.2	10.1	9.6 - 10.6	60.1	58.8 - 61.2	9.2	8.7 - 9.7
96	Iran, Islamic Republic of	60.5	61.3	60.2 - 62.3	11.9	11.3 - 12.5	59.8	58.6 - 61.1	10.9	10.2 - 11.6
97	Samoa	60.5	58.7	57.5 - 59.8	9.5	9.0 - 10.1	62.3	60.9 - 63.6	12.3	11.7 - 13.0
98	Guyana	60.2	57.1	55.8 - 58.6	15.4	14.5 - 16.4	63.3	61.9 - 64.7	16.8	15.8 - 17.8
99	Thailand	60.2	58.4	57.1 - 59.6	13.7	12.9 - 14.5	62.1	60.9 - 63.3	13.9	13.1 - 14.7
100	Uzbekistan	60.2	58.0	57.4 - 58.8	11.5	11.3 - 12.2	62.3	61.6 - 63.1	13.4	13.1 - 14.3
101	Jordan	60.0	60.7	59.8 - 61.5	9.5	9.1 - 10.0	59.3	58.2 - 60.4	8.9	8.5 - 9.4
102	Albania	60.0	56.5	55.8 - 57.4	10.1	9.9 - 10.9	63.4	62.7 - 64.4	13.9	13.6 - 14.7
103	Indonesia	59.7	58.8	57.5 - 60.1	16.3	15.3 - 17.2	60.6	59.3 - 61.8	15.8	15.0 - 16.6
104	Micronesia, Federated States of	59.6	58.7	57.2 - 60.0	11.1	10.4 - 11.8	60.6	59.0 - 62.0	11.5	10.7 - 12.4
105	Peru	59.4	58.0	56.9 - 59.0	12.3	11.7 - 13.0	60.8	59.6 - 62.0	13.1	12.3 - 13.9
106	Fiji	59.4	57.7	56.1 - 59.1	8.3	8.0 - 9.1	61.1	59.8 - 62.3	9.8	9.5 - 10.8
107	Libyan Arab Jamahiriya	59.3	59.7	58.7 - 60.7	9.7	9.2 - 10.2	58.9	57.6 - 60.2	9.3	8.7 - 10.0

Expectation of disability at birth (years)		Percentage of lifespan lived with disability		DISTRIBUTION[b] Equality of child survival[c]			
Males	Females	Males	Females	Rank	Member State	Index	Uncertainty interval
6.5	7.3	9.4	9.8	54	Kuwait	0.876	0.784 - 0.971
8.6	9.6	12.2	12.4	55	Qatar	0.874	0.781 - 0.969
7.9	8.6	11.0	11.5	56	Latvia	0.872	0.776 - 0.967
5.9	7.0	8.5	9.5	57	Paraguay	0.871	0.821 - 0.917
5.8	8.7	8.2	12.0	58	Antigua and Barbuda	0.861	0.759 - 0.963
10.9	14.3	14.6	18.0	59	Oman	0.861	0.757 - 0.964
6.3	7.1	9.3	9.4	60	Argentina	0.859	0.756 - 0.962
6.8	8.7	9.7	11.8	61	Georgia	0.859	0.755 - 0.963
5.9	7.2	9.0	9.6	62	United Arab Emirates	0.858	0.749 - 0.964
6.4	10.4	9.5	13.3	63	Armenia	0.858	0.756 - 0.962
8.0	8.5	11.4	11.5	64	Republic of Moldova	0.858	0.757 - 0.962
7.2	8.6	10.6	11.4	65	Mexico	0.858	0.810 - 0.906
7.4	11.8	10.3	15.8	66	Palau	0.858	0.755 - 0.962
7.0	8.8	10.1	12.0	67	Bahamas	0.857	0.753 - 0.961
8.9	11.9	12.4	15.8	68	Uruguay	0.856	0.730 - 0.969
6.3	7.2	9.8	9.5	69	Russian Federation	0.852	0.746 - 0.960
5.8	6.9	9.1	9.3	70	Saudi Arabia	0.847	0.736 - 0.958
8.9	8.8	12.9	11.8	71	Fiji	0.846	0.737 - 0.957
8.6	9.7	12.2	13.1	72	Bahrain	0.845	0.734 - 0.956
5.7	8.1	8.2	11.6	73	Seychelles	0.845	0.734 - 0.957
7.8	8.6	11.5	11.6	74	Thailand	0.845	0.786 - 0.908
6.8	8.6	10.0	11.8	75	Trinidad and Tobago	0.844	0.774 - 0.915
6.5	7.1	9.9	9.7	76	Venezuela, Bolivarian Republic of	0.840	0.726 - 0.953
7.9	8.3	11.6	11.3	77	Mauritius	0.837	0.723 - 0.952
7.7	7.7	11.6	10.4	78	Romania	0.837	0.722 - 0.953
9.2	9.9	12.9	13.6	79	Bosnia and Herzegovina	0.834	0.720 - 0.950
6.4	7.6	9.8	10.4	80	Sri Lanka	0.833	0.716 - 0.949
6.9	8.0	10.2	11.2	81	Samoa	0.830	0.710 - 0.948
6.5	7.4	10.2	9.9	82	Grenada	0.829	0.711 - 0.949
6.2	7.3	9.9	9.9	83	Jordan	0.824	0.704 - 0.945
5.7	8.1	8.4	11.7	84	Tonga	0.823	0.702 - 0.946
7.3	8.7	10.7	12.2	85	The former Yugoslav Republic of Macedonia	0.821	0.700 - 0.944
6.3	6.8	9.7	9.5	86	Saint Lucia	0.818	0.696 - 0.940
8.3	8.5	12.4	11.6	87	Jamaica	0.811	0.686 - 0.936
6.3	7.4	9.7	10.3	88	Lebanon	0.810	0.685 - 0.938
6.3	8.3	9.4	11.9	89	Saint Vincent and the Grenadines	0.808	0.682 - 0.934
5.0	7.2	7.4	10.6	90	Yugoslavia	0.807	0.682 - 0.936
6.6	7.6	10.5	10.3	91	Saint Kitts and Nevis	0.806	0.679 - 0.935
8.2	8.5	12.0	12.0	92	Cook Islands	0.805	0.662 - 0.942
7.5	8.2	11.1	11.6	93	Panama	0.804	0.675 - 0.936
11.1	11.6	15.9	15.5	94	Suriname	0.798	0.668 - 0.929
5.1	7.2	7.7	10.7	95	Belize	0.796	0.665 - 0.927
5.5	8.1	8.2	11.9	96	Nicaragua	0.796	0.755 - 0.839
6.7	8.4	10.2	11.9	97	Dominican Republic	0.789	0.723 - 0.854
8.4	8.9	12.9	12.3	98	Zimbabwe	0.785	0.718 - 0.856
7.6	8.3	11.6	11.8	99	Azerbaijan	0.784	0.649 - 0.920
7.7	8.9	11.7	12.6	100	Niue	0.783	0.649 - 0.921
5.6	8.2	8.4	12.1	101	China	0.782	0.648 - 0.918
8.6	9.3	13.3	12.8	102	Libyan Arab Jamahiriya	0.782	0.647 - 0.919
7.8	8.4	11.7	12.2	103	Peru	0.779	0.745 - 0.812
7.8	9.5	11.7	13.5	104	Viet Nam	0.779	0.643 - 0.918
7.6	8.2	11.6	11.9	105	Senegal	0.773	0.713 - 0.831
6.3	8.1	9.8	11.7	106	Guatemala	0.764	0.716 - 0.813
5.3	8.1	8.2	12.1	107	Syrian Arab Republic	0.764	0.624 - 0.905

Annex Table 5 Health attainment, level and distribution in all Member States, estimates for 1997 and 1999

									LEVEL[a]	
					Disability-adjusted life expectancy (years)					
		Total population		Males				Females		
Rank	Member State	At birth	At birth	Uncertainty interval	At age 60	Uncertainty interval	At birth	Uncertainty interval	At age 60	Uncertainty interval
108	Seychelles	59.3	56.4	55.7 - 57.3	8.6	8.3 - 9.4	62.1	61.5 - 63.0	11.7	11.4 - 12.4
109	Bahamas	59.1	56.7	55.1 - 58.1	11.3	10.5 - 12.1	61.6	59.9 - 63.4	13.0	12.0 - 14.0
110	Morocco	59.1	58.7	57.9 - 59.6	11.5	11.0 - 12.0	59.4	58.4 - 60.4	11.4	10.8 - 12.0
111	Brazil	59.1	55.2	54.4 - 56.1	11.8	11.5 - 12.7	62.9	62.2 - 63.9	14.8	14.4 - 15.8
112	Palau	59.0	57.4	56.1 - 58.5	8.0	7.5 - 8.5	60.7	59.2 - 61.9	9.7	9.1 - 10.4
113	Philippines	58.9	57.1	56.0 - 58.1	10.3	9.7 - 10.9	60.7	59.4 - 61.9	12.4	11.6 - 13.1
114	Syrian Arab Republic	58.8	58.8	57.7 - 59.9	9.7	9.2 - 10.2	58.9	57.6 - 60.2	10.0	9.4 - 10.6
115	Egypt	58.5	58.6	57.7 - 59.5	11.8	11.2 - 12.2	58.3	57.1 - 59.6	11.7	11.1 - 12.4
116	Viet Nam	58.2	56.7	55.6 - 57.9	9.7	9.1 - 10.4	59.6	58.4 - 60.9	10.8	10.1 - 11.5
117	Nicaragua	58.1	56.4	55.3 - 57.4	11.1	10.4 - 11.8	59.9	58.7 - 61.1	12.5	11.7 - 13.2
118	Cape Verde	57.6	54.6	53.0 - 56.2	11.4	10.6 - 12.3	60.6	58.8 - 62.4	15.3	14.2 - 16.4
119	Tuvalu	57.4	57.1	55.7 - 58.3	10.3	9.7 - 10.9	57.6	56.2 - 58.8	9.4	8.8 - 10.0
120	Tajikistan	57.3	55.1	53.5 - 56.5	12.3	11.4 - 13.2	59.4	57.9 - 60.9	15.6	14.7 - 16.4
121	Marshall Islands	56.8	56.0	54.4 - 57.4	10.7	10.0 - 11.4	57.6	55.9 - 59.0	11.1	10.3 - 12.0
122	Kazakhstan	56.4	51.5	50.9 - 52.2	8.8	8.7 - 9.5	61.2	60.8 - 62.0	13.1	12.8 - 13.9
123	Kyrgyzstan	56.3	53.4	52.6 - 54.2	9.6	9.4 - 10.4	59.1	58.3 - 60.1	12.4	12.1 - 13.3
124	Pakistan	55.9	55.0	53.8 - 56.3	11.3	10.5 - 12.1	56.8	54.6 - 57.9	12.6	11.9 - 13.2
125	Kiribati	55.3	53.9	52.4 - 55.3	9.4	8.7 - 10.1	56.6	55.0 - 58.0	11.0	10.3 - 11.7
126	Iraq	55.3	55.4	54.4 - 56.4	9.2	8.7 - 9.8	55.1	53.9 - 56.2	8.2	7.6 - 8.8
127	Solomon Islands	54.9	54.5	53.0 - 55.8	8.8	8.2 - 9.5	55.3	53.7 - 56.7	9.2	8.6 - 9.9
128	Turkmenistan	54.3	51.9	50.6 - 53.3	9.0	8.7 - 10.0	56.7	55.3 - 58.0	10.9	10.6 - 11.8
129	Guatemala	54.3	52.1	51.1 - 53.1	9.1	8.6 - 9.8	56.4	55.4 - 57.5	10.1	9.5 - 10.7
130	Maldives	53.9	54.4	53.0 - 55.9	12.1	11.3 - 13.0	53.3	51.8 - 54.7	11.5	10.8 - 12.2
131	Mongolia	53.8	51.3	49.7 - 52.7	11.8	11.0 - 14.4	56.3	54.7 - 57.7	14.3	13.4 - 15.1
132	Sao Tome and Principe	53.5	52.1	51.1 - 53.3	11.4	11.1 - 12.5	54.8	53.8 - 55.8	11.7	11.4 - 12.6
133	Bolivia	53.3	52.5	51.3 - 53.7	11.6	10.9 - 12.3	54.1	52.8 - 55.2	11.2	10.6 - 11.9
134	India	53.2	52.8	52.1 - 53.5	10.6	10.4 - 11.3	53.5	52.8 - 54.3	12.1	11.8 - 12.8
135	Vanuatu	52.8	51.3	49.8 - 52.7	8.0	7.4 - 8.6	54.4	52.8 - 55.8	9.2	8.5 - 9.8
136	Nauru	52.5	49.8	48.7 - 50.9	3.6	3.1 - 4.0	55.1	53.8 - 56.2	5.9	5.4 - 6.4
137	Democratic People's Republic of Korea	52.3	51.4	49.8 - 53.1	9.6	8.7 - 10.6	53.1	51.3 - 55.0	11.6	10.7 - 12.6
138	Bhutan	51.8	51.4	50.0 - 52.7	11.4	10.7 - 12.0	52.2	50.7 - 53.6	12.6	12.0 - 13.3
139	Myanmar	51.6	51.4	50.0 - 52.6	12.5	11.7 - 13.3	51.9	50.5 - 53.2	12.3	11.6 - 12.9
140	Bangladesh	49.9	50.1	48.7 - 51.3	9.9	9.2 - 10.5	49.8	48.3 - 51.2	10.5	9.8 - 11.1
141	Yemen	49.7	49.7	48.1 - 51.1	8.5	7.9 - 9.2	49.7	48.2 - 51.1	8.2	7.5 - 8.8
142	Nepal	49.5	49.4	48.1 - 50.7	10.3	9.6 - 10.9	49.5	48.2 - 50.9	10.0	9.4 - 10.7
143	Gambia	48.3	47.2	46.3 - 48.2	9.9	9.3 - 10.6	49.4	48.4 - 50.4	11.7	11.2 - 12.4
144	Gabon	47.8	46.6	45.4 - 47.6	10.3	9.8 - 10.8	49.0	47.8 - 50.1	12.3	11.8 - 12.8
145	Papua New Guinea	47.0	45.5	44.3 - 46.8	8.2	7.5 - 8.9	48.5	47.1 - 49.8	8.7	8.0 - 9.4
146	Comoros	46.8	46.1	45.1 - 47.1	8.9	8.3 - 9.6	47.5	46.5 - 48.5	9.8	9.4 - 10.4
147	Lao People's Democratic Republic	46.1	45.0	43.5 - 46.5	8.9	8.0 - 9.7	47.1	45.5 - 48.6	8.8	7.9 - 9.6
148	Cambodia	45.7	43.9	42.6 - 45.1	7.4	6.6 - 8.2	47.5	46.1 - 48.9	9.3	8.7 - 10.0
149	Ghana	45.5	45.0	43.8 - 46.2	9.9	9.3 - 10.6	46.0	44.8 - 47.2	10.2	9.6 - 10.8
150	Congo	45.1	44.3	43.1 - 45.5	10.7	10.0 - 11.3	45.9	44.6 - 47.1	12.8	12.2 - 13.4
151	Senegal	44.6	43.5	42.5 - 44.5	8.8	8.1 - 9.5	45.6	44.6 - 46.7	11.3	10.6 - 11.9
152	Equatorial Guinea	44.1	42.8	41.7 - 43.9	9.4	8.9 - 10	45.4	44.4 - 46.6	11.0	10.5 - 11.7
153	Haiti	43.8	42.4	41.0 - 43.6	7.4	6.8 - 8.0	45.2	43.7 - 46.7	8.0	7.3 - 8.7
154	Sudan	43.0	42.6	41.2 - 43.7	5.6	5.1 - 6.0	43.5	42.1 - 44.6	6.0	5.6 - 6.5
155	Côte d'Ivoire	42.8	42.2	41.2 - 43.3	11.9	11.5 - 12.5	43.3	42.3 - 44.4	12.7	12.2 - 13.2
156	Cameroon	42.2	41.5	40.4 - 42.5	9.6	9.0 - 10.2	43.0	41.8 - 44.2	11.9	11.3 - 12.5
157	Benin	42.2	41.9	40.9 - 42.9	9.6	9.0 - 10.3	42.6	41.5 - 43.6	10.6	9.9 - 11.2
158	Mauritania	41.4	40.2	39.2 - 41.2	9.2	8.6 - 9.9	42.5	41.5 - 43.5	11.0	10.3 - 11.7
159	Togo	40.7	40.0	38.8 - 41.3	9.5	8.8 - 10.1	41.4	40.1 - 42.6	11.0	10.5 - 11.6
160	South Africa	39.8	38.6	37.7 - 39.5	6.8	6.4 - 7.3	41.0	39.9 - 42.1	9.3	8.9 - 9.8

Expectation of disability at birth (years)		Percentage of lifespan lived with disability				DISTRIBUTION[b]		
						Equality of child survival[c]		
Males	Females	Males	Females	Rank	Member State	Index	Uncertainty interval	
8.4	8.4	13.0	11.9	108	Brazil	0.762	0.702 - 0.823	
10.3	12.0	15.4	16.3	109	Turkey	*0.759*	*0.616 - 0.902*	
6.4	7.4	9.8	11.0	110	Algeria	*0.753*	*0.607 - 0.897*	
8.5	8.8	13.3	12.3	111	Morocco	0.748	0.685 - 0.809	
7.1	9.0	11.0	13.0	112	Micronesia, Federated States of	*0.747*	*0.602 - 0.893*	
7.1	8.7	11.0	12.5	113	Iran, Islamic Republic of	*0.745*	*0.600 - 0.891*	
5.8	8.2	8.9	12.3	114	Tunisia	0.744	0.678 - 0.817	
5.6	7.5	8.8	11.4	115	El Salvador	*0.741*	*0.596 - 0.887*	
8.0	9.2	12.3	13.3	116	Tuvalu	*0.732*	*0.584 - 0.881*	
8.4	8.9	13.0	13.0	117	Solomon Islands	*0.728*	*0.585 - 0.873*	
9.6	11.2	15.0	15.5	118	Bolivia	*0.725*	*0.661 - 0.792*	
6.8	7.9	10.6	12.1	119	Honduras	*0.723*	*0.575 - 0.873*	
10.1	10.6	15.5	15.2	120	Marshall Islands	*0.712*	*0.562 - 0.866*	
7.9	9.5	12.4	14.2	121	Kiribati	*0.706*	*0.556 - 0.860*	
7.2	8.7	12.3	12.4	122	Kyrgyzstan	*0.699*	*0.545 - 0.856*	
8.2	9.9	13.3	14.3	123	Cape Verde	*0.694*	*0.543 - 0.848*	
7.6	8.2	12.1	12.6	124	Tajikistan	*0.694*	*0.540 - 0.850*	
7.4	8.9	12.1	13.6	125	Bangladesh	0.692	0.626 - 0.763	
6.2	7.7	10.0	12.2	126	Guyana	*0.691*	*0.537 - 0.846*	
7.5	8.7	12.2	13.7	127	Vanuatu	*0.686*	*0.537 - 0.837*	
9.1	8.6	14.9	13.2	128	South Africa	*0.685*	*0.531 - 0.840*	
8.1	8.3	13.4	12.8	129	Albania	*0.684*	*0.536 - 0.832*	
8.9	9.3	14.0	14.9	130	Iraq	*0.684*	*0.535 - 0.832*	
7.7	8.5	13.0	13.1	131	Turkmenistan	*0.684*	*0.528 - 0.843*	
10.0	10.1	16.1	15.5	132	Benin	0.680	0.594 - 0.763	
8.3	8.1	13.6	13.1	133	Ecuador	0.679	0.590 - 0.772	
6.8	7.7	11.3	12.5	134	Maldives	*0.671*	*0.518 - 0.826*	
7.4	8.6	12.7	13.7	135	Kenya	0.660	0.595 - 0.723	
6.6	8.1	11.6	12.9	136	Gabon	*0.656*	*0.501 - 0.810*	
6.6	7.6	11.3	12.5	137	Burkina Faso	0.654	0.576 - 0.731	
8.2	8.7	13.8	14.2	138	Uganda	0.653	0.572 - 0.732	
7.1	7.4	12.1	12.4	139	Sao Tome and Principe	*0.650*	*0.500 - 0.803*	
7.4	8.3	12.9	14.3	140	Swaziland	*0.645*	*0.489 - 0.801*	
7.6	8.3	13.2	14.3	141	Egypt	0.643	0.598 - 0.688	
7.9	8.3	13.7	14.3	142	Congo	*0.635*	*0.480 - 0.792*	
8.8	9.5	15.7	16.1	143	Comoros	0.633	0.521 - 0.753	
8.0	8.5	14.6	14.8	144	Uzbekistan	0.632	0.530 - 0.731	
7.8	8.1	14.7	14.3	145	Democratic People's Republic of Korea	*0.631*	*0.478 - 0.785*	
9.9	10.6	17.7	18.3	146	Botswana	*0.624*	*0.472 - 0.776*	
9.0	9.5	16.6	16.7	147	Lao People's Democratic Republic	*0.624*	*0.464 - 0.789*	
8.3	7.9	15.8	14.2	148	Mongolia	*0.624*	*0.467 - 0.784*	
9.2	9.6	16.9	17.2	149	Ghana	0.610	0.513 - 0.711	
9.3	9.3	17.4	16.9	150	Cambodia	*0.606*	*0.450 - 0.763*	
10.0	10.6	18.7	18.8	151	Equatorial Guinea	*0.604*	*0.448 - 0.762*	
8.6	9.9	16.7	17.9	152	Haiti	0.602	0.500 - 0.704	
8.2	9.8	16.2	17.8	153	India	0.601	0.578 - 0.622	
10.5	11.2	19.8	20.5	154	Burundi	0.599	0.490 - 0.699	
5.1	5.0	10.8	10.3	155	Gambia	*0.599*	*0.446 - 0.755*	
8.4	9.0	16.9	17.3	156	Indonesia	0.599	0.562 - 0.637	
9.4	10.7	18.4	20.1	157	Papua New Guinea	*0.599*	*0.446 - 0.754*	
9.3	10.5	18.8	19.7	158	Bhutan	*0.598*	*0.445 - 0.752*	
8.9	9.4	18.2	18.6	159	Sudan	0.595	0.525 - 0.666	
8.7	8.8	18.4	17.6	160	Cameroon	0.593	0.503 - 0.690	

Annex Table 5 Health attainment, level and distribution in all Member States, estimates for 1997 and 1999

							LEVEL[a]			
			Disability-adjusted life expectancy (years)							
		Total population		Males			Females			
Rank	Member State	At birth	At birth	Uncertainty interval	At age 60	Uncertainty interval	At birth	Uncertainty interval	At age 60	Uncertainty interval
161	Chad	39.4	38.6	37.2 - 39.8	9.2	8.6 - 9.9	40.2	38.8 - 41.5	10.6	10.0 - 11.2
162	Kenya	39.3	39.0	37.9 - 40.2	9.2	8.6 - 13.4	39.6	38.4 - 41.0	12.0	11.5 - 12.5
163	Nigeria	38.3	38.1	36.9 - 39.2	8.7	8.1 - 9.4	38.4	37.1 - 39.6	10.1	9.5 - 10.7
164	Swaziland	38.1	37.8	36.5 - 39.0	8.1	7.7 - 8.6	38.4	36.9 - 39.9	9.5	9.0 - 10.0
165	Angola	38.0	37.0	35.7 - 38.1	8.9	8.3 - 9.6	38.9	37.7 - 40.0	10.8	10.1 - 11.4
166	Djibouti	37.9	37.7	36.2 - 38.8	6.9	6.4 - 7.4	38.1	36.6 - 39.3	7.9	7.6 - 8.2
167	Guinea	37.8	37.0	36.1 - 38.0	8.5	7.9 - 9.2	38.5	37.5 - 39.5	9.6	9.0 - 10.3
168	Afghanistan	37.7	36.7	34.9 - 38.5	7.9	7.0 - 8.8	38.7	36.9 - 40.5	7.9	7.2 - 8.7
169	Eritrea	37.7	38.5	37.6 - 39.5	8.2	7.6 - 8.7	36.9	35.9 - 37.9	7.9	7.4 - 8.4
170	Guinea-Bissau	37.2	36.8	35.6 - 37.9	9.1	8.5 - 13.4	37.5	36.4 - 38.6	10.0	9.4 - 10.6
171	Lesotho	36.9	36.6	35.3 - 38.0	9.9	9.3 - 10.4	37.2	35.7 - 38.7	11.3	10.8 - 11.9
172	Madagascar	36.6	36.5	35.5 - 37.4	6.7	6.1 - 7.2	36.8	35.7 - 37.7	6.6	6.0 - 7.2
173	Somalia	36.4	35.9	34.4 - 37.2	6.1	5.6 - 6.5	36.9	35.3 - 38.1	7.5	7.2 - 7.9
174	Democratic Republic of the Congo	36.3	36.4	35.5 - 37.3	7.3	6.8 - 7.9	36.2	35.4 - 37.3	7.8	7.3 - 8.4
175	Central African Republic	36.0	35.6	34.6 - 36.7	8.8	8.3 - 9.3	36.5	35.3 - 37.7	10.6	10.1 - 11.1
176	United Republic of Tanzania	36.0	35.9	35.1 - 36.8	7.8	7.2 - 8.4	36.1	35.2 - 37.1	9.2	8.7 - 9.8
177	Namibia	35.6	35.8	34.3 - 37.4	9.8	9.3 - 10.4	35.4	33.8 - 37.4	12.1	11.5 - 12.6
178	Burkina Faso	35.5	35.3	34.1 - 36.6	7.9	7.3 - 8.5	35.7	34.4 - 37.0	9.1	8.5 - 9.8
179	Burundi	34.6	34.6	33.0 - 36.2	7.6	6.9 - 8.3	34.6	32.8 - 36.3	9.4	8.8 - 10.0
180	Mozambique	34.4	33.7	32.3 - 35.3	8.3	7.7 - 8.9	35.1	33.5 - 36.9	10.7	10.1 - 11.4
181	Liberia	34.0	33.8	32.7 - 34.9	7.3	6.7 - 8.0	34.2	33.1 - 35.3	8.3	7.7 - 8.9
182	Ethiopia	33.5	33.5	32.5 - 34.5	7.5	7.0 - 8.1	33.5	32.3 - 34.7	8.6	8.0 - 9.2
183	Mali	33.1	32.6	31.6 - 33.7	7.7	7.1 - 8.3	33.5	32.5 - 34.5	9.0	8.4 - 9.7
184	Zimbabwe	32.9	33.4	32.3 - 34.5	8.8	8.3 - 9.4	32.4	31.3 - 33.7	10.1	9.6 - 10.6
185	Rwanda	32.8	32.9	31.6 - 34.3	6.9	6.2 - 7.6	32.7	31.3 - 34.3	7.4	6.9 - 8.1
186	Uganda	32.7	32.9	32.1 - 33.9	6.2	5.6 - 6.9	32.5	31.6 - 33.5	7.4	6.8 - 8.0
187	Botswana	32.3	32.3	31.7 - 32.9	6.1	5.6 - 6.6	32.2	31.6 - 33.0	9.7	9.3 - 10.0
188	Zambia	30.3	30.0	28.9 - 30.9	7.6	6.9 - 8.3	30.7	29.5 - 31.7	10.7	10.1 - 11.4
189	Malawi	29.4	29.3	28.3 - 30.2	6.8	6.2 - 7.5	29.4	28.4 - 30.4	8.3	7.7 - 8.9
190	Niger	29.1	28.1	27.1 - 29.0	6.6	5.8 - 7.4	30.1	29.0 - 31.1	9.6	8.8 - 10.6
191	Sierra Leone	25.9	25.8	24.5 - 26.8	6.0	5.4 - 6.7	26.0	24.8 - 27.1	6.0	5.3 - 6.7

[a] 1999.

[b] 1997.

[c] Figures in italics are based on estimates.

Expectation of disability at birth (years)		Percentage of lifespan lived with disability				DISTRIBUTION[b]		
						Equality of child survival[c]		
Males	Females	Males	Females		Rank	Member State	Index	Uncertainty interval
8.7	9.9	18.4	19.8		161	Nepal	0.586	0.513 - 0.663
8.4	8.5	17.7	17.6		162	Myanmar	*0.579*	*0.426 - 0.733*
8.7	9.7	18.5	20.2		163	Mauritania	*0.573*	*0.415 - 0.732*
8.0	8.4	17.5	17.9		164	Lesotho	*0.570*	*0.418 - 0.724*
9.3	10.2	20.0	20.7		165	Yemen	0.558	0.492 - 0.626
7.3	7.0	16.2	15.5		166	Guinea	*0.549*	*0.392 - 0.707*
9.2	10.4	19.9	21.2		167	Eritrea	*0.544*	*0.390 - 0.702*
8.5	8.4	18.9	17.9		168	Madagascar	0.544	0.459 - 0.630
8.2	9.6	17.5	20.6		169	Djibouti	*0.543*	*0.389 - 0.698*
8.2	9.5	18.1	20.2		170	Togo	0.535	0.463 - 0.603
7.5	8.0	17.0	17.7		171	Zambia	0.535	0.448 - 0.633
8.5	10.9	19.0	22.9		172	United Republic of Tanzania	0.530	0.448 - 0.611
8.2	7.8	18.6	17.4		173	Namibia	0.529	0.430 - 0.629
8.7	10.3	19.3	22.1		174	Democratic Republic of the Congo	*0.527*	*0.374 - 0.683*
7.7	8.4	17.7	18.7		175	Chad	*0.520*	*0.368 - 0.675*
8.5	9.5	19.1	20.8		176	Ethiopia	*0.510*	*0.358 - 0.665*
7.5	7.6	17.4	17.7		177	Guinea-Bissau	*0.510*	*0.357 - 0.665*
8.8	10.0	19.9	21.9		178	Angola	*0.509*	*0.357 - 0.664*
8.6	9.2	19.9	21.1		179	Somalia	0.495	0.341 - 0.650
8.1	8.9	19.3	20.3		180	Mali	0.489	0.428 - 0.556
8.7	10.7	20.4	23.8		181	Côte d'Ivoire	0.472	0.395 - 0.549
7.9	9.5	19.1	22.1		182	Afghanistan	*0.470*	*0.317 - 0.625*
8.7	10.5	21.0	23.8		183	Pakistan	0.460	0.395 - 0.526
7.5	7.6	18.4	18.9		184	Niger	0.457	0.374 - 0.540
8.4	9.6	20.3	22.6		185	Rwanda	0.437	0.356 - 0.526
9.0	9.9	21.4	23.4		186	Sierra Leone	*0.433*	*0.278 - 0.591*
7.2	7.1	18.2	18.0		187	Malawi	0.378	0.266 - 0.492
8.0	8.3	21.1	21.3		188	Nigeria	0.336	0.262 - 0.410
8.0	9.0	21.3	23.3		189	Central African Republic	0.301	0.198 - 0.406
9.0	10.5	24.3	25.8		190	Mozambique	0.261	0.171 - 0.358
7.4	9.5	22.4	26.7		191	Liberia	0.245	0.136 - 0.364

Annex Table 6 Responsiveness of health systems, level and distribution in all Member States, WHO indexes, estimates for 1999[a]

Rank	Member State	Index	Uncertainty interval	Rank	Member State	Index	Uncertainty interval
	LEVEL				**DISTRIBUTION**		
1	United States of America	8.10	7.32 – 8.96	1	United Arab Emirates	1.000	1.000 – 1.000
2	Switzerland	7.44	6.79 – 8.13	2	Bulgaria	0.996	0.994 – 0.997
3	Luxembourg	7.37	6.73 – 8.06	3 – 38	Argentina	0.995	0.992 – 0.997
4	Denmark	7.12	6.55 – 7.73	3 – 38	Australia	0.995	0.993 – 0.997
5	Germany	7.10	6.52 – 7.72	3 – 38	Austria	0.995	0.993 – 0.997
6	Japan	7.00	6.43 – 7.61	3 – 38	Bahamas	0.995	0.992 – 0.997
7 – 8	Canada	6.98	6.44 – 7.54	3 – 38	Bahrain	0.995	0.992 – 0.997
7 – 8	Norway	6.98	6.40 – 7.60	3 – 38	Barbados	0.995	0.993 – 0.997
9	Netherlands	6.92	6.38 – 7.49	3 – 38	Belgium	0.995	0.993 – 0.997
10	Sweden	6.90	6.35 – 7.47	3 – 38	Brunei Darrusalam	0.995	0.993 – 0.997
11	Cyprus	6.88	6.76 – 7.00	3 – 38	Canada	0.995	0.993 – 0.997
12 – 13	Australia	6.86	6.34 – 7.40	3 – 38	Denmark	0.995	0.993 – 0.997
12 – 13	Austria	6.86	6.31 – 7.45	3 – 38	Finland	0.995	0.993 – 0.997
14	Monaco	6.85	6.32 – 7.44	3 – 38	France	0.995	0.993 – 0.997
15	Iceland	6.84	6.31 – 7.42	3 – 38	Germany	0.995	0.993 – 0.997
16 – 17	Belgium	6.82	6.29 – 7.39	3 – 38	Greece	0.995	0.993 – 0.997
16 – 17	France	6.82	6.27 – 7.42	3 – 38	Iceland	0.995	0.993 – 0.997
18	Bahamas	6.77	6.28 – 7.29	3 – 38	Ireland	0.995	0.993 – 0.997
19	Finland	6.76	6.26 – 7.29	3 – 38	Israel	0.995	0.993 – 0.997
20 – 21	Israel	6.70	6.22 – 7.22	3 – 38	Italy	0.995	0.993 – 0.997
20 – 21	Singapore	6.70	6.16 – 7.25	3 – 38	Japan	0.995	0.993 – 0.997
22 – 23	Italy	6.65	6.13 – 7.20	3 – 38	Kuwait	0.995	0.993 – 0.997
22 – 23	New Zealand	6.65	6.18 – 7.15	3 – 38	Luxembourg	0.995	0.993 – 0.997
24	Brunei Darussalam	6.59	6.11 – 7.07	3 – 38	Malta	0.995	0.993 – 0.997
25	Ireland	6.52	6.03 – 7.02	3 – 38	Mauritius	0.995	0.992 – 0.997
26 – 27	Qatar	6.51	6.02 – 7.00	3 – 38	Monaco	0.995	0.993 – 0.997
26 – 27	United Kingdom	6.51	6.01 – 7.05	3 – 38	Netherlands	0.995	0.993 – 0.997
28	Andorra	6.44	5.97 – 6.93	3 – 38	New Zealand	0.995	0.993 – 0.997
29	Kuwait	6.34	5.84 – 6.82	3 – 38	Norway	0.995	0.993 – 0.997
30	United Arab Emirates	6.33	6.24 – 6.41	3 – 38	Qatar	0.995	0.993 – 0.997
31	Malaysia	6.32	6.21 – 6.42	3 – 38	Saint Kitts and Nevis	0.995	0.993 – 0.997
32	San Marino	6.30	5.84 – 6.79	3 – 38	San Marino	0.995	0.993 – 0.997
33	Thailand	6.23	6.11 – 6.35	3 – 38	Singapore	0.995	0.993 – 0.997
34	Spain	6.18	5.74 – 6.63	3 – 38	Spain	0.995	0.992 – 0.997
35	Republic of Korea	6.12	5.99 – 6.24	3 – 38	Sweden	0.995	0.993 – 0.997
36	Greece	6.05	5.63 – 6.48	3 – 38	Switzerland	0.995	0.993 – 0.997
37	Slovenia	6.04	5.62 – 6.48	3 – 38	United Kingdom	0.995	0.993 – 0.997
38	Portugal	6.00	5.58 – 6.44	3 – 38	United States of America	0.995	0.993 – 0.997
39	Barbados	5.98	5.57 – 6.41	39 – 42	Andorra	0.994	0.992 – 0.996
40	Argentina	5.93	5.53 – 6.34	39 – 42	Antigua and Barbuda	0.994	0.992 – 0.996
41	Uruguay	5.87	5.47 – 6.28	39 – 42	Nauru	0.994	0.992 – 0.996
42	Nauru	5.83	5.41 – 6.25	39 – 42	Palau	0.994	0.992 – 0.996
43 – 44	Bahrain	5.82	5.38 – 6.24	43	Republic of Korea	0.992	0.990 – 0.994
43 – 44	Malta	5.82	5.42 – 6.24	44	Cyprus	0.991	0.988 – 0.994
45	Chile	5.81	5.41 – 6.21	45 – 47	Belarus	0.987	0.984 – 0.990
46	Mongolia	5.79	5.67 – 5.92	45 – 47	Czech Republic	0.987	0.984 – 0.990
47 – 48	Antigua and Barbuda	5.78	5.37 – 6.17	45 – 47	Lithuania	0.987	0.984 – 0.990
47 – 48	Czech Republic	5.78	5.38 – 6.19	48	Philippines	0.986	0.982 – 0.987
49	Philippines	5.75	5.64 – 5.87	49	Oman	0.983	0.979 – 0.987
50	Poland	5.73	5.61 – 5.85	50 – 52	Algeria	0.982	0.977 – 0.985
51	Viet Nam	5.70	5.59 – 5.81	50 – 52	Saudi Arabia	0.982	0.978 – 0.986
52	Palau	5.69	5.27 – 6.09	50 – 52	Thailand	0.982	0.973 – 0.990
53 – 54	Mexico	5.66	5.25 – 6.07	53 – 57	Jordan	0.981	0.976 – 0.985
53 – 54	Saint Kitts and Nevis	5.66	5.26 – 6.06	53 – 57	Latvia	0.981	0.977 – 0.985
55	Lebanon	5.61	5.20 – 6.01	53 – 57	Portugal	0.981	0.977 – 0.985

LEVEL				DISTRIBUTION			
Rank	Member State	Index	Uncertainty interval	Rank	Member State	Index	Uncertainty interval
56	Mauritius	5.57	5.15 – 5.96	53 – 57	Slovenia	0.981	0.977 – 0.985
57 – 58	Fiji	5.53	5.10 – 5.93	53 – 57	Uruguay	0.981	0.977 – 0.985
57 – 58	Libyan Arab Jamahiriya	5.53	5.10 – 5.93	58	Hungary	0.980	0.976 – 0.985
59	Panama	5.52	5.11 – 5.90	59	Egypt	0.979	0.968 – 0.988
60	Slovakia	5.51	5.37 – 5.66	60 – 61	Kazakhstan	0.976	0.972 – 0.981
61	Tonga	5.49	5.07 – 5.89	60 – 61	Tunisia	0.976	0.971 – 0.981
62	Hungary	5.47	5.36 – 5.59	62	Malaysia	0.975	0.965 – 0.983
63 – 64	Grenada	5.46	5.04 – 5.85	63 – 64	Slovakia	0.973	0.968 – 0.978
63 – 64	Indonesia	5.46	5.35 – 5.57	63 – 64	Ukraine	0.973	0.968 – 0.978
65	Cook Islands	5.45	5.05 – 5.85	65	Poland	0.970	0.964 – 0.976
66	Estonia	5.44	5.04 – 5.84	66	Turkey	0.969	0.964 – 0.974
67	Saudi Arabia	5.40	4.97 – 5.78	67 – 68	Morocco	0.967	0.960 – 0.973
68	Costa Rica	5.39	4.99 – 5.77	67 – 68	Romania	0.967	0.961 – 0.972
69 – 72	Latvia	5.37	4.97 – 5.77	69	Estonia	0.963	0.957 – 0.968
69 – 72	Russian Federation	5.37	4.97 – 5.76	70	Indonesia	0.961	0.948 – 0.973
69 – 72	Syrian Arab Republic	5.37	4.94 – 5.76	71	Uzbekistan	0.960	0.953 – 0.965
69 – 72	Venezuela, Bolivarian Republic of	5.37	4.98 – 5.75	72	Dominican Republic	0.959	0.952 – 0.966
73 – 74	Romania	5.35	4.96 – 5.76	73 – 74	Fiji	0.956	0.950 – 0.962
73 – 74	South Africa	5.35	5.21 – 5.49	73 – 74	Jamaica	0.956	0.950 – 0.962
75	Seychelles	5.34	4.94 – 5.73	75	Seychelles	0.955	0.948 – 0.961
76 – 79	Belarus	5.32	4.92 – 5.72	76	Libyan Arab Jamahiriya	0.953	0.947 – 0.960
76 – 79	Botswana	5.32	5.15 – 5.49	77 – 78	Dominica	0.949	0.942 – 0.955
76 – 79	Croatia	5.32	4.93 – 5.71	77 – 78	Sri Lanka	0.949	0.941 – 0.956
76 – 79	Ecuador	5.32	5.15 – 5.49	79 – 81	Lebanon	0.947	0.940 – 0.954
80 – 81	Lithuania	5.31	4.90 – 5.71	79 – 81	Suriname	0.947	0.940 – 0.953
80 – 81	Samoa	5.31	4.88 – 5.72	79 – 81	Syrian Arab Republic	0.947	0.940 – 0.954
82	Colombia	5.30	4.92 – 5.68	82	Saint Lucia	0.946	0.938 – 0.953
83	Oman	5.27	4.85 – 5.65	83	Croatia	0.945	0.939 – 0.952
84 – 86	Dominica	5.25	4.86 – 5.64	84 – 85	Brazil	0.944	0.942 – 0.968
84 – 86	Jordan	5.25	4.83 – 5.63	84 – 85	Grenada	0.944	0.937 – 0.951
84 – 86	Saint Lucia	5.25	4.84 – 5.63	86 – 87	Costa Rica	0.943	0.936 – 0.950
87	Suriname	5.23	4.82 – 5.62	86 – 87	Russian Federation	0.943	0.936 – 0.950
88 – 89	China	5.20	4.79 – 5.58	88	Panama	0.939	0.932 – 0.946
88 – 89	Turkmenistan	5.20	4.78 – 5.59	89	Cook Islands	0.938	0.929 – 0.946
90 – 91	Algeria	5.19	4.77 – 5.57	90	Belize	0.937	0.929 – 0.944
90 – 91	Kazakhstan	5.19	4.80 – 5.58	91	Mongolia	0.934	0.916 – 0.952
92	Armenia	5.18	4.77 – 5.57	92	Venezuela, Bolivarian Republic of	0.933	0.925 – 0.941
93	Turkey	5.16	4.74 – 5.53	93 – 94	Colombia	0.931	0.923 – 0.939
94	Tunisia	5.15	4.75 – 5.52	93 – 94	Iran, Islamic Republic of	0.931	0.923 – 0.939
95	Dominican Republic	5.14	4.74 – 5.51	95	The former Yugoslav Republic of Macedonia	0.926	0.915 – 0.935
96	Ukraine	5.13	4.72 – 5.52	96	Kyrgyzstan	0.925	0.915 – 0.933
97	Paraguay	5.12	4.74 – 5.50	97	Tonga	0.921	0.910 – 0.932
98 – 99	Maldives	5.11	4.69 – 5.49	98 – 100	Cuba	0.920	0.909 – 0.930
98 – 99	Marshall Islands	5.11	4.70 – 5.52	98 – 100	Saint Vincent and the Grenadines	0.920	0.911 – 0.929
100	Iran, Islamic Republic of	5.10	4.71 – 5.48	98 – 100	Samoa	0.920	0.908 – 0.930
101	Sri Lanka	5.08	4.69 – 5.47	101 – 102	Gabon	0.919	0.909 – 0.928
102	Egypt	5.06	4.94 – 5.17	101 – 102	Maldives	0.919	0.909 – 0.928
103 – 104	Iraq	5.05	4.63 – 5.43	103	Chile	0.918	0.902 – 0.933
103 – 104	Saint Vincent and the Grenadines	5.05	4.66 – 5.43	104	Senegal	0.914	0.889 – 0.928
105 – 107	Belize	5.03	4.63 – 5.40	105 – 106	China	0.911	0.899 – 0.922
105 – 107	Jamaica	5.03	4.65 – 5.41	105 – 106	Guyana	0.911	0.900 – 0.921
105 – 107	Uzbekistan	5.03	4.62 – 5.42	107	Republic of Moldova	0.910	0.899 – 0.919
108 – 110	Bosnia and Herzegovina	5.02	4.64 – 5.40	108 – 109	Mexico	0.909	0.888 – 0.924
108 – 110	India	5.02	4.61 – 5.41	108 – 109	Trinidad and Tobago	0.909	0.894 – 0.925
108 – 110	Swaziland	5.02	4.61 – 5.40	110	Swaziland	0.908	0.897 – 0.918

Annex Table 6 Responsiveness of health systems, level and distribution in all Member States, WHO indexes, estimates for 1999[a]

	LEVEL				DISTRIBUTION		
Rank	Member State	Index	Uncertainty interval	Rank	Member State	Index	Uncertainty interval
111	The former Yugoslav Republic of Macedonia	5.01	4.62 – 5.40	111 – 112	Armenia	0.905	0.891 – 0.917
112	Micronesia, Federated States of	5.00	4.60 – 5.38	111 – 112	Botswana	0.905	0.877 – 0.932
113	Namibia	4.99	4.62 – 5.37	113	Turkmenistan	0.899	0.886 – 0.912
114	Guyana	4.98	4.58 – 5.36	114	Iraq	0.898	0.883 – 0.912
115 – 117	Cuba	4.97	4.57 – 5.36	115	Pakistan	0.897	0.883 – 0.909
115 – 117	Guatemala	4.97	4.81 – 5.12	116	Yugoslavia	0.895	0.882 – 0.907
115 – 117	Yugoslavia	4.97	4.59 – 5.36	117	Albania	0.894	0.878 – 0.910
118 – 119	Gabon	4.96	4.57 – 5.32	118	Equatorial Guinea	0.892	0.877 – 0.906
118 – 119	Senegal	4.96	4.83 – 5.09	119	Papua New Guinea	0.891	0.875 – 0.906
120 – 121	Kiribati	4.95	4.54 – 5.35	120	Solomon Islands	0.890	0.875 – 0.903
120 – 121	Pakistan	4.95	4.54 – 5.32	121	Viet Nam	0.884	0.870 – 0.900
122	Zimbabwe	4.94	4.82 – 5.05	122	Kiribati	0.883	0.864 – 0.901
123	Republic of Moldova	4.92	4.54 – 5.30	123	Mauritania	0.882	0.840 – 0.919
124	Kyrgyzstan	4.91	4.51 – 5.29	124	Bosnia and Herzegovina	0.881	0.866 – 0.895
125	Tajikistan	4.90	4.49 – 5.29	125	Azerbaijan	0.878	0.863 – 0.893
126	Niue	4.87	4.48 – 5.25	126	Sao Tome and Principe	0.877	0.857 – 0.895
127	Vanuatu	4.85	4.46 – 5.22	127	India	0.876	0.856 – 0.895
128	El Salvador	4.84	4.47 – 5.22	128 – 129	El Salvador	0.874	0.854 – 0.892
129	Honduras	4.82	4.45 – 5.19	128 – 129	Micronesia, Federated States of	0.874	0.858 – 0.889
130 – 131	Azerbaijan	4.81	4.43 – 5.19	130 – 131	Democratic Peoples' Republic of Korea	0.873	0.852 – 0.892
130 – 131	Brazil	4.81	4.68 – 4.94	130 – 131	Guinea	0.873	0.842 – 0.902
132 – 135	Ghana	4.80	4.69 – 4.92	132	Vanuatu	0.872	0.854 – 0.887
132 – 135	Solomon Islands	4.80	4.40 – 5.18	133	Paraguay	0.871	0.848 – 0.892
132 – 135	Tuvalu	4.80	4.40 – 5.18	134 – 135	Cape Verde	0.866	0.847 – 0.882
132 – 135	Zambia	4.80	4.40 – 5.18	134 – 135	Marshall Islands	0.866	0.848 – 0.882
136	Albania	4.79	4.39 – 5.17	136	Tajikistan	0.864	0.845 – 0.881
137 – 138	Cambodia	4.77	4.37 – 5.15	137 – 138	Bhutan	0.861	0.840 – 0.881
137 – 138	Congo	4.77	4.39 – 5.15	137 – 138	Cambodia	0.861	0.836 – 0.884
139	Democratic People's Republic of Korea	4.76	4.36 – 5.14	139	Nicaragua	0.860	0.840 – 0.878
140	Nicaragua	4.75	4.36 – 5.11	140	Djibouti	0.858	0.834 – 0.880
141	Trinidad and Tobago	4.73	4.60 – 4.86	141	Georgia	0.855	0.835 – 0.874
142	Democratic Republic of the Congo	4.72	4.34 – 5.10	142	Kenya	0.852	0.830 – 0.871
143	Equatorial Guinea	4.71	4.33 – 5.07	143 – 144	Lao People's Democratic Republic	0.850	0.778 – 0.912
144	Kenya	4.67	4.28 – 5.05	143 – 144	Rwanda	0.850	0.824 – 0.875
145 – 147	Lao People's Democratic Republic	4.62	4.23 – 5.00	145	Niue	0.848	0.824 – 0.871
145 – 147	Lesotho	4.62	4.23 – 4.99	146	Ghana	0.847	0.811 – 0.882
145 – 147	Rwanda	4.62	4.22 – 5.01	147	South Africa	0.844	0.811 – 0.869
148	Sao Tome and Principe	4.61	4.21 – 4.99	148 – 149	Lesotho	0.842	0.818 – 0.863
149	Nigeria	4.60	4.22 – 4.98	148 – 149	Sudan	0.842	0.818 – 0.863
150	Papua New Guinea	4.59	4.18 – 4.96	150	United Republic of Tanzania	0.836	0.808 – 0.862
151 – 153	Bolivia	4.58	4.46 – 4.70	151	Congo	0.834	0.780 – 0.881
151 – 153	Morocco	4.58	4.20 – 4.94	152	Malawi	0.831	0.804 – 0.855
151 – 153	Myanmar	4.58	4.21 – 4.95	153 – 155	Comoros	0.830	0.801 – 0.856
154	Cape Verde	4.56	4.17 – 4.92	153 – 155	Côte d'Ivoire	0.830	0.804 – 0.857
155	Togo	4.54	4.16 – 4.91	153 – 155	Tuvalu	0.830	0.804 – 0.856
156	Cameroon	4.50	4.13 – 4.87	156	Namibia	0.828	0.802 – 0.854
157 – 160	Comoros	4.46	4.06 – 4.83	157	Gambia	0.825	0.797 – 0.850
157 – 160	Côte d'Ivoire	4.46	4.08 – 4.83	158	Myanmar	0.822	0.785 – 0.856
157 – 160	Haiti	4.46	4.10 – 4.84	159	Guatemala	0.812	0.787 – 0.837
157 – 160	United Republic of Tanzania	4.46	4.06 – 4.84	160	Benin	0.811	0.776 – 0.843
161	Bulgaria	4.43	4.30 – 4.57	161	Peru	0.808	0.793 – 0.850
162	Malawi	4.42	4.03 – 4.80	162	Togo	0.803	0.771 – 0.835
163	Bhutan	4.35	3.96 – 4.72	163	Honduras	0.800	0.757 – 0.841
164	Sudan	4.34	3.96 – 4.71	164	Burkina Faso	0.799	0.751 – 0.847
165 – 167	Gambia	4.33	3.95 – 4.70	165	Uganda	0.796	0.751 – 0.818

LEVEL				DISTRIBUTION			
Rank	Member State	Index	Uncertainty interval	Rank	Member State	Index	Uncertainty interval
165 – 167	Georgia	4.33	4.18 – 4.48	166 – 167	Nepal	0.792	0.757 – 0.825
165 – 167	Mauritania	*4.33*	*3.97 – 4.69*	166 – 167	Zimbabwe	0.792	0.747 – 0.814
168 – 169	Guinea	*4.29*	*3.92 – 4.64*	168	Burundi	*0.790*	*0.750 – 0.825*
168 – 169	Madagascar	*4.29*	*3.92 – 4.65*	169 – 170	Democratic Republic of the Congo	*0.783*	*0.743 – 0.817*
170	Djibouti	*4.28*	*3.87 – 4.66*	169 – 170	Eritrea	*0.783*	*0.743 – 0.822*
171	Burundi	*4.25*	*3.86 – 4.64*	171	Zambia	*0.781*	*0.739 – 0.816*
172	Peru	4.24	4.12 – 4.36	172 – 173	Afghanistan	*0.776*	*0.729 – 0.819*
173	Sierra Leone	*4.23*	*3.86 – 4.61*	172 – 173	Haiti	*0.776*	*0.726 – 0.823*
174	Burkina Faso	4.18	4.06 – 4.31	174	Guinea-Bissau	*0.762*	*0.703 – 0.818*
175 – 176	Benin	*4.14*	*3.75 – 4.50*	175	Mozambique	*0.758*	*0.703 – 0.810*
175 – 176	Liberia	*4.14*	*3.77 – 4.50*	176	Liberia	*0.753*	*0.680 – 0.822*
177	Angola	*4.10*	*3.74 – 4.46*	177	Nigeria	*0.746*	*0.696 – 0.792*
178	Bangladesh	4.07	3.94 – 4.20	178	Bolivia	0.745	0.723 – 0.768
179	Ethiopia	*4.00*	*3.62 – 4.38*	179 – 180	Ethiopia	*0.733*	*0.665 – 0.797*
180	Yemen	*3.98*	*3.61 – 4.35*	179 – 180	Madagascar	*0.733*	*0.665 – 0.798*
181 – 182	Afghanistan	*3.96*	*3.57 – 4.33*	181	Bangladesh	0.728	0.699 – 0.756
181 – 182	Chad	*3.96*	*3.59 – 4.31*	182	Ecuador	0.723	0.709 – 0.821
183	Central African Republic	*3.94*	*3.57 – 4.30*	183	Cameroon	*0.710*	*0.564 – 0.827*
184	Guinea-Bissau	*3.89*	*3.52 – 4.26*	184	Niger	*0.690*	*0.591 – 0.781*
185	Nepal	3.83	3.69 – 3.98	185	Chad	*0.688*	*0.573 – 0.792*
186	Eritrea	*3.75*	*3.36 – 4.13*	186	Sierra Leone	*0.686*	*0.595 – 0.771*
187 – 188	Mali	*3.74*	*3.36 – 4.13*	187	Mali	*0.685*	*0.601 – 0.763*
187 – 188	Uganda	3.74	3.61 – 3.87	188	Angola	*0.683*	*0.549 – 0.797*
189 – 190	Mozambique	*3.73*	*3.34 – 4.12*	189	Yemen	*0.673*	*0.489 – 0.820*
189 – 190	Niger	*3.73*	*3.35 – 4.12*	190	Somalia	*0.621*	*0.440 – 0.772*
191	Somalia	*3.69*	*3.31 – 4.07*	191	Central African Republic	*0.414*	*0.006 – 0.733*

ª Figures in italics are based on estimates.

Annex Table 7 Fairness of financial contribution to health systems in all Member States, WHO index, estimates for 1997[a]

Rank	Member State	Index	Uncertainty interval
1	Colombia	0.992	0.990 – 0.994
2	Luxembourg	0.981	0.967 – 0.992
3 – 5	Belgium	0.979	0.964 – 0.991
3 – 5	Djibouti	0.979	0.965 – 0.990
3 – 5	Denmark	0.979	0.964 – 0.991
6 – 7	Ireland	0.978	0.965 – 0.989
6 – 7	Germany	0.978	0.964 – 0.989
8 – 11	Norway	0.977	0.962 – 0.990
8 – 11	Japan	0.977	0.961 – 0.990
8 – 11	Finland	0.977	0.961 – 0.990
8 – 11	United Kingdom	0.977	0.963 – 0.988
12 – 15	Austria	0.976	0.959 – 0.991
12 – 15	Libyan Arab Jamahiriya	0.976	0.961 – 0.988
12 – 15	Sweden	0.976	0.959 – 0.990
12 – 15	Iceland	0.976	0.961 – 0.988
16	Kiribati	0.975	0.959 – 0.987
17 – 19	Solomon Islands	0.974	0.959 – 0.987
17 – 19	Nauru	0.974	0.958 – 0.987
17 – 19	Canada	0.974	0.959 – 0.986
20 – 22	Marshall Islands	0.973	0.957 – 0.986
20 – 22	Netherlands	0.973	0.959 – 0.985
20 – 22	United Arab Emirates	0.973	0.958 – 0.985
23 – 25	New Zealand	0.972	0.956 – 0.985
23 – 25	Cuba	0.972	0.957 – 0.984
23 – 25	Micronesia, Federated States of	0.972	0.956 – 0.985
26 – 29	Spain	0.971	0.956 – 0.984
26 – 29	France	0.971	0.956 – 0.983
26 – 29	Tuvalu	0.971	0.954 – 0.984
26 – 29	Australia	0.971	0.956 – 0.983
30 – 32	San Marino	0.970	0.953 – 0.984
30 – 32	Kuwait	0.970	0.955 – 0.982
30 – 32	Palau	0.970	0.954 – 0.983
33 – 34	Andorra	0.969	0.952 – 0.984
33 – 34	Samoa	0.969	0.953 – 0.982
35 – 36	Niue	0.968	0.952 – 0.982
35 – 36	Uruguay	0.968	0.950 – 0.983
37	Saudi Arabia	0.965	0.950 – 0.978
38 – 40	Switzerland	0.964	0.948 – 0.979
38 – 40	Israel	0.964	0.949 – 0.978
38 – 40	Mozambique	0.964	0.948 – 0.977
41	Greece	0.963	0.946 – 0.978
42 – 44	Monaco	0.962	0.941 – 0.980
42 – 44	India	0.962	0.949 – 0.966
42 – 44	Malta	0.962	0.940 – 0.980
45 – 47	Guyana	0.961	0.952 – 0.968
45 – 47	Cook Islands	0.961	0.945 – 0.975
45 – 47	Italy	0.961	0.935 – 0.981
48	United Republic of Tanzania	0.959	0.956 – 0.968
49 – 50	Turkey	0.958	0.941 – 0.973
49 – 50	Jordan	0.958	0.942 – 0.973
51 – 52	Bangladesh	0.956	0.955 – 0.961
51 – 52	Maldives	0.956	0.939 – 0.972
53	Republic of Korea	0.955	0.931 – 0.974

Rank	Member State	Index	Uncertainty interval
54 – 55	United States of America	0.954	0.929 – 0.974
54 – 55	Fiji	0.954	0.938 – 0.969
56 – 57	Iraq	0.952	0.932 – 0.970
56 – 57	Oman	0.952	0.935 – 0.967
58 – 60	Chad	0.951	0.927 – 0.972
58 – 60	Rwanda	0.951	0.920 – 0.975
58 – 60	Portugal	0.951	0.932 – 0.968
61	Bahrain	0.950	0.933 – 0.966
62 – 63	Vanuatu	0.949	0.932 – 0.965
62 – 63	Pakistan	0.949	0.941 – 0.967
64 – 65	Seychelles	0.948	0.923 – 0.969
64 – 65	Costa Rica	0.948	0.921 – 0.970
66 – 67	Saint Lucia	0.947	0.929 – 0.965
66 – 67	Sao Tome and Principe	0.947	0.922 – 0.968
68	Bolivia	0.946	0.928 – 0.964
69	Trinidad and Tobago	0.945	0.926 – 0.962
70	Qatar	0.944	0.924 – 0.962
71 – 72	Czech Republic	0.943	0.894 – 0.981
71 – 72	Papua New Guinea	0.943	0.906 – 0.971
73	Indonesia	0.942	0.918 – 0.963
74 – 75	Algeria	0.941	0.916 – 0.963
74 – 75	Ghana	0.941	0.910 – 0.966
76 – 78	Guinea	0.940	0.919 – 0.958
76 – 78	Sri Lanka	0.940	0.910 – 0.964
76 – 78	Panama	0.940	0.908 – 0.966
79 – 81	Comoros	0.939	0.913 – 0.962
79 – 81	Romania	0.939	0.912 – 0.961
79 – 81	Kenya	0.939	0.917 – 0.959
82 – 83	Slovenia	0.938	0.887 – 0.977
82 – 83	Bosnia and Herzegovina	0.938	0.890 – 0.976
84 – 86	Liberia	0.937	0.911 – 0.960
84 – 86	Gabon	0.937	0.911 – 0.960
84 – 86	Belarus	0.937	0.878 – 0.980
87	Senegal	0.936	0.914 – 0.954
88	Ecuador	0.935	0.912 – 0.955
89 – 95	Bhutan	0.934	0.904 – 0.960
89 – 95	Botswana	0.934	0.909 – 0.957
89 – 95	Brunei Darussalam	0.934	0.890 – 0.968
89 – 95	Malawi	0.934	0.909 – 0.957
89 – 95	Argentina	0.934	0.899 – 0.963
89 – 95	Lesotho	0.934	0.882 – 0.975
89 – 95	Cape Verde	0.934	0.908 – 0.957
96	Slovakia	0.933	0.864 – 0.981
97	Mongolia	0.932	0.881 – 0.972
98	Venezuela, Bolivarian Republic of	0.931	0.898 – 0.960
99 – 100	Dominica	0.930	0.895 – 0.960
99 – 100	Saint Vincent and the Grenadines	0.930	0.895 – 0.960
101 – 102	Singapore	0.929	0.880 – 0.967
101 – 102	Lebanon	0.929	0.899 – 0.954
103 – 104	Angola	0.928	0.900 – 0.953
103 – 104	Afghanistan	0.928	0.890 – 0.958
105 – 106	Hungary	0.927	0.875 – 0.970

Annex Table 7 Fairness of financial contribution to health systems in all Member States, WHO index, estimates for 1997[a]

Rank	Member State	Index	Uncertainty interval
105 – 106	Georgia	0.927	0.876 – 0.969
107	Barbados	0.926	0.890 – 0.957
108 – 111	Croatia	0.925	0.869 – 0.970
108 – 111	Tunisia	0.925	0.896 – 0.949
108 – 111	Eritrea	0.925	0.896 – 0.951
108 – 111	Tonga	0.925	0.896 – 0.950
112 – 113	Tajikistan	0.923	0.871 – 0.966
112 – 113	Iran, Islamic Republic of	0.923	0.890 – 0.951
114	Burundi	0.922	0.876 – 0.958
115	Jamaica	0.921	0.861 – 0.923
116 – 120	Madagascar	0.919	0.889 – 0.946
116 – 120	Azerbaijan	0.919	0.863 – 0.964
116 – 120	Côte d'Ivoire	0.919	0.879 – 0.952
116 – 120	Antigua and Barbuda	0.919	0.882 – 0.952
116 – 120	The former Yugoslav Republic of Macedonia	0.919	0.867 – 0.963
121	Turkmenistan	0.918	0.859 – 0.966
122 – 123	Guinea-Bissau	0.917	0.854 – 0.966
122 – 123	Malaysia	0.917	0.881 – 0.948
124	Mauritius	0.916	0.885 – 0.945
125 – 127	Namibia	0.915	0.884 – 0.944
125 – 127	Egypt	0.915	0.848 – 0.966
125 – 127	Morocco	0.915	0.878 – 0.945
128 – 130	Thailand	0.913	0.913 – 0.926
128 – 130	Philippines	0.913	0.880 – 0.943
128 – 130	Uganda	0.913	0.875 – 0.946
131 – 133	Lithuania	0.912	0.857 – 0.958
131 – 133	Cyprus	0.912	0.870 – 0.946
131 – 133	Uzbekistan	0.912	0.858 – 0.957
134	Equatorial Guinea	0.911	0.877 – 0.942
135	Yemen	0.910	0.870 – 0.944
136 – 137	Somalia	0.909	0.855 – 0.952
136 – 137	Saint Kitts and Nevis	0.909	0.867 – 0.945
138 – 139	Bahamas	0.906	0.863 – 0.944
138 – 139	Ethiopia	0.906	0.863 – 0.942
140 – 141	Benin	0.905	0.868 – 0.938
140 – 141	Ukraine	0.905	0.849 – 0.952
142 – 143	Syrian Arab Republic	0.904	0.856 – 0.944
142 – 143	South Africa	0.904	0.822 – 0.967
144	Mexico	0.903	0.880 – 0.905
145	Estonia	0.902	0.846 – 0.949
146	Belize	0.901	0.856 – 0.941
147	Grenada	0.900	0.853 – 0.940
148	Republic of Moldova	0.898	0.841 – 0.946
149	Gambia	0.897	0.854 – 0.935
150 – 151	Mali	0.896	0.846 – 0.940
150 – 151	Poland	0.896	0.838 – 0.946
152	Togo	0.895	0.853 – 0.933
153	Mauritania	0.893	0.840 – 0.938
154	Dominican Republic	0.892	0.842 – 0.934
155	Zambia	0.891	0.881 – 0.917
156	Swaziland	0.890	0.797 – 0.962
157	Guatemala	0.889	0.797 – 0.959
158	Yugoslavia	0.886	0.827 – 0.939

Rank	Member State	Index	Uncertainty interval
159	Lao People's Democratic Republic	*0.885*	*0.814 – 0.943*
160 – 161	Sudan	*0.883*	*0.802 – 0.946*
160 – 161	Niger	*0.883*	*0.822 – 0.933*
162	Congo	*0.881*	*0.827 – 0.926*
163	Haiti	*0.875*	*0.814 – 0.925*
164 – 165	Nicaragua	0.874	0.812 – 0.894
164 – 165	Latvia	*0.874*	*0.805 – 0.931*
166	Central African Republic	*0.872*	*0.761 – 0.958*
167	Kazakhstan	0.867	*0.803 – 0.921*
168	Chile	*0.864*	*0.771 – 0.937*
169	Democratic Republic of the Congo	*0.857*	*0.786 – 0.918*
170	Bulgaria	0.856	0.839 – 0.873
171	Kyrgyzstan	0.854	0.853 – 0.894
172	Suriname	*0.853*	*0.774 – 0.917*
173 – 174	Albania	*0.851*	*0.765 – 0.921*
173 – 174	Burkina Faso	*0.851*	*0.775 – 0.915*
175	Zimbabwe	*0.850*	*0.746 – 0.932*
176	El Salvador	*0.846*	*0.755 – 0.918*
177	Paraguay	0.842	0.827 – 0.848
178	Honduras	*0.834*	*0.728 – 0.917*
179	Democratic People's Republic of Korea	*0.829*	*0.752 – 0.893*
180	Nigeria	*0.827*	*0.726 – 0.907*
181	Armenia	*0.822*	*0.707 – 0.913*
182	Cameroon	*0.821*	*0.719 – 0.907*
183	Cambodia	*0.814*	*0.676 – 0.916*
184	Peru	0.805	0.792 – 0.820
185	Russian Federation	0.802	0.776 – 0.836
186	Nepal	0.714	0.696 – 0.732
187	Viet Nam	0.643	0.632 – 0.672
188	China	*0.638*	*0.472 – 0.774*
189	Brazil	0.623	0.620 – 0.683
190	Myanmar	*0.582*	*0.306 – 0.793*
191	Sierra Leone	*0.468*	*0.000 – 0.853*

[a] Figures in italics are based on estimates.

Annex Table 8 Selected national health accounts indicators for all Member States, estimates for 1997[a]

Member State	HEALTH EXPENDITURE (%)							PER CAPITA HEALTH EXPENDITURE (US$)				
	Total expenditure on health as % of GDP	Public expenditure as % of total expenditure on health	Private expenditure as % of total health expenditure	Out-of-pocket expenditure as % of total expenditure on health	Tax-funded and other public expenditure as % of public expenditure on health	Social security expenditure as % of public expenditure on health	Public expenditure on health as % of total public expenditure	Total expenditure at official exchange rate	Out-of-pocket expenditure at official exchange rate	Total expenditure in international dollars	Public expenditure in international dollars	Out-of-pocket expenditure in international dollars[b]
Afghanistan	3.2	40.6	59.4	59.4	100	...	...	2	1	28	11	17
Albania	3.5	77.7	22.3	22.3	82.5	17.5	9.5	26	6	63	49	14
Algeria	3.1	50.8	49.2	49.2	100	...	4.9	44	22	122	62	60
Andorra	7.5	86.7	13.3	13.3	100	...	38.5	1 368	182	1 216	1 055	162
Angola	3.6	59.6	40.4	40.4	100	...	18.2	...	...	47	28	19
Antigua and Barbuda	6.4	57.3	42.7	39.3	100	...	16.0	775	305	598	343	235
Argentina	8.2	57.5	42.5	32.6	39.6	60.4	21.6	676	220	823	473	268
Armenia	7.9	41.5	58.5	58.5	100	...	13.1	36	21	152	63	89
Australia	7.8	72.0	28.0	16.6	100	...	15.5	1 730	287	1 601	1 153	266
Austria	9.0	67.3	32.7	23.6	12.4	87.6	11.9	2 277	536	1 960	1 320	462
Azerbaijan	2.9	79.3	20.7	20.7	100	...	13.3	20	4	48	38	10
Bahamas	5.9	49.9	50.1	46.4	100	...	13.7	785	364	1 230	614	571
Bahrain	4.4	58.5	41.5	37.7	100	...	9.6	478	180	539	315	204
Bangladesh	4.9	46.0	54.0	54.0	100	...	9.1	13	7	70	32	38
Barbados	7.3	62.5	37.5	34.6	100	...	13.7	596	206	814	509	281
Belarus	5.9	82.6	17.4	17.4	100	...	10.0	78	14	253	209	44
Belgium	8.0	83.2	16.8	14.7	18.7	81.3	13.2	1 918	282	1 738	1 446	255
Belize	4.7	51.6	48.4	48.3	100	...	8.2	176	85	212	109	103
Benin	3.0	47.2	52.8	52.8	100	...	5.7	12	6	39	18	21
Bhutan	7.0	46.2	53.8	53.8	100	...	10.1	14	8	82	38	44
Bolivia	5.8	59.1	41.0	33.8	42.7	57.3	10.4	59	20	153	90	52
Bosnia and Herzegovina	7.6	92.6	7.5	7.5	100	...	...	77	6	145	135	11
Botswana	4.2	61.0	39.0	36.4	100	...	5.9	132	48	219	133	80
Brazil	6.5	48.7	51.3	45.6	100	...	9.4	319	145	428	208	195
Brunei Darussalam	5.4	40.6	59.4	59.4	100	...	4.5	...	...	857	348	509
Bulgaria	4.8	81.9	18.1	16.9	99.9	0.1	10.0	59	10	193	158	33
Burkina Faso	4.2	30.9	69.1	69.1	100	...	5.3	8	6	37	12	26
Burundi	4.0	35.6	64.4	64.4	19.2	80.8	6.6	6	4	26	9	17
Cambodia	7.2	9.4	90.6	90.6	100	...	7.0	21	19	73	7	66
Cameroon	5.0	20.1	79.9	79.9	100	...	0.7	31	24	86	17	69
Canada	8.6	72.0	28.0	17.0	98.9	1.1	15.3	1 783	304	1 836	1 322	313
Cape Verde	2.8	63.8	36.2	36.2	100	...	4.2	34	12	60	38	22
Central African Republic	2.9	68.9	31.1	31.1	100	...	6.4	8	3	34	23	10
Chad	4.3	79.3	20.7	20.7	100	...	13.2	7	1	35	28	7
Chile	6.1	49.0	51.0	48.6	24.0	76.0	13.5	315	153	581	285	282
China	2.7	24.9	75.1	75.1	100	...	5.5	20	15	74	18	55
Colombia	9.3	54.5	45.6	25.9	62.5	37.5	17.2	247	64	507	276	131
Comoros	4.5	68.2	31.8	31.8	100	...	8.7	14	4	47	32	15
Congo	5.0	36.6	63.4	63.4	100	...	4.6	58	37	101	37	64
Cook Islands	7.4	76.7	23.3	23.3	100	...	8.6	389	91	345	264	80
Costa Rica	8.7	77.1	23.0	22.3	16.2	83.8	20.1	226	50	489	377	109
Côte d'Ivoire	3.2	38.4	61.6	61.6	100	...	3.3	23	14	57	22	35
Croatia	8.1	79.7	20.3	20.3	2.4	97.6	22.3	352	71	410	327	83
Cuba	6.3	87.5	12.5	12.5	100	...	10.0	131	16	109	96	14
Cyprus	5.9	38.8	61.2	63.1	7.9	92.1	5.6	648	408	731	256	461
Czech Republic	7.6	92.3	7.7	7.7	17.6	82.4	15.9	391	30	640	591	50
Democratic People's Republic of Korea	3.0	83.7	16.4	16.4	100	...	...	37	6	39	33	6
Democratic Republic of the Congo	3.7	0.9	99.1	90.1	100	...	0.1	...	...	22	1	20
Denmark	8.0	84.3	15.7	15.7	100	...	12.9	2 574	403	1 940	1 636	304
Djibouti	2.8	72.9	27.1	27.1	100	...	5.7	23	6	48	35	13
Dominica	6.0	65.0	35.0	31.9	100	...	10.3	282	90	286	186	91
Dominican Republic	4.9	38.5	61.5	36.8	73.0	27.0	10.5	91	33	202	78	74
Ecuador	4.6	52.8	47.2	38.8	59.4	40.6	8.9	75	29	186	98	72
Egypt	3.7	27.0	73.1	73.1	100	...	3.3	44	32	118	32	86
El Salvador	7.0	37.2	62.8	62.8	48.5	51.5	21.2	182	114	228	85	143

Member State	HEALTH EXPENDITURE (%)							PER CAPITA HEALTH EXPENDITURE (US$)				
	Total expenditure on health as % of GDP	Public expenditure as % of total expenditure on health	Private expenditure as % of total health expenditure	Out-of-pocket expenditure as % of total expenditure on health	Tax-funded and other public expenditure as % of public expenditure on health	Social security expenditure as % of public expenditure on health	Public expenditure on health as % of total public expenditure	Total expenditure at official exchange rate	Out-of-pocket expenditure at official exchange rate	Total expenditure in international dollars	Public expenditure in international dollars	Out-of-pocket expenditure in international dollars[b]
Equatorial Guinea	3.5	57.2	42.9	42.9	100	...	7.9	40	17	89	51	38
Eritrea	3.4	55.7	44.3	44.3	100	...	3.4	6	3	24	13	11
Estonia	6.4	78.9	21.2	21.2	8.4	91.6	10.5	204	43	346	273	73
Ethiopia	3.8	36.2	63.8	63.8	100	...	6.1	4	3	20	7	13
Fiji	4.2	69.2	30.8	30.8	100	...	8.3	115	35	214	148	66
Finland	7.6	73.7	26.3	19.3	80.4	19.6	10.7	1 789	345	1 539	1 134	297
France	9.8	76.9	23.1	20.4	3.3	96.7	13.8	2 369	482	2 125	1 634	433
Gabon	3.0	66.5	33.5	33.5	100	...	6.2	138	46	196	130	66
Gambia	4.5	45.9	54.1	54.1	100	...	7.3	12	6	52	24	28
Georgia	4.4	8.6	91.4	91.4	100	...	3.4	45	41	94	8	86
Germany	10.5	77.5	22.5	11.3	23.4	76.6	14.7	2 713	306	2 365	1 832	267
Ghana	3.1	47.0	53.0	53.0	100	...	6.9	11	6	45	21	24
Greece	8.0	65.8	34.2	31.7	64.8	35.2	12.6	905	287	964	634	306
Grenada	6.3	46.6	53.4	49.2	100	...	10.2	305	150	298	139	147
Guatemala	2.4	62.5	37.5	29.9	53.7	46.3	12.2	41	12	87	55	26
Guinea	3.5	57.2	42.8	42.8	100	...	9.7	19	8	52	30	22
Guinea-Bissau	5.7	75.6	24.4	24.4	100	...	38.8	13	3	54	41	13
Guyana	5.1	79.1	21.0	19.7	100	...	11.1	45	9	130	103	26
Haiti	4.6	33.6	66.4	62.5	100	...	13.8	18	11	55	18	34
Honduras	7.5	36.0	64.0	60.1	74.6	25.5	13.0	59	35	156	56	94
Hungary	5.3	84.9	15.1	15.1	58.9	41.1	9.2	236	36	372	316	56
Iceland	7.9	83.8	16.2	16.2	68.8	31.2	18.9	2 149	347	1 757	1 473	284
India	5.2	13.0	87.0	84.6	100	...	3.9	23	19	84	11	71
Indonesia	1.7	36.8	63.2	47.4	100	...	3.0	18	8	56	21	26
Iran, Islamic Republic of	4.4	42.8	57.2	57.2	83.0	17.1	7.2	108	62	200	86	114
Iraq	4.2	58.9	41.1	41.1	100	...	...	251	103	110	65	45
Ireland	6.2	77.3	22.7	...	100	...	17.1	1 326	...	1 200	928	...
Israel	8.2	75.0	25.0	19.1	66.3	33.7	12.8	1 385	264	1 402	1 051	267
Italy	9.3	57.1	42.9	41.8	100	...	10.5	1 855	774	1 824	1 042	762
Jamaica	6.0	56.5	43.5	23.3	100	...	8.9	149	35	212	120	49
Japan	7.1	80.2	19.9	19.9	15.3	84.7	16.2	2 373	471	1 759	1 410	349
Jordan	5.2	67.2	32.8	32.8	100	...	8.5	59	19	178	119	58
Kazakhstan	3.9	63.6	36.4	36.4	57.6	42.4	10.3	62	22	127	81	46
Kenya	4.6	64.1	35.9	35.9	100	...	11.2	17	6	58	37	21
Kiribati	9.9	99.3	0.7	0.7	100	...	14.0	122	1	152	151	1
Kuwait	3.3	87.4	12.6	12.6	100	...	8.4	572	72	605	529	76
Kyrgyzstan	4.0	69.6	30.4	30.4	95.3	4.7	9.7	15	5	66	46	20
Lao People's Democratic Republic	3.6	62.7	37.3	37.3	100	...	8.6	13	5	53	33	20
Latvia	6.1	61.0	39.0	39.0	48.3	51.7	9.0	140	54	246	150	96
Lebanon	10.1	29.6	70.4	53.8	100	...	7.8	461	248	563	167	303
Lesotho	5.6	72.6	27.4	27.4	100	...	12.4	28	8	100	73	27
Liberia	3.0	66.7	33.3	33.3	100	...	6.7	31	10	33	22	11
Libyan Arab Jamahiriya	3.4	54.2	45.8	45.8	100	...	2.7	296	136	221	120	102
Lithuania	6.4	75.7	24.3	24.3	18.7	81.3	11.4	167	40	273	207	66
Luxembourg	6.6	91.4	8.6	7.2	17.1	83.0	13.0	2 580	185	1 985	1 815	142
Madagascar	2.1	53.8	46.2	46.2	100	...	6.6	5	2	18	10	8
Malawi	5.8	59.2	40.8	36.7	100	...	13.3	15	5	49	29	18
Malaysia	2.4	57.6	42.4	42.4	100	...	5.1	110	46	202	116	85
Maldives	8.2	63.9	36.1	36.1	100	...	11.0	107	39	248	159	90
Mali	4.2	45.8	54.2	48.7	100	...	7.9	10	5	34	15	16
Malta	6.3	58.9	41.1	38.0	1.5	98.5	8.9	551	209	755	445	287
Marshall Islands	9.0	74.3	25.7	25.7	100	...	13.1	253	65	238	177	61
Mauritania	5.6	30.3	69.7	69.7	100	...	6.6	24	17	73	22	51
Mauritius	3.5	52.9	47.1	47.1	100	...	7.7	129	61	288	152	136
Mexico	5.6	41.0	59.1	52.9	26.4	73.6	6.0	240	127	421	172	222

Annex Table 8 Selected national health accounts indicators for all Member States, estimates for 1997[a]

Member State	HEALTH EXPENDITURE (%)							PER CAPITA HEALTH EXPENDITURE (US$)				
	Total expenditure on health as % of GDP	Public expenditure as % of total expenditure on health	Private expenditure as % of total health expenditure	Out-of-pocket expenditure as % of total expenditure on health	Tax-funded and other public expenditure as % of public expenditure on health	Social security expenditure as % of public expenditure on health	Public expenditure on health as % of total public expenditure	Total expenditure at official exchange rate	Out-of-pocket expenditure at official exchange rate	Total expenditure in international dollars	Public expenditure in international dollars	Out-of-pocket expenditure in international dollars[b]
Micronesia, Federated States of	7.4	92.3	7.8	7.8	100	...	46.3	242	19	234	216	18
Monaco	8.0	62.5	37.5	37.5	26.0	74.0	...	1 264	474	1 799	1 124	675
Mongolia	4.3	82.0	18.0	4.9	84.7	15.3	13.3	16	1	69	56	3
Morocco	5.3	40.7	59.3	59.3	48.8	51.2	6.5	66	39	159	65	95
Mozambique	5.8	71.3	28.7	19.6	100	...	9.3	5	1	50	36	10
Myanmar	2.6	12.6	87.4	87.4	100	...	3.7	100	88	78	10	69
Namibia	7.5	51.7	48.3	48.3	100	...	10.2	153	74	312	161	150
Nauru	5.0	99.0	1.0	1.0	100	...	9.1	593	6	602	596	6
Nepal	3.7	26.0	74.0	74.0	100	...	5.3	8	6	41	11	30
Netherlands	8.8	70.7	29.3	16.8	100	...	12.7	2 041	343	1 911	1 351	321
New Zealand	8.2	71.7	28.3	22.0	100	...	12.7	1 416	312	1 393	999	307
Nicaragua	8.0	53.3	46.7	39.9	80.1	20.0	13.0	35	14	150	80	60
Niger	3.5	46.6	53.4	53.4	100	...	6.0	5	3	27	13	14
Nigeria	3.1	28.2	71.8	71.8	100	...	5.4	30	22	35	10	25
Niue	5.7	87.6	12.4	12.4	100	...	...	91	11	92	81	11
Norway	6.5	82.0	18.0	18.0	100	...	12.1	2 283	412	1 708	1 400	308
Oman	3.9	54.5	45.5	35.9	...	...	5.6	370	133	334	182	120
Pakistan	4.0	22.9	77.1	77.1	100	...	2.9	17	13	71	16	55
Palau	6.0	90.0	10.0	10.0	100	...	15.0	552	55	559	503	56
Panama	7.5	74.0	26.0	26.0	44.5	55.5	20.7	238	62	449	332	117
Papua New Guinea	3.1	77.6	22.4	22.4	100	...	7.5	36	8	77	59	17
Paraguay	5.6	35.6	64.4	55.4	49.8	50.2	14.6	106	59	206	73	114
Peru	5.6	39.7	60.3	50.2	44.2	55.8	13.0	149	75	246	98	123
Philippines	3.4	48.5	51.5	49.1	100	...	7.2	40	19	100	48	49
Poland	6.2	71.6	28.4	28.4	100	...	10.1	229	65	392	281	111
Portugal	8.2	57.5	42.5	40.9	100	...	10.8	845	345	1 060	609	433
Qatar	6.5	57.5	42.5	42.5	100	...	7.6	1 042	443	1 105	635	470
Republic of Korea	6.7	37.8	62.3	43.0	72.1	27.9	12.4	700	301	862	325	371
Republic of Moldova	8.3	75.1	24.9	24.9	100	...	12.4	35	9	133	100	33
Romania	3.8	60.3	39.8	39.8	100	...	6.7	59	23	136	82	54
Russian Federation	5.4	76.8	23.2	23.2	100	...	22.9	158	37	251	193	58
Rwanda	4.3	50.1	49.9	49.9	100	...	17.7	13	7	35	18	18
Saint Kitts and Nevis	6.0	51.5	48.5	44.7	100	...	10.4	404	181	489	252	219
Saint Lucia	4.0	65.1	34.9	32.2	100	...	9.0	211	68	218	142	70
Saint Vincent and the Grenadines	5.9	66.5	33.5	31.4	100	...	9.5	211	68	210	138	67
Samoa	3.8	88.9	11.1	11.1	100	...	9.1	47	5	108	96	12
San Marino	7.5	73.5	26.5	26.5	33.3	66.7	15.0	2 257	598	1 301	956	345
Sao Tome and Principe	4.0	75.0	25.0	25.0	100	...	4.3	13	3	45	34	11
Saudi Arabia	3.5	80.2	19.8	6.3	100	...	9.4	260	27	332	297	35
Senegal	4.5	55.7	44.3	44.3	100	...	13.2	23	10	71	40	32
Seychelles	5.9	76.2	23.8	23.8	100	...	8.4	424	101	470	358	112
Sierra Leone	4.9	9.7	90.3	90.3	100	...	3.1	11	10	31	3	28
Singapore	3.1	35.8	64.2	64.2	100	...	5.5	876	563	750	268	481
Slovakia	8.6	81.8	18.2	18.2	0.3	99.7	14.1	311	57	574	470	105
Slovenia	9.4	80.8	19.2	10.2	13.0	87.0	16.6	857	87	996	805	101
Solomon Islands	3.2	99.3	0.7	0.7	100	...	5.2	19	...	83	83	1
Somalia	1.5	71.4	28.6	28.6	100	...	...	11	3	11	8	3
South Africa	7.1	46.5	53.5	46.3	100	...	9.8	268	124	396	184	183
Spain	8.0	70.6	29.4	20.4	41.0	59.0	13.3	1 071	218	1 211	855	247
Sri Lanka	3.0	45.4	54.7	51.8	100	...	5.2	25	13	77	35	40
Sudan	3.5	20.9	79.1	79.1	100	...	9.6	13	10	43	9	34
Suriname	7.6	34.0	66.0	66.0	100	...	5.0	114	75	257	87	169
Swaziland	3.4	72.3	27.7	27.7	100	...	8.2	49	13	118	86	33
Sweden	9.2	78.0	22.0	22.0	100	...	11.5	2 456	540	1 943	1 516	427
Switzerland	10.1	69.3	30.7	29.7	22.1	77.9	13.3	3 564	1 057	2 644	1 833	784

Member State	HEALTH EXPENDITURE (%)							PER CAPITA HEALTH EXPENDITURE (US$)				
	Total expenditure on health as % of GDP	Public expenditure as % of total expenditure on health	Private expenditure as % of total health expenditure	Out-of-pocket expenditure as % of total expenditure on health	Tax-funded and other public expenditure as % of public expenditure on health	Social security expenditure as % of public expenditure on health	Public expenditure on health as % of total public expenditure	Total expenditure at official exchange rate	Out-of-pocket expenditure at official exchange rate	Total expenditure in international dollars	Public expenditure in international dollars	Out-of-pocket expenditure in international dollars[b]
Syrian Arab Republic	2.5	33.6	66.4	66.4	100	...	2.9	151	101	109	37	72
Tajikistan	7.6	87.8	12.2	12.2	100	...	39.6	11	1	94	82	11
Thailand	5.7	33.0	67.0	65.4	88.7	11.3	10.2	133	92	327	108	214
The former Yugoslav Republic of Macedonia	6.1	84.8	15.2	15.2	100	...	15.6	120	18	141	119	21
Togo	2.8	42.8	57.2	57.2	100	...	4.3	9	5	34	15	20
Tonga	7.8	46.0	54.0	54.0	100	...	13.2	141	76	257	118	139
Trinidad and Tobago	4.3	58.6	41.4	38.2	100	...	8.8	197	75	325	190	124
Tunisia	5.4	41.7	58.3	53.0	59.6	40.4	7.2	111	59	239	100	127
Turkey	3.9	74.0	26.0	23.3	65.1	34.9	10.9	118	27	231	171	54
Turkmenistan	4.3	86.0	14.0	14.0	100	...	13.9	24	3	90	77	13
Tuvalu	5.9	91.5	8.5	8.5	100	...	12.7	813	69	59	54	5
Uganda	4.1	35.1	64.9	48.2	100	...	9.9	14	9	44	17	27
Ukraine	5.6	75.5	24.5	24.5	100	...	9.6	54	13	128	96	31
United Arab Emirates	4.2	35.4	64.6	3.8	100	...	12.6	900	42	816	262	38
United Kingdom	5.8	96.9	3.1	3.1	100	...	14.3	1 303	40	1 193	1 156	37
United Republic of Tanzania	4.8	60.7	39.3	39.3	100	...	27.2	12	5	36	22	14
United States of America	13.7	44.1	55.9	16.6	57.9	42.1	18.5	4 187	696	3 724	1 643	619
Uruguay	10.0	20.3	79.7	21.4	89.0	11.0	6.0	660	141	849	172	182
Uzbekistan	4.2	80.9	19.1	19.1	100	...	10.3	24	5	109	88	21
Vanuatu	3.3	64.3	35.8	35.8	100	...	9.6	47	17	85	55	30
Venezuela, Bolivarian Republic of	3.9	67.4	32.6	32.6	66.6	33.4	10.5	150	49	298	201	97
Viet Nam	4.8	20.0	80.0	80.0	100	...	4.4	17	14	65	13	52
Yemen	3.4	37.9	62.1	62.1	100	...	3.3	12	7	33	12	20
Yugoslavia	4.5	64.8	35.2	35.2	100	...	...	127	28	127	98	28
Zambia	5.9	38.2	61.8	42.4	100	...	9.7	27	11	64	34	25
Zimbabwe	6.2	43.4	56.6	38.2	100	...	10.2	46	24	130	62	67

[a] Normal typeface indicates complete data with high reliability.

Italics indicate incomplete data with high to medium reliability.

Grey figures indicate incomplete data with low reliability.

Measured expenditure and orders of magnitude only. All estimates are preliminary. As in every systems accounting build-up, the "first-round data" are likely to be substantially modified in subsequent stages of the system's developmental process.

[b] Out-of-pocket expenditure in international dollars does not include voluntary health insurance and other private expenditures.

... Data not available or not applicable.

Annex Table 9 Overall health system attainment in all Member States, WHO index, estimates for 1997

Rank	Uncertainty interval	Member State	Index	Uncertainty interval
1	1	Japan	93.4	92.6 – 94.3
2	2 – 8	Switzerland	92.2	91.2 – 93.3
3	2 – 6	Norway	92.2	91.4 – 93.1
4	2 – 11	Sweden	92.0	91.1 – 93.0
5	2 – 11	Luxembourg	92.0	91.0 – 93.0
6	3 – 11	France	91.9	91.0 – 92.9
7	4 – 14	Canada	91.7	90.8 – 92.6
8	4 – 15	Netherlands	91.6	90.7 – 92.5
9	6 – 13	United Kingdom	91.6	90.9 – 92.3
10	6 – 18	Austria	91.5	90.5 – 92.4
11	7 – 21	Italy	91.4	90.5 – 92.2
12	7 – 19	Australia	91.3	90.4 – 92.2
13	7 – 18	Belgium	91.3	90.2 – 92.3
14	8 – 20	Germany	91.3	90.4 – 92.2
15	7 – 24	United States of America	91.1	89.9 – 92.3
16	10 – 23	Iceland	91.0	90.0 – 92.1
17	9 – 23	Andorra	91.0	90.1 – 92.0
18	9 – 23	Monaco	91.0	90.0 – 92.0
19	12 – 23	Spain	91.0	90.1 – 91.8
20	13 – 24	Denmark	90.9	90.0 – 91.8
21	12 – 24	San Marino	90.9	90.0 – 91.7
22	13 – 25	Finland	90.8	89.8 – 91.7
23	17 – 25	Greece	90.5	89.7 – 91.3
24	18 – 26	Israel	90.5	89.6 – 91.3
25	20 – 26	Ireland	90.2	89.3 – 91.1
26	22 – 26	New Zealand	90.1	89.3 – 91.0
27	26 – 30	Singapore	88.9	87.4 – 90.3
28	27 – 31	Cyprus	88.6	87.4 – 89.6
29	27 – 32	Slovenia	87.9	86.5 – 89.2
30	28 – 33	Czech Republic	87.8	86.9 – 88.7
31	29 – 32	Malta	87.7	86.9 – 88.5
32	29 – 32	Portugal	87.6	86.3 – 88.9
33	30 – 42	Chile	86.0	84.6 – 87.2
34	33 – 37	Poland	85.8	85.0 – 86.6
35	33 – 37	Republic of Korea	85.7	83.4 – 87.7
36	35 – 41	Croatia	85.1	83.8 – 86.4
37	34 – 40	Brunei Darussalam	84.9	83.4 – 86.3
38	34 – 41	Barbados	84.9	83.7 – 86.0
39	35 – 43	Slovakia	84.7	83.0 – 86.0
40	38 – 41	Cuba	84.2	83.5 – 85.0
41	37 – 45	Colombia	83.8	82.6 – 84.9
42	39 – 46	Dominica	83.4	82.0 – 84.6
43	39 – 47	Hungary	83.4	82.2 – 84.4
44	42 – 50	United Arab Emirates	82.8	81.8 – 83.7
45	42 – 48	Costa Rica	82.5	81.7 – 83.4
46	44 – 52	Kuwait	82.3	81.2 – 83.3
47	43 – 52	Qatar	82.2	81.2 – 83.2
48	44 – 55	Estonia	81.7	80.2 – 83.1
49	46 – 56	Argentina	81.6	80.4 – 82.7
50	46 – 63	Uruguay	81.2	79.7 – 82.8
51	45 – 60	Mexico	81.1	79.2 – 82.7
52	48 – 60	Lithuania	81.0	79.5 – 82.5
53	49 – 62	Belarus	81.0	80.0 – 82.0

Rank	Uncertainty interval	Member State	Index	Uncertainty interval
54	48 – 61	Philippines	80.9	79.6 – 82.0
55	48 – 59	Malaysia	80.8	79.2 – 82.2
56	46 – 65	Trinidad and Tobago	80.8	79.2 – 82.5
57	45 – 64	Thailand	80.7	78.8 – 82.5
58	53 – 61	Bahrain	80.4	79.3 – 81.3
59	54 – 62	Oman	80.2	79.2 – 81.1
60	53 – 66	Ukraine	80.1	78.5 – 81.5
61	55 – 63	Saudi Arabia	80.0	79.0 – 80.9
62	55 – 81	Kazakhstan	79.0	76.7 – 81.1
63	61 – 70	Palau	78.8	77.8 – 79.8
64	60 – 78	Bahamas	78.6	77.2 – 80.0
65	62 – 74	Venezuela, Bolivarian Republic of	78.5	77.4 – 79.6
66	58 – 90	Dominican Republic	78.1	76.0 – 80.3
67	63 – 88	Latvia	78.0	76.2 – 79.9
68	63 – 86	Grenada	77.9	76.8 – 78.9
69	64 – 84	Jamaica	77.9	76.4 – 79.4
70	65 – 85	Panama	77.9	76.9 – 78.8
71	64 – 84	Antigua and Barbuda	77.9	76.6 – 79.1
72	65 – 82	Romania	77.8	75.9 – 79.5
73	60 – 90	Paraguay	77.8	76.5 – 79.0
74	66 – 85	Bulgaria	77.6	76.9 – 78.4
75	69 – 83	Nauru	77.6	75.6 – 79.6
76	66 – 89	Georgia	77.5	76.6 – 78.4
77	62 – 92	Tunisia	77.5	76.4 – 78.5
78	69 – 86	Fiji	77.4	76.0 – 78.7
79	67 – 90	Bosnia and Herzegovina	77.3	75.8 – 78.7
80	70 – 89	Sri Lanka	77.3	76.1 – 78.3
81	64 – 105	Armenia	77.0	76.0 – 77.9
82	73 – 91	Samoa	76.9	75.9 – 78.0
83	74 – 90	Seychelles	76.8	75.8 – 77.8
84	75 – 91	Jordan	76.7	74.2* – 79.2
85	74 – 94	Tonga	76.7	75.6 – 77.8
86	65 – 101	Albania	76.7	73.7 – 79.2
87	75 – 93	Saint Lucia	76.7	75.5 – 77.9
88	72 – 101	Cook Islands	76.5	74.4 – 78.1
89	76 – 97	The former Yugoslav Republic of Macedonia	76.4	74.9 – 77.7
90	79 – 97	Mauritius	76.2	75.0 – 77.3
91	78 – 99	Republic of Moldova	76.1	74.6 – 77.6
92	82 – 100	Saint Vincent and the Grenadines	75.9	74.5 – 77.1
93	84 – 100	Lebanon	75.7	74.5 – 76.9
94	76 – 104	Morocco	75.7	73.8 – 77.5
95	82 – 104	Yugoslavia	75.5	73.7 – 77.2
96	88 – 104	Turkey	75.4	74.1 – 76.6
97	87 – 103	Libyan Arab Jamahiriya	75.3	73.9 – 76.5
98	90 – 107	Saint Kitts and Nevis	74.8	73.2 – 76.2
99	95 – 110	Algeria	74.4	73.6 – 75.2
100	96 – 107	Russian Federation	74.3	72.9 – 75.8
101	92 – 110	Nicaragua	74.2	72.7 – 75.5
102	96 – 110	Niue	74.1	72.6 – 75.4
103	95 – 112	Azerbaijan	74.0	72.1 – 75.7
104	96 – 112	Belize	74.0	71.7 – 76.5
105	93 – 113	Suriname	73.9	72.7 – 75.0

**Annex Table 9 Overall health system attainment in all Member States, WHO index,
estimates for 1997**

Rank	Uncertainty interval	Member State	Index	Uncertainty interval
106	98 – 110	Indonesia	73.8	71.8 – 75.8
107	87 – 114	Ecuador	73.8	72.3 – 75.3
108	99 – 113	Solomon Islands	73.7	70.8 – 76.5
109	88 – 117	Uzbekistan	73.5	71.6 – 75.4
110	95 – 114	Egypt	73.5	71.8 – 74.9
111	106 – 116	Micronesia, Federated States of	72.4	70.9 – 73.8
112	105 – 117	Syrian Arab Republic	72.4	70.7 – 74.0
113	102 – 123	Guatemala	72.3	70.7 – 73.9
114	106 – 118	Iran, Islamic Republic of	72.0	69.5 – 74.2
115	110 – 120	Peru	71.5	70.3 – 72.7
116	111 – 125	Guyana	71.0	69.0 – 72.5
117	112 – 125	Bolivia	70.7	69.1 – 72.5
118	113 – 126	Senegal	70.5	68.9 – 72.1
119	115 – 127	Marshall Islands	70.3	68.6 – 71.6
120	115 – 127	Tuvalu	70.2	68.6 – 71.6
121	117 – 124	India	70.1	69.3 – 71.0
122	114 – 133	El Salvador	69.6	67.1 – 71.9
123	117 – 131	Kiribati	69.5	67.7 – 70.9
124	120 – 133	Iraq	69.0	67.4 – 70.6
125	118 – 133	Brazil	68.9	67.1 – 70.4
126	122 – 137	Cape Verde	68.3	66.1 – 70.1
127	121 – 136	Tajikistan	68.3	66.2 – 70.1
128	124 – 136	Maldives	68.0	66.2 – 69.5
129	121 – 140	Honduras	67.8	66.0 – 69.8
130	124 – 139	Turkmenistan	67.7	64.9 – 70.4
131	122 – 138	Bangladesh	67.6	65.8 – 69.4
132	118 – 145	China	67.5	65.2 – 69.6
133	124 – 138	Pakistan	67.3	63.0 – 70.9
134	128 – 139	Vanuatu	67.1	64.7 – 69.1
135	128 – 140	Kyrgyzstan	67.0	65.2 – 68.5
136	125 – 141	Mongolia	67.0	65.2 – 68.5
137	123 – 145	Comoros	66.4	63.4 – 69.6
138	132 – 143	Sao Tome and Principe	65.9	64.0 – 67.6
139	127 – 145	Ghana	65.8	63.2 – 68.6
140	133 – 142	Viet Nam	65.8	64.6 – 66.9
141	138 – 148	Gabon	64.5	62.7 – 66.2
142	137 – 147	Kenya	64.3	62.4 – 66.0
143	136 – 150	Benin	64.2	61.5 – 66.6
144	141 – 153	Bhutan	63.1	61.1 – 64.8
145	138 – 157	Haiti	62.8	59.7 – 66.2
146	140 – 160	Yemen	62.3	59.7 – 64.8
147	141 – 159	Zimbabwe	62.3	59.1 – 65.3
148	141 – 158	Sudan	62.3	59.4 – 65.0
149	142 – 159	Democratic People's Republic of Korea	62.2	59.5 – 64.4
150	144 – 159	Papua New Guinea	62.0	59.7 – 63.8
151	146 – 164	South Africa	61.0	58.4 – 63.1
152	151 – 164	Equatorial Guinea	60.2	58.0 – 61.9
153	150 – 165	Gambia	60.2	58.1 – 62.5
154	147 – 168	Lao People's Democratic Republic	60.1	57.9 – 62.1
155	151 – 165	Congo	60.1	57.9 – 62.2
156	149 – 165	Togo	60.0	57.3 – 62.5
157	148 – 165	Côte d'Ivoire	60.0	57.7 – 62.1
158	148 – 166	United Republic of Tanzania	60.0	58.0 – 62.1

Rank	Uncertainty interval	Member State	Index	Uncertainty interval
159	149 – 170	Burkina Faso	59.4	57.5 – 61.4
160	151 – 168	Nepal	59.3	56.4 – 62.1
161	149 – 170	Burundi	59.3	56.4 – 62.1
162	152 – 169	Uganda	59.3	56.4 – 62.1
163	148 – 173	Cameroon	59.1	54.9 – 62.8
164	152 – 172	Swaziland	59.0	56.7 – 61.3
165	149 – 170	Namibia	58.8	55.7 – 61.3
166	153 – 175	Cambodia	58.2	54.3 – 61.3
167	157 – 173	Madagascar	57.8	55.3 – 60.2
168	161 – 173	Botswana	57.4	55.5 – 58.9
169	162 – 174	Mauritania	57.2	55.0 – 59.2
170	163 – 175	Djibouti	56.8	54.9 – 58.4
171	162 – 177	Rwanda	56.5	54.1 – 58.9
172	167 – 176	Guinea	56.3	53.9 – 58.3
173	164 – 177	Lesotho	56.0	54.0 – 57.7
174	163 – 180	Zambia	55.6	53.0 – 58.4
175	162 – 190	Myanmar	53.7	51.3 – 56.0
176	173 – 183	Eritrea	53.7	51.5 – 55.5
177	172 – 183	Chad	53.6	46.7 – 59.2
178	174 – 183	Mali	53.3	50.9 – 55.6
179	176 – 186	Democratic Republic of the Congo	52.6	49.7 – 55.7
180	175 – 186	Guinea-Bissau	52.4	49.8 – 54.8
181	176 – 186	Angola	52.4	49.7 – 54.6
182	173 – 187	Malawi	52.3	49.5 – 54.7
183	177 – 186	Afghanistan	52.1	49.8 – 54.0
184	176 – 188	Nigeria	51.7	48.5 – 54.7
185	178 – 189	Mozambique	50.6	48.2 – 53.2
186	182 – 189	Ethiopia	50.5	47.8 – 53.3
187	179 – 189	Liberia	50.4	48.0 – 52.4
188	180 – 189	Niger	50.1	47.0 – 53.4
189	183 – 189	Somalia	49.4	46.1 – 52.4
190	184 – 190	Central African Republic	45.9	39.0 – 52.0
191	191	Sierra Leone	35.7	23.7 – 43.8

Annex Table 10 Health system performance in all Member States, WHO indexes, estimates for 1997

	PERFORMANCE ON HEALTH LEVEL (DALE)					OVERALL PERFORMANCE			
Rank	Uncertainty interval	Member State	Index	Uncertainty interval	Rank	Uncertainty interval	Member State	Index	Uncertainty interval
1	1 – 5	Oman	0.992	0.975 – 1.000	1	1 – 5	France	0.994	0.982 – 1.000
2	1 – 4	Malta	0.989	0.968 – 1.000	2	1 – 5	Italy	0.991	0.978 – 1.000
3	2 – 7	Italy	0.976	0.957 – 0.994	3	1 – 6	San Marino	0.988	0.973 – 1.000
4	2 – 7	France	0.974	0.953 – 0.994	4	2 – 7	Andorra	0.982	0.966 – 0.997
5	2 – 7	San Marino	0.971	0.949 – 0.988	5	3 – 7	Malta	0.978	0.965 – 0.993
6	3 – 8	Spain	0.968	0.948 – 0.989	6	2 – 11	Singapore	0.973	0.947 – 0.998
7	4 – 9	Andorra	0.964	0.942 – 0.980	7	4 – 8	Spain	0.972	0.959 – 0.985
8	3 – 12	Jamaica	0.956	0.928 – 0.986	8	4 – 14	Oman	0.961	0.938 – 0.985
9	7 – 11	Japan	0.945	0.926 – 0.963	9	7 – 12	Austria	0.959	0.946 – 0.972
10	8 – 15	Saudi Arabia	0.936	0.915 – 0.959	10	8 – 11	Japan	0.957	0.948 – 0.965
11	9 – 13	Greece	0.936	0.920 – 0.951	11	8 – 12	Norway	0.955	0.947 – 0.964
12	9 – 16	Monaco	0.930	0.908 – 0.948	12	10 – 15	Portugal	0.945	0.931 – 0.958
13	10 – 15	Portugal	0.929	0.911 – 0.945	13	10 – 16	Monaco	0.943	0.929 – 0.957
14	10 – 15	Singapore	0.929	0.909 – 0.942	14	13 – 19	Greece	0.933	0.921 – 0.945
15	13 – 17	Austria	0.914	0.896 – 0.931	15	12 – 20	Iceland	0.932	0.917 – 0.948
16	13 – 23	United Arab Emirates	0.907	0.883 – 0.932	16	14 – 21	Luxembourg	0.928	0.914 – 0.942
17	14 – 22	Morocco	0.906	0.886 – 0.925	17	14 – 21	Netherlands	0.928	0.914 – 0.942
18	16 – 23	Norway	0.897	0.878 – 0.914	18	16 – 21	United Kingdom	0.925	0.913 – 0.937
19	17 – 24	Netherlands	0.893	0.875 – 0.911	19	14 – 22	Ireland	0.924	0.909 – 0.939
20	15 – 31	Solomon Islands	0.892	0.863 – 0.920	20	17 – 24	Switzerland	0.916	0.903 – 0.930
21	18 – 26	Sweden	0.890	0.870 – 0.907	21	18 – 24	Belgium	0.915	0.903 – 0.926
22	19 – 28	Cyprus	0.885	0.865 – 0.898	22	14 – 29	Colombia	0.910	0.881 – 0.939
23	19 – 30	Chile	0.884	0.864 – 0.903	23	20 – 26	Sweden	0.908	0.893 – 0.921
24	21 – 28	United Kingdom	0.883	0.866 – 0.900	24	16 – 30	Cyprus	0.906	0.879 – 0.932
25	18 – 32	Costa Rica	0.882	0.859 – 0.898	25	22 – 27	Germany	0.902	0.890 – 0.914
26	21 – 31	Switzerland	0.879	0.860 – 0.891	26	22 – 32	Saudi Arabia	0.894	0.872 – 0.916
27	21 – 31	Iceland	0.879	0.861 – 0.897	27	23 – 33	United Arab Emirates	0.886	0.861 – 0.911
28	23 – 30	Belgium	0.878	0.860 – 0.894	28	26 – 32	Israel	0.884	0.870 – 0.897
29	23 – 33	Venezuela, Bolivarian Republic of	0.873	0.853 – 0.891	29	18 – 39	Morocco	0.882	0.834 – 0.925
30	23 – 37	Bahrain	0.867	0.843 – 0.890	30	27 – 32	Canada	0.881	0.868 – 0.894
31	28 – 35	Luxembourg	0.864	0.847 – 0.881	31	27 – 33	Finland	0.881	0.866 – 0.895
32	29 – 38	Ireland	0.859	0.840 – 0.870	32	28 – 34	Australia	0.876	0.861 – 0.891
33	27 – 40	Turkey	0.858	0.835 – 0.878	33	22 – 43	Chile	0.870	0.816 – 0.918
34	25 – 48	Belize	0.853	0.821 – 0.884	34	32 – 36	Denmark	0.862	0.848 – 0.874
35	33 – 40	Canada	0.849	0.832 – 0.864	35	31 – 41	Dominica	0.854	0.824 – 0.883
36	32 – 42	Cuba	0.849	0.830 – 0.866	36	33 – 40	Costa Rica	0.849	0.825 – 0.871
37	30 – 49	El Salvador	0.846	0.817 – 0.873	37	35 – 44	United States of America	0.838	0.817 – 0.859
38	28 – 52	Saint Vincent and the Grenadines	0.845	0.812 – 0.876	38	34 – 46	Slovenia	0.838	0.813 – 0.859
39	35 – 43	Australia	0.844	0.826 – 0.861	39	36 – 44	Cuba	0.834	0.816 – 0.852
40	36 – 44	Israel	0.841	0.825 – 0.858	40	36 – 48	Brunei Darussalam	0.829	0.808 – 0.849
41	39 – 47	Germany	0.836	0.819 – 0.852	41	38 – 45	New Zealand	0.827	0.815 – 0.840
42	33 – 54	Dominican Republic	0.834	0.806 – 0.863	42	37 – 48	Bahrain	0.824	0.804 – 0.845
43	37 – 53	Egypt	0.829	0.811 – 0.849	43	39 – 53	Croatia	0.812	0.782 – 0.837
44	41 – 50	Finland	0.829	0.812 – 0.844	44	41 – 51	Qatar	0.812	0.793 – 0.831
45	38 – 55	Algeria	0.829	0.808 – 0.850	45	41 – 52	Kuwait	0.810	0.790 – 0.830
46	41 – 55	Tunisia	0.824	0.803 – 0.844	46	41 – 53	Barbados	0.808	0.779 – 0.834
47	38 – 58	Yugoslavia	0.824	0.798 – 0.848	47	36 – 59	Thailand	0.807	0.759 – 0.852
48	40 – 61	Honduras	0.820	0.793 – 0.844	48	43 – 54	Czech Republic	0.805	0.781 – 0.825
49	37 – 63	Grenada	0.819	0.789 – 0.850	49	42 – 55	Malaysia	0.802	0.772 – 0.830
50	42 – 59	Uruguay	0.819	0.794 – 0.842	50	45 – 59	Poland	0.793	0.762 – 0.819
51	41 – 64	Colombia	0.814	0.787 – 0.843	51	38 – 67	Dominican Republic	0.789	0.735 – 0.845
52	42 – 65	Paraguay	0.813	0.785 – 0.842	52	41 – 67	Tunisia	0.785	0.741 – 0.832
53	43 – 64	Qatar	0.813	0.786 – 0.839	53	47 – 62	Jamaica	0.782	0.754 – 0.809
54	43 – 69	Saint Lucia	0.809	0.781 – 0.837	54	50 – 64	Venezuela, Bolivarian Republic of	0.775	0.745 – 0.803
55	41 – 70	Cape Verde	0.808	0.776 – 0.842	55	41 – 75	Albania	0.774	0.709 – 0.834

PERFORMANCE ON HEALTH LEVEL (DALE)

Rank	Uncertainty interval	Member State	Index	Uncertainty interval
56	47 – 64	Armenia	0.806	0.785 – 0.823
57	51 – 61	Croatia	0.805	0.789 – 0.821
58	48 – 65	Iran, Islamic Republic of	0.805	0.783 – 0.827
59	45 – 73	Dominica	0.804	0.774 – 0.833
60	49 – 67	Azerbaijan	0.803	0.781 – 0.820
61	52 – 65	China	0.800	0.782 – 0.813
62	55 – 66	Slovenia	0.797	0.781 – 0.813
63	56 – 73	Mexico	0.789	0.771 – 0.808
64	55 – 76	Albania	0.789	0.766 – 0.808
65	61 – 72	Denmark	0.785	0.769 – 0.801
66	57 – 80	Sri Lanka	0.783	0.761 – 0.807
67	57 – 80	Panama	0.783	0.759 – 0.807
68	56 – 83	Kuwait	0.782	0.753 – 0.808
69	61 – 78	The former Yugoslav Republic of Macedonia	0.781	0.761 – 0.796
70	59 – 83	Bosnia and Herzegovina	0.780	0.754 – 0.803
71	65 – 76	Argentina	0.779	0.762 – 0.794
72	67 – 78	United States of America	0.774	0.758 – 0.789
73	61 – 86	Bhutan	0.773	0.748 – 0.797
74	63 – 84	Nicaragua	0.772	0.750 – 0.793
75	65 – 84	Iraq	0.770	0.752 – 0.791
76	67 – 85	Brunei Darussalam	0.768	0.749 – 0.787
77	61 – 88	Suriname	0.768	0.740 – 0.798
78	66 – 88	Brazil	0.767	0.745 – 0.787
79	70 – 84	Trinidad and Tobago	0.767	0.750 – 0.780
80	72 – 83	New Zealand	0.766	0.750 – 0.780
81	73 – 83	Czech Republic	0.765	0.749 – 0.779
82	66 – 91	Yemen	0.761	0.733 – 0.789
83	72 – 88	Seychelles	0.759	0.739 – 0.778
84	73 – 91	Georgia	0.758	0.736 – 0.776
85	73 – 89	Pakistan	0.757	0.738 – 0.777
86	75 – 92	Malaysia	0.751	0.731 – 0.771
87	77 – 92	Barbados	0.749	0.730 – 0.770
88	85 – 92	Slovakia	0.742	0.729 – 0.757
89	84 – 94	Poland	0.742	0.723 – 0.758
90	79 – 98	Indonesia	0.741	0.715 – 0.766
91	85 – 99	Syrian Arab Republic	0.733	0.712 – 0.755
92	89 – 96	Bulgaria	0.733	0.717 – 0.747
93	89 – 103	Lithuania	0.724	0.705 – 0.742
94	89 – 104	Libyan Arab Jamahiriya	0.723	0.699 – 0.746
95	89 – 105	Cook Islands	0.722	0.696 – 0.746
96	89 – 104	Ecuador	0.721	0.700 – 0.742
97	91 – 105	Lebanon	0.719	0.697 – 0.740
98	93 – 107	Nepal	0.714	0.691 – 0.736
99	93 – 107	Guatemala	0.714	0.691 – 0.735
100	94 – 107	Jordan	0.711	0.689 – 0.732
101	97 – 104	Ukraine	0.711	0.695 – 0.726
102	93 – 111	Thailand	0.710	0.682 – 0.736
103	93 – 109	Bangladesh	0.709	0.684 – 0.735
104	92 – 115	Guyana	0.704	0.672 – 0.738
105	101 – 111	Hungary	0.698	0.682 – 0.714
106	102 – 111	Republic of Moldova	0.696	0.680 – 0.710
107	100 – 113	Republic of Korea	0.694	0.674 – 0.711
108	93 – 121	Niue	0.693	0.650 – 0.731

OVERALL PERFORMANCE

Rank	Uncertainty interval	Member State	Index	Uncertainty interval
56	51 – 63	Seychelles	0.773	0.747 – 0.797
57	47 – 77	Paraguay	0.761	0.714 – 0.806
58	55 – 67	Republic of Korea	0.759	0.740 – 0.776
59	50 – 78	Senegal	0.756	0.711 – 0.800
60	53 – 73	Philippines	0.755	0.720 – 0.789
61	52 – 74	Mexico	0.755	0.719 – 0.789
62	54 – 73	Slovakia	0.754	0.721 – 0.781
63	49 – 81	Egypt	0.752	0.707 – 0.798
64	50 – 80	Kazakhstan	0.752	0.699 – 0.802
65	55 – 80	Uruguay	0.745	0.702 – 0.782
66	59 – 74	Hungary	0.743	0.713 – 0.768
67	53 – 81	Trinidad and Tobago	0.742	0.695 – 0.784
68	59 – 75	Saint Lucia	0.740	0.717 – 0.765
69	58 – 81	Belize	0.736	0.697 – 0.772
70	60 – 81	Turkey	0.734	0.698 – 0.764
71	58 – 83	Nicaragua	0.733	0.696 – 0.770
72	64 – 84	Belarus	0.723	0.691 – 0.750
73	65 – 82	Lithuania	0.722	0.690 – 0.750
74	63 – 83	Saint Vincent and the Grenadines	0.722	0.686 – 0.754
75	66 – 81	Argentina	0.722	0.695 – 0.747
76	68 – 84	Sri Lanka	0.716	0.692 – 0.740
77	68 – 85	Estonia	0.714	0.684 – 0.741
78	57 – 99	Guatemala	0.713	0.642 – 0.774
79	70 – 88	Ukraine	0.708	0.674 – 0.734
80	68 – 93	Solomon Islands	0.705	0.664 – 0.739
81	70 – 92	Algeria	0.701	0.669 – 0.730
82	75 – 88	Palau	0.700	0.679 – 0.719
83	75 – 88	Jordan	0.698	0.675 – 0.720
84	75 – 91	Mauritius	0.691	0.665 – 0.719
85	74 – 96	Grenada	0.689	0.652 – 0.723
86	76 – 93	Antigua and Barbuda	0.688	0.657 – 0.718
87	79 – 96	Libyan Arab Jamahiriya	0.683	0.655 – 0.707
88	69 – 111	Bangladesh	0.675	0.618 – 0.732
89	83 – 107	The former Yugoslav Republic of Macedonia	0.664	0.630 – 0.695
90	84 – 106	Bosnia and Herzegovina	0.664	0.632 – 0.694
91	85 – 104	Lebanon	0.664	0.638 – 0.688
92	85 – 107	Indonesia	0.660	0.632 – 0.689
93	83 – 110	Iran, Islamic Republic of	0.659	0.620 – 0.693
94	87 – 108	Bahamas	0.657	0.625 – 0.687
95	87 – 107	Panama	0.656	0.627 – 0.686
96	90 – 106	Fiji	0.653	0.630 – 0.674
97	78 – 123	Benin	0.647	0.573 – 0.710
98	94 – 107	Nauru	0.647	0.630 – 0.664
99	92 – 110	Romania	0.645	0.624 – 0.666
100	90 – 113	Saint Kitts and Nevis	0.643	0.611 – 0.678
101	92 – 114	Republic of Moldova	0.639	0.600 – 0.672
102	94 – 113	Bulgaria	0.639	0.617 – 0.660
103	91 – 117	Iraq	0.637	0.597 – 0.669
104	86 – 126	Armenia	0.630	0.566 – 0.682
105	94 – 118	Latvia	0.630	0.589 – 0.665
106	94 – 120	Yugoslavia	0.629	0.586 – 0.664
107	95 – 121	Cook Islands	0.628	0.583 – 0.664
108	94 – 120	Syrian Arab Republic	0.628	0.589 – 0.661

Annex Table 10 Health system performance in all Member States, WHO indexes, estimates for 1997

Rank	Uncertainty interval	Member State	Index	Uncertainty interval	Rank	Uncertainty interval	Member State	Index	Uncertainty interval
		PERFORMANCE ON HEALTH LEVEL (DALE)					**OVERALL PERFORMANCE**		
109	103 – 116	Gambia	0.687	0.671 – 0.704	109	93 – 122	Azerbaijan	0.626	0.582 – 0.665
110	100 – 121	Micronesia, Federated States of	0.684	0.656 – 0.717	110	91 – 123	Suriname	0.623	0.571 – 0.671
111	107 – 117	Romania	0.682	0.668 – 0.696	111	88 – 125	Ecuador	0.619	0.565 – 0.684
112	107 – 119	Uzbekistan	0.681	0.662 – 0.700	112	105 – 118	India	0.617	0.599 – 0.638
113	105 – 120	Mauritius	0.679	0.657 – 0.702	113	95 – 127	Cape Verde	0.617	0.561 – 0.664
114	105 – 121	Tonga	0.677	0.651 – 0.704	114	103 – 121	Georgia	0.615	0.583 – 0.642
115	107 – 119	Estonia	0.677	0.657 – 0.694	115	94 – 130	El Salvador	0.608	0.544 – 0.667
116	109 – 119	Belarus	0.676	0.657 – 0.692	116	106 – 121	Tonga	0.607	0.582 – 0.632
117	109 – 121	Sao Tome and Principe	0.671	0.651 – 0.691	117	92 – 134	Uzbekistan	0.599	0.532 – 0.668
118	112 – 120	India	0.670	0.654 – 0.683	118	86 – 139	Comoros	0.592	0.509 – 0.689
119	111 – 123	Peru	0.665	0.643 – 0.686	119	114 – 126	Samoa	0.589	0.564 – 0.612
120	108 – 123	Vanuatu	0.665	0.639 – 0.689	120	92 – 140	Yemen	0.587	0.497 – 0.672
121	115 – 125	Latvia	0.655	0.631 – 0.677	121	114 – 129	Niue	0.584	0.549 – 0.614
122	114 – 127	Saint Kitts and Nevis	0.650	0.621 – 0.679	122	109 – 132	Pakistan	0.583	0.541 – 0.626
123	115 – 131	Antigua and Barbuda	0.641	0.606 – 0.678	123	114 – 131	Micronesia, Federated States of	0.579	0.543 – 0.610
124	120 – 133	Fiji	0.632	0.600 – 0.662	124	111 – 136	Bhutan	0.575	0.520 – 0.618
125	121 – 131	Palau	0.632	0.606 – 0.656	125	111 – 136	Brazil	0.573	0.526 – 0.619
126	122 – 131	Philippines	0.630	0.608 – 0.653	126	112 – 135	Bolivia	0.571	0.526 – 0.615
127	124 – 131	Russian Federation	0.623	0.606 – 0.638	127	118 – 138	Vanuatu	0.559	0.512 – 0.594
128	123 – 134	Tuvalu	0.618	0.594 – 0.644	128	119 – 140	Guyana	0.554	0.504 – 0.593
129	124 – 137	Myanmar	0.612	0.584 – 0.641	129	122 – 138	Peru	0.547	0.517 – 0.577
130	125 – 136	Viet Nam	0.611	0.587 – 0.634	130	126 – 136	Russian Federation	0.544	0.527 – 0.563
131	127 – 139	Samoa	0.602	0.579 – 0.626	131	115 – 145	Honduras	0.544	0.471 – 0.611
132	128 – 138	Senegal	0.601	0.584 – 0.620	132	114 – 147	Burkina Faso	0.543	0.472 – 0.611
133	129 – 139	Côte d'Ivoire	0.598	0.580 – 0.617	133	124 – 144	Sao Tome and Principe	0.535	0.482 – 0.575
134	128 – 140	Kyrgyzstan	0.598	0.575 – 0.620	134	119 – 151	Sudan	0.524	0.447 – 0.594
135	129 – 138	Kazakhstan	0.598	0.581 – 0.615	135	118 – 150	Ghana	0.522	0.452 – 0.596
136	129 – 139	Benin	0.596	0.576 – 0.616	136	130 – 145	Tuvalu	0.518	0.481 – 0.551
137	127 – 142	Bahamas	0.593	0.564 – 0.624	137	124 – 149	Côte d'Ivoire	0.517	0.463 – 0.572
138	132 – 144	Mongolia	0.581	0.555 – 0.607	138	120 – 152	Haiti	0.517	0.439 – 0.595
139	134 – 143	Haiti	0.580	0.561 – 0.599	139	129 – 149	Gabon	0.511	0.456 – 0.553
140	131 – 144	Marshall Islands	0.579	0.549 – 0.609	140	130 – 148	Kenya	0.505	0.461 – 0.549
141	137 – 145	Comoros	0.570	0.550 – 0.590	141	133 – 147	Marshall Islands	0.504	0.469 – 0.534
142	137 – 145	Bolivia	0.567	0.544 – 0.590	142	135 – 150	Kiribati	0.495	0.455 – 0.529
143	139 – 146	Gabon	0.559	0.538 – 0.579	143	125 – 157	Burundi	0.494	0.411 – 0.572
144	138 – 148	Kiribati	0.554	0.525 – 0.581	144	125 – 162	China	0.485	0.375 – 0.567
145	140 – 148	Tajikistan	0.551	0.523 – 0.580	145	134 – 154	Mongolia	0.483	0.429 – 0.531
146	141 – 149	Papua New Guinea	0.546	0.520 – 0.572	146	135 – 154	Gambia	0.482	0.427 – 0.533
147	144 – 154	Maldives	0.524	0.496 – 0.555	147	138 – 154	Maldives	0.477	0.430 – 0.516
148	146 – 153	Eritrea	0.521	0.504 – 0.538	148	137 – 159	Papua New Guinea	0.467	0.400 – 0.522
149	146 – 154	Sudan	0.519	0.496 – 0.543	149	136 – 158	Uganda	0.464	0.404 – 0.526
150	146 – 155	Afghanistan	0.517	0.488 – 0.547	150	138 – 159	Nepal	0.457	0.400 – 0.516
151	147 – 153	Mauritania	0.517	0.501 – 0.533	151	143 – 157	Kyrgyzstan	0.455	0.410 – 0.490
152	145 – 158	Turkmenistan	0.513	0.479 – 0.546	152	142 – 158	Togo	0.449	0.398 – 0.501
153	147 – 156	Democratic People's Republic of Korea	0.510	0.485 – 0.536	153	143 – 161	Turkmenistan	0.443	0.390 – 0.490
154	148 – 157	Somalia	0.506	0.480 – 0.530	154	147 – 163	Tajikistan	0.428	0.381 – 0.470
155	152 – 160	Lao People's Democratic Republic	0.489	0.466 – 0.510	155	143 – 167	Zimbabwe	0.427	0.352 – 0.497
156	154 – 162	Guinea-Bissau	0.481	0.462 – 0.499	156	145 – 166	United Republic of Tanzania	0.422	0.368 – 0.479
157	153 – 162	Cambodia	0.481	0.460 – 0.501	157	149 – 168	Djibouti	0.414	0.355 – 0.459
158	153 – 162	Ghana	0.479	0.457 – 0.500	158	152 – 170	Eritrea	0.399	0.339 – 0.446
159	155 – 164	Togo	0.472	0.452 – 0.492	159	149 – 170	Madagascar	0.397	0.329 – 0.463
160	157 – 164	Guinea	0.469	0.455 – 0.483	160	155 – 166	Viet Nam	0.393	0.366 – 0.420
161	156 – 165	Chad	0.465	0.444 – 0.487	161	155 – 170	Guinea	0.385	0.334 – 0.425
162	157 – 166	Burkina Faso	0.463	0.441 – 0.483	162	154 – 172	Mauritania	0.384	0.328 – 0.431

	PERFORMANCE ON HEALTH LEVEL (DALE)					OVERALL PERFORMANCE			
Rank	Uncertainty interval	Member State	Index	Uncertainty interval	Rank	Uncertainty interval	Member State	Index	Uncertainty interval
163	158 – 167	Djibouti	0.457	0.434 – 0.479	163	156 – 176	Mali	0.361	0.284 – 0.429
164	160 – 166	Central African Republic	0.454	0.436 – 0.470	164	150 – 181	Cameroon	0.357	0.246 – 0.458
165	159 – 167	Angola	0.453	0.433 – 0.473	165	157 – 178	Lao People's Democratic Republic	0.356	0.298 – 0.410
166	162 – 168	Nauru	0.444	0.424 – 0.464	166	160 – 176	Congo	0.354	0.302 – 0.401
167	164 – 170	Congo	0.433	0.411 – 0.454	167	157 – 180	Democratic People's Republic of Korea	0.353	0.278 – 0.414
168	164 – 172	Mozambique	0.424	0.399 – 0.450	168	158 – 180	Namibia	0.340	0.268 – 0.413
169	167 – 171	Ethiopia	0.418	0.400 – 0.435	169	164 – 179	Botswana	0.338	0.288 – 0.373
170	168 – 172	Mali	0.410	0.393 – 0.426	170	158 – 180	Niger	0.337	0.266 – 0.416
171	168 – 174	Burundi	0.403	0.374 – 0.435	171	163 – 180	Equatorial Guinea	0.337	0.277 – 0.384
172	169 – 174	Cameroon	0.399	0.375 – 0.421	172	161 – 182	Rwanda	0.327	0.268 – 0.389
173	170 – 174	Madagascar	0.394	0.378 – 0.410	173	164 – 181	Afghanistan	0.325	0.262 – 0.376
174	172 – 175	Equatorial Guinea	0.377	0.355 – 0.400	174	161 – 184	Cambodia	0.322	0.234 – 0.392
175	174 – 176	Nigeria	0.353	0.331 – 0.375	175	164 – 182	South Africa	0.319	0.251 – 0.374
176	175 – 178	Liberia	0.337	0.318 – 0.355	176	164 – 183	Guinea-Bissau	0.314	0.239 – 0.375
177	176 – 178	Niger	0.323	0.306 – 0.340	177	166 – 184	Swaziland	0.305	0.234 – 0.369
178	176 – 178	Kenya	0.320	0.298 – 0.343	178	167 – 183	Chad	0.303	0.231 – 0.363
179	179 – 180	Uganda	0.280	0.264 – 0.295	179	167 – 186	Somalia	0.286	0.199 – 0.369
180	179 – 180	United Republic of Tanzania	0.279	0.260 – 0.298	180	173 – 185	Ethiopia	0.276	0.215 – 0.326
181	181 – 185	Rwanda	0.240	0.214 – 0.265	181	172 – 186	Angola	0.275	0.198 – 0.343
182	181 – 185	South Africa	0.232	0.209 – 0.251	182	170 – 186	Zambia	0.269	0.204 – 0.339
183	181 – 185	Sierra Leone	0.230	0.213 – 0.247	183	174 – 186	Lesotho	0.266	0.205 – 0.319
184	181 – 186	Swaziland	0.229	0.205 – 0.255	184	170 – 187	Mozambique	0.260	0.186 – 0.339
185	182 – 187	Democratic Republic of the Congo	0.217	0.198 – 0.235	185	171 – 188	Malawi	0.251	0.174 – 0.332
186	183 – 188	Lesotho	0.211	0.187 – 0.236	186	180 – 189	Liberia	0.200	0.117 – 0.282
187	186 – 188	Malawi	0.196	0.181 – 0.211	187	183 – 189	Nigeria	0.176	0.094 – 0.251
188	187 – 189	Botswana	0.183	0.172 – 0.194	188	185 – 189	Democratic Republic of the Congo	0.171	0.100 – 0.232
189	185 – 189	Namibia	0.183	0.152 – 0.214	189	179 – 190	Central African Republic	0.156	0.000 – 0.306
190	190	Zambia	0.112	0.095 – 0.129	190	175 – 191	Myanmar	0.138	0.000 – 0.311
191	191	Zimbabwe	0.080	0.057 – 0.103	191	190 – 191	Sierra Leone	0.000	0.000 – 0.079

LIST OF MEMBER STATES BY
WHO REGION AND MORTALITY STRATUM

African Region (AFR)

Algeria – High child, high adult
Angola – High child, high adult
Benin – High child, high adult
Botswana – High child, very high adult
Burkina Faso – High child, high adult
Burundi – High child, very high adult
Cameroon – High child, high adult
Cape Verde – High child, high adult
Central African Republic – High child, very high adult
Chad – High child, high adult
Comoros – High child, high adult
Congo – High child, very high adult
Côte d'Ivoire – High child, very high adult
Democratic Republic of the Congo – High child, very high adult
Equatorial Guinea – High child, high adult
Eritrea – High child, very high adult
Ethiopia – High child, very high adult
Gabon – High child, high adult
Gambia – High child, high adult
Ghana – High child, high adult
Guinea – High child, high adult
Guinea-Bissau – High child, high adult
Kenya – High child, very high adult
Lesotho – High child, very high adult
Liberia – High child, high adult
Madagascar – High child, high adult
Malawi – High child, very high adult
Mali – High child, high adult
Mauritania – High child, high adult
Mauritius – High child, high adult
Mozambique – High child, very high adult
Namibia – High child, very high adult
Niger – High child, high adult

Nigeria – High child, high adult
Rwanda – High child, very high adult
Sao Tome and Principe – High child, high adult
Senegal – High child, high adult
Seychelles – High child, high adult
Sierra Leone – High child, high adult
South Africa – High child, very high adult
Swaziland – High child, very high adult
Togo – High child, high adult
Uganda – High child, very high adult
United Republic of Tanzania – High child, very high adult
Zambia – High child, very high adult
Zimbabwe – High child, very high adult

Region of the Americas (AMR)

Antigua and Barbuda – Low child, low adult
Argentina – Low child, low adult
Bahamas – Low child, low adult
Barbados – Low child, low adult
Belize – Low child, low adult
Bolivia – High child, high adult
Brazil – Low child, low adult
Canada – Very low child, very low adult
Chile – Low child, low adult
Colombia – Low child, low adult
Costa Rica – Low child, low adult
Cuba – Very low child, very low adult
Dominica – Low child, low adult
Dominican Republic – Low child, low adult
Ecuador – High child, high adult
El Salvador – Low child, low adult
Grenada – Low child, low adult
Guatemala – High child, high adult
Guyana – Low child, low adult

Haiti – High child, high adult
Honduras – Low child, low adult
Jamaica – Low child, low adult
Mexico – Low child, low adult
Nicaragua – High child, high adult
Panama – Low child, low adult
Paraguay – Low child, low adult
Peru – High child, high adult
Saint Kitts and Nevis – Low child, low adult
Saint Lucia – Low child, low adult
Saint Vincent and the Grenadines – Low child, low adult
Suriname – Low child, low adult
Trinidad and Tobago – Low child, low adult
United States of America – Very low child, very low adult
Uruguay – Low child, low adult
Venezuela, Bolivarian Republic of – Low child, low adult

Eastern Mediterranean Region (EMR)

Afghanistan – High child, high adult
Bahrain – Low child, low adult
Cyprus – Low child, low adult
Djibouti – High child, high adult
Egypt – High child, high adult
Iran, Islamic Republic of – Low child, low adult
Iraq – High child, high adult
Jordan – Low child, low adult
Kuwait – Low child, low adult
Lebanon – Low child, low adult
Libyan Arab Jamahiriya – Low child, low adult
Morocco – High child, high adult
Oman – Low child, low adult

Pakistan – High child, high adult
Qatar – Low child, low adult
Saudi Arabia – Low child, low adult
Somalia – High child, high adult
Sudan – High child, high adult
Syrian Arab Republic – Low child, low adult
Tunisia – Low child, low adult
United Arab Emirates – Low child, low adult
Yemen – High child, high adult

European Region (EUR)

Albania – Low child, low adult
Andorra – Very low child, very low adult
Armenia – Low child, low adult
Austria – Very low child, very low adult
Azerbaijan – Low child, low adult
Belarus – Low child, high adult
Belgium – Very low child, very low adult
Bosnia and Herzegovina – Low child, low adult
Bulgaria – Low child, low adult
Croatia – Very low child, very low adult
Czech Republic – Very low child, very low adult
Denmark – Very low child, very low adult
Estonia – Low child, high adult
Finland – Very low child, very low adult
France – Very low child, very low adult
Georgia – Low child, low adult
Germany – Very low child, very low adult
Greece – Very low child, very low adult
Hungary – Low child, high adult
Iceland – Very low child, very low adult
Ireland – Very low child, very low adult
Israel – Very low child, very low adult
Italy – Very low child, very low adult
Kazakhstan – Low child, high adult

Kyrgyzstan – Low child, low adult
Latvia – Low child, high adult
Lithuania – Low child, high adult
Luxembourg – Very low child, very low adult
Malta – Very low child, very low adult
Monaco – Very low child, very low adult
Netherlands – Very low child, very low adult
Norway – Very low child, very low adult
Poland – Low child, low adult
Portugal – Very low child, very low adult
Republic of Moldova – Low child, high adult
Romania – Low child, low adult
Russian Federation – Low child, high adult
San Marino – Very low child, very low adult
Slovakia – Low child, low adult
Slovenia – Very low child, very low adult
Spain – Very low child, very low adult
Sweden – Very low child, very low adult
Switzerland – Very low child, very low adult
Tajikistan – Low child, low adult
The former Yugoslav Republic of Macedonia – Low child, low adult
Turkey – Low child, low adult
Turkmenistan – Low child, low adult
Ukraine – Low child, high adult
United Kingdom – Very low child, very low adult
Uzbekistan – Low child, low adult
Yugoslavia – Low child, low adult

South-East Asia Region (SEAR)

Bangladesh – High child, high adult
Bhutan – High child, high adult
Democratic People's Republic of Korea – High child, high adult
India – High child, high adult
Indonesia – Low child, low adult

Maldives – High child, high adult
Myanmar – High child, high adult
Nepal – High child, high adult
Sri Lanka – Low child, low adult
Thailand – Low child, low adult

Western Pacific Region (WPR)

Australia – Very low child, very low adult
Brunei Darussalam – Very low child, very low adult
Cambodia – Low child, low adult
China – Low child, low adult
Cook Islands – Low child, low adult
Fiji – Low child, low adult
Japan – Very low child, very low adult
Kiribati – Low child, low adult
Lao People's Democratic Republic – Low child, low adult
Malaysia – Low child, low adult
Marshall Islands – Low child, low adult
Micronesia, Federated States of – Low child, low adult
Mongolia – Low child, low adult
Nauru – Low child, low adult
New Zealand – Very low child, very low adult
Niue – Low child, low adult
Palau – Low child, low adult
Papua New Guinea – Low child, low adult
Philippines – Low child, low adult
Republic of Korea – Low child, low adult
Samoa – Low child, low adult
Singapore – Very low child, very low adult
Solomon Islands – Low child, low adult
Tonga – Low child, low adult
Tuvalu – Low child, low adult
Vanuatu – Low child, low adult
Viet Nam – Low child, low adult

ACKNOWLEDGEMENTS

Headquarters Advisory Group

Anarfi Asamoa-Baah
James Banda
Jamie Bartram
Rafael Bengoa
Andrew Cassels
David Evans
Pamela Hartigan
Hans Hogerzeil
Katja Janovsky
Sergio Spinaci
Jim Tulloch
Eva Wallstam
Hilary Wild
Derek Yach

Regional Reference Group

Daniel López Acuña, AMRO
Alastair Dingwall, WPRO
Josep Figueras, EURO
Martin Mckee, EURO
Abdel Aziz Saleh, EURO
U Than Sein, SEARO
Leonard Tapsoba, AFRO

Working Groups

Basic demography
Omar Ahmad
Alan Lopez
Doris Ma Fat
Christopher Murray
Joshua Salomon

Causes of death
Christina Biller
Cynthia Boschi Pinto
Mie Inoue
Alan Lopez
Rafael Lozano
Christopher Murray
Eduardo Sabate
Joshua Salomon
Toshihiko Satoh
Lana Tomaskovic

Burden of disease
Cynthia Boschi Pinto
Somnath Chatterji
Brodie Ferguson
Mie Inoue
Alan Lopez
Rafael Lozano
Colin Mathers
Christopher Murray
Anthony Rodgers

Eduardo Sabate
Toshihiko Satoh
Lana Tomaskovic
Bedirhan Üstün
Voranuch Wangsuphachart

Disability-adjusted life expectancy
Brodie Ferguson
Alan Lopez
Colin Mathers
Christopher Murray
Ritu Sadana
Joshua Salomon

Health inequalities
Brodie Ferguson
Julio Frenk
Emmanuela Gakidou
Gary King
Christopher Murray
Lana Tomaskovic

Responsiveness
Charles Darby
Amala de Silva
Kei Kawabata
Christopher Murray
Nicole Valentine

Fairness of financial contribution
Carmen Elisa Florez
Jürgen John
Kei Kawabata
Felicia Knaul
Patrick Lydon
Christopher Murray
Philip Musgrove
Juan Pablo Ortiz de Iturbide
Wibulpolprasert Suwit
Aysit Tansel
Hugh Waters
Ke Xu

Health system preferences
Julio Frenk
Emmanuela Gakidou
Christopher Murray

National health accounts and profiles
Dominique Freire
Patricia Hernández
Catharina Hjortsberg
Chandika Indikadahena
Jack Langenbrunner
Jean-Pierre Poullier
Phyllida Travis
Naoko Watanabe

Performance analysis
Lydia Bendib
David Evans
Jeremy Lauer
Christopher Murray
Ajay Tandon

Basic economic data
Yukiko Asada
Lydia Bendib
Steeve Ebener
David Evans
Raymond Hutubessy
Jeremy Lauer
Christopher Murray
Tessa Tan-Torres Edejer
Ajay Tandon

Other contributors
Gabriella Covino
Dan Wikler
Marie Windsor-Leutke

Participants at Consultative Meeting of Health System Experts
(Geneva, December 1999)

Walid Ammar
   (Ministry of Health, Lebanon)
Anders Anell
   (The Swedish Institute for Health Economics, Sweden)
Peter Berman
   (Harvard School of Public Health, United States)
Jonathan Broomberg
   (Praxis Capital, South Africa)
Richard Feachem
   (Editor-in-Chief, Bulletin of WHO)
Toshihiko Hasegawa
   (Institute of Health Services Management, Japan)
William Hsiao
   (Harvard School of Public Health, United States)
Jeremy Hurst
   (Organization for Economic Co-operation and Development, France)
Barbara McPake
   (London School of Hygiene and Tropical Medicine, United Kingdom)
Abdelhay Mechbal
   (WHO Regional Office for the Eastern Mediterranean)
Ingrid Petersson
   (Swedish National Insurance Board, Sweden)

Alexander Preker
   (The World Bank, United States)
Neelam Sekhri Feachem
   (Healthcare Redesign Group of Companies, United States)
Suwit Wibulpolprasert
   (Ministry of Public Health, Thailand)
Beatriz Zurita
   (Mexican Health Foundation, Mexico)

Participants at Meeting of Key Informants
(Geneva, December 1999)

Jeannette Aguirre de Abruzzese (Bolivia)
Robert Basaza (Uganda)
Aleksandra Banaszewska (Poland)
Edgar Barillas (Guatemala)
Gilbert Buckle (Ghana)
Vung Nguyen Dang (Viet Nam)
Charles Darby (United States)
Jose de Noronha (Brazil)
Damani de Silva (Sri Lanka)
Orkhon Dontor (Mongolia)
Andras Fogarsi (Hungary)
Samy Gadalla (Egypt)
Zora Gerova (Slovak Republic)
David Gzirishvili (Georgia)
Jorge Hermida (Ecuador)
Gilbert Hiawalyer (Papua New Guinea)
Pimonpan Isarabhakdi (Thailand)
Saroj Jayasinghe (Sri Lanka)
Mohd. Ab. Kadar bin Marikar (Malaysia)
Shereen Khan (Bangladesh)
Shixue Li (China)
Marilyn Lorenzo (Philippines)
Gillian Moalosi (Botswana)
Ok Ryun Moon (Republic of Korea)
Grace Murindwa (Uganda)
Lipika Nanda (India)
Kai Hong Phua (Singapore)
Bhojraj Pokharel (Nepal)
Andreas Polynikis (Cyprus)
Farba Sall (Senegal)
Dragomira Shuleva (Bulgaria)
Agus Suwandono (Indonesia)
Karl Theodore (Trinidad and Tobago)
Martin Valdivia (Peru)
Marcos Vergara (Chile)
Gohar Wajid (United Arab Emirates)
David Whittaker (South Africa)
Yazoume Ye (Burkino Faso)
Thomas Zigora (Zimbabwe)
Beatriz Zurita (Mexico)

INDEX

Page numbers in **bold** type indicate main discussions.

CPSIA information can be obtained
at www.ICGtesting.com
Printed in the USA
LVHW061800050921
697042LV00007B/79